Clinical Manual of
Emergency Psychiatry

Clinical Manual of Emergency Psychiatry

Edited by

Michelle B. Riba, M.D., M.S.

Divy Ravindranath, M.D., M.S.

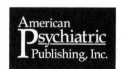

American Psychiatric Publishing, Inc.

Washington, DC
London, England

If you would like to buy between 25 and 99 copies of this or any other APPI title, you are eligible for a 20% discount; please contact APPI Customer Service at appi@psych.org or 800-368-5777. If you wish to buy 100 or more copies of the same title, please e-mail us at bulksales@psych.org for a price quote.

Copyright © 2010 American Psychiatric Publishing, Inc.
ALL RIGHTS RESERVED

Manufactured in the United States of America on acid-free paper
14 13 12 11 10   5 4 3 2 1
First Edition

Typeset in Adobe's Formata and AGaramond.

American Psychiatric Publishing, Inc.
1000 Wilson Boulevard
Arlington, VA 22209-3901
www.appi.org

WM
401
C6405
2010

Library of Congress Cataloging-in-Publication Data
Clinical manual of emergency psychiatry / edited by Michelle B. Riba, Divy Ravindranath. — 1st ed.
     p. ; cm.
   Includes bibliographical references and index.
   ISBN 978-1-58562-295-5 (pbk. : alk. paper)
   1. Psychiatric emergencies—Handbooks, manuals, etc. I. Riba, Michelle B.
II. Ravindranath, Divy, 1977–
   [DNLM: 1. Emergency Services, Psychiatric—methods. 2. Emergency Services, Psychiatric—organization & administration. 3. Mental Disorders—diagnosis.
4. Mental Disorders—therapy. WM 401 C6405 2010]
   RC480.6.C55 2010
   616.89'025—dc22

                                                                2009051640

British Library Cataloguing in Publication Data
A CIP record is available from the British Library.

Contents

1 **Approach to Psychiatric Emergencies** 1

Katherine Maloy, M.D.
Kishor Malavade, M.D.

2 **The Suicidal Patient** **33**

Felicia Kuo Wong, M.D.
Ana Wolanin, M.S., R.N.
Patrick Smallwood, M.D.

10 Child and Adolescent Emergency Psychiatry 207

B. Harrison Levine, M.D., M.P.H.
Julia E. Najara, M.D.

11 Seclusion and Restraint in Emergency Settings 233

Wanda K. Mohr, Ph.D., A.P.R.N., F.A.A.N.
Gem Lucas, D.O.

12 Legal and Ethical Issues in Emergency Psychiatry 261

Nancy Byatt, D.O., M.B.A.
Debra A. Pinals, M.D.

List of Tables

List of Figures

Contributors

James Abelson, M.D., Ph.D.
Professor, Department of Psychiatry, University of Michigan, Ann Arbor, Michigan

Iyad Alkhouri, M.D.
Assistant Professor, Department of Psychiatry, University of Michigan Medical School, Ann Arbor, Michigan

Amin Azzam, M.D., M.A.
Department of Psychiatry, University of California—San Francisco, San Francisco, California

James A. Bourgeois, O.D., M.D., F.A.P.M.
Professor and Vice Chair, Education, Department of Psychiatry and Behavioural Neurosciences, Faculty of Health Sciences, McMaster University, Michael G. DeGroote School of Medicine, Hamilton, Ontario, Canada

Philippe-Edouard Boursiquot, M.D.
Resident in Psychiatry, Department of Psychiatry and Behavioural Neurosciences, McMaster University, Hamilton, Ontario, Canada

Jennifer S. Brasch, M.D.
Associate Professor, Department of Psychiatry and Behavioural Neurosciences, McMaster University; Medical Director, Psychiatric Emergency Service, St. Joseph's Healthcare Hamilton, Ontario, Canada

Kirk Brower, M.D.
Professor, Department of Psychiatry, University of Michigan Medical School, Ann Arbor, Michigan

Nancy Byatt, D.O., M.B.A.
Assistant Professor of Psychiatry, University of Massachusetts Medical School; Attending Psychiatrist, Psychosomatic Medicine and Emergency Mental Health, UMass Memorial Medical Center, Worcester, Massachusetts

M. Justin Coffey, M.D.
Chief Resident in Psychiatry, Department of Psychiatry, University of Michigan, Ann Arbor, Michigan

Gregory W. Dalack, M.D.
Associate Professor and Interim Chair, Department of Psychiatry, University of Michigan Medical School, Ann Arbor, Michigan

Tamara Gay, M.D.
Assistant Professor, Department of Psychiatry, University of Michigan Medical School, Ann Arbor, Michigan

Patrick Gibbons, D.O., M.S.W.
Research Fellow, Department of Psychiatry, University of Michigan Medical School, Ann Arbor, Michigan

Rachel L. Glick, M.D.
Professor, Department of Psychiatry, University of Michigan Medical School, Ann Arbor, Michigan

Fadi Haddad, M.D.
Director of Child Psychiatric Emergency Services, Bellevue Hospital Center; Clinical Assistant Professor of Child and Adolescent Psychiatry, NYU School of Medicine, New York, New York

Laura Hirshbein, M.D., Ph.D.
Assistant Professor, Department of Psychiatry, University of Michigan Medical School, Ann Arbor, Michigan

Erick Hung, M.D.
Department of Psychiatry, University of California—San Francisco, San Francisco, California

B. Harrison Levine, M.D., M.P.H.
Assistant Professor, Department of Psychiatry, University of Colorado School of Medicine; Medical Director, Psychiatric Consultation Liaison and Emergency Services, The Children's Hospital, Aurora, Colorado

Gem Lucas, D.O.
Child and Adolescent Psychiatry Fellow, Division of Child/Adolescent Psychiatry, UMDNJ–Robert Wood Johnson Medical School, Piscataway, New Jersey

Kishor Malavade, M.D.
Clinical Assistant Professor, New York University School of Medicine, NYU Langone Medical Center, New York, New York

Katherine Maloy, M.D.
Attending Psychiatrist, Comprehensive Psychiatric Emergency Program, Bellevue Hospital; Clinical Assistant Professor, New York University School of Medicine, NYU Langone Medical Center, New York, New York

Tracy McCarthy, M.D.
Resident in Psychiatry, Department of Psychiatry and Behavioral Sciences, University of California, Davis Medical Center, Sacramento, California

Wanda K. Mohr, Ph.D., A.P.R.N., F.A.A.N.
Professor, Psychiatric Mental Health Nursing, University of Medicine and Dentistry of New Jersey, New Hope, Pennsylvania

Julia E. Najara, M.D.
Private practice; formerly Assistant Clinical Professor of Psychiatry, Columbia University; Director, Comprehensive Emergency Service, Pediatric Psychiatry Division, Morgan Stanley Children's Hospital of New York Presbyterian, New York, New York

Debra A. Pinals, M.D.
Director, Forensic Education, Law and Psychiatry Program; Associate Professor, Department of Psychiatry, University of Massachusetts Medical School, Worcester, Massachusetts

Ernest Poortinga, M.D.
Adjunct Clinical Assistant Professor of Psychiatry, University of Michigan Medical School; Forensic Psychiatry and Consulting Forensic Examiner, Center for Forensic Psychiatry, Saline, Michigan

Vasilis K. Pozios, M.D.
House Officer, Department of Psychiatry, University of Michigan, Ann Arbor, Michigan

Melanie Quintero, Ph.D.
Senior Psychologist, CPEP Interim Crisis Clinic, New York, New York

Divy Ravindranath, M.D., M.S.
Psychosomatic Medicine Fellow, Department of Psychiatry, University of Michigan, Ann Arbor, Michigan

Michelle B. Riba, M.D., M.S.
Professor and Associated Chair for Integrated Medicine and Psychiatric Services, Department of Psychiatry, University of Michigan, Ann Arbor, Michigan

Patricia Schwartz, M.D.
Clinical Assistant Professor, Department of Psychiatry, New York University School of Medicine, New York, New York

Zoya Simakhodskaya, Ph.D.
Clinical Instructor of Psychiatry, NYU School of Medicine, New York, New York

Patrick Smallwood, M.D.
Assistant Professor of Psychiatry, University of Massachusetts Medical School; Medical Director, Psychosomatic Medicine and Emergency Mental Health, UMass Memorial Medical Center, Worcester, Massachusetts

Michael Alan Taylor, M.D.
Adjunct Clinical Professor of Psychiatry, Department of Psychiatry, University of Michigan, Ann Arbor, Michigan

Mary Weathers, M.D.
Resident in Psychiatry, New York University School of Medicine/Bellevue Hospital, New York, New York

Ana Wolanin, M.S., R.N.
University of Massachusetts Medical School, Director of Psychiatric Services, UMass Memorial Medical Center, Worcester, Massachusetts

Felicia Kuo Wong, M.D.
Resident in Psychiatry, University of Massachusetts Medical School, UMass Memorial Medical Center, Worcester, Massachusetts

The following contributors to this book have indicated a financial interest in or other affiliation with a commercial supporter, a manufacturer of a commercial product, a provider of a commercial service, a nongovernmental organization, and/or a government agency, as listed below:

Amin Azzam, M.D., M.A.—The author served as one of two primary editors for *First Aid for the Psychiatry Boards,* published by the McGraw-Hill Companies, Inc., Publishing Group, and receives a 10% royalty share on all domestic print or electronic copies sold and a 5% royalty share on all foreign sales, direct marketing sales, and/or specialty sales.

Kishor Malavade, M.D.—*Speaker:* Eli Lilly USA Lecture Bureau

The following contributors have no competing interests to report:

James Abelson, M.D., Ph.D.
Iyad Alkhouri, M.D.
James A. Bourgeois, O.D., M.D., F.A.P.M.
Philippe-Edouard Boursiquot, M.D.
Nancy Byatt, D.O., M.B.A.
M. Justin Coffey, M.D.
Gregory W. Dalack, M.D.
Tamara Gay, M.D.
Patrick Gibbons, D.O., M.S.W.
Fadi Haddad, M.D.
Laura Hirshbein, M.D., Ph.D.
Erick Hung, M.D.
Katherine Maloy, M.D.

Wanda K. Mohr, Ph.D., A.P.R.N., F.A.A.N.

Vasilis K. Pozios, M.D.

Melanie Quintero, Ph.D.

Divy Ravindranath, M.D., M.S.

Michelle B. Riba, M.D., M.S.

Patricia Schwartz, M.D.

Zoya Simakhodskaya, Ph.D.

Patrick Smallwood, M.D.

Michael Alan Taylor, M.D.

Mary Weathers, M.D.

Ana Wolanin, M.S., R.N.

Felicia Kuo Wong, M.D.

Preface

One of the most challenging clinical settings in psychiatry is the psychiatric emergency department. Taking care of patients who are acutely ill in a timely manner takes incredible skill and ability. Making the incorrect assessment can have life-and-death implications. In addition, family members are very much a part of the clinical situation and are often themselves frightened and worried. Besides facing the acuity of the clinical issues, trainees working in this very difficult and high-stress setting at times have only backup supervision by phone rather than in-person oversight. Busy psychiatric emergency departments where first-year and second-year psychiatry residents are trying to quickly understand complicated clinical situations from patients who are quite ill makes for very challenging work indeed.

In this book, we have sought to provide trainees and clinicians with an understanding and the background of psychiatric emergency services in a format that can be easily read and highlighted. Each chapter was cowritten by a trainee or junior faculty member as well as a senior faculty member at an academic medical center. We chose topics that are generally the most important and practical in any busy psychiatric emergency department. Case vignettes are also included to contextualize the information provided and allow readers to envision the applicable clinical scenario even if they are not actively seeing patients in the emergency department setting. This is not meant to be a textbook but rather a first pass at what psychiatrists often confront when working in this type of setting. Our hope was to make this a reader-friendly and useful clinical manual that reflects widespread practices in various academic centers and that can be read by trainees in many different disciplines.

With this in mind, we arranged many of the chapters by chief complaint (e.g., suicidal ideation) rather than by psychiatric diagnosis (e.g., borderline personality disorder). Many psychiatric conditions can result in the same psychiatric emergency. Moreover, the emergency department is one of the few arenas where patients do not arrive "prelabeled." Therefore, we felt that organizing the book based on chief complaints would give the reader the greatest opportunity to review the key points, as needed, just before seeing a patient.

This book also includes chapters on supervision and the role of medical students and teaching in the psychiatric emergency department. These chapters provide guidance both for supervisors, with regard to how to maximize the learning potential of the emergency department, and for trainees, with regard to what to expect from their supervisors and how to maximize the supervision they receive. Legal and ethical issues in emergency psychiatry, disposition and resource options, and moving patients from the clinic to the emergency room are also considered in separate chapters.

We hope that readers will let us know what was helpful or not in this first edition of the clinical manual. For subsequent editions, we are open to changes based on constructive comments. We recognize that due to the ongoing development of newer treatments and options, future editions might also address pharmacological and psychotherapeutic updates.

We appreciate the opportunity to have our respected colleagues participate in the writing and editing of this clinical manual. We hope that our undertaking of this book will allow us to be better clinicians and teachers and thereby provide improved service and care to our patients and their families.

Our sincere thanks and appreciation to Linda Gacioch, the administrative manager for this clinical manual. Linda did an excellent job of organizing and making sure that this project was done in a thoroughly professional and systematic manner.

Michelle B. Riba, M.D., M.S.
Divy Ravindranath, M.D., M.S.

Acknowledgments

The volume editors extend their appreciation to the following faculty, residents, and fellows for their expert chapter reviews and editorial assistance:

Prachi Agarwala, M.D., Child and Adolescent Psychiatry Fellow, University of Michigan

Sara Bobak, M.D., Child and Adolescent Psychiatry Fellow, University of Michigan

M. Justin Coffey, M.D., Chief Resident in Psychiatry, University of Michigan

Daniel Gih, M.D., Child and Adolescent Psychiatry Fellow, University of Michigan

Katie Hecksel, M.D., Child and Adolescent Psychiatry Fellow, Mayo Clinic

Brian Mickey, M.D., Attending Psychiatrist, University of Michigan

Richard W. Miller, M.D., Resident in Psychiatry, University of Michigan

Sara Mohiuddin, M.D., Attending Psychiatrist, University of Michigan

Christina Mueller, M.D., Child and Adolescent Psychiatry Fellow, University of Michigan

Jennifer Seibert, M.D., Staff Psychiatrist, Salisbury NC VAMC, Charlotte Community-Based Outpatient Clinic

Lizette Solis, M.D., Resident in Psychiatry, University of Michigan

Drs. Riba and Ravindranath also extend their sincere appreciation to Linda Gacioch for her excellent administrative, organizational, and editorial assistance.

Approach to Psychiatric Emergencies

Katherine Maloy, M.D.
Kishor Malavade, M.D.

Although the vast majority of psychiatric practice takes place outside of the hospital setting, the proportion of visits to emergency departments for psychiatric reasons is increasing. In 2004, the 4.3 million psychiatric emergency visits accounted for approximately 5.4% of total emergency department visits (Hazlett et al. 2004). According to a 2008 utilization study, uninsured patients with psychiatric disorders were more likely to have multiple emergency department visits and hospitalizations than insured patients (Baillargeon et al. 2008). As the ranks of uninsured individuals rise, psychiatric emergency services are likely to experience an increasing demand. Many common medical illnesses present with behavioral pathology and can cause changes in thinking and mood, and as the population ages, the prevalence of dementia and medical illnesses is escalating, further increasing demand for psychiatric emergency services (Walsh et al. 2008). Also, patients who come to the emergency department solely for medical reasons can present with personality traits and maladaptive coping skills that may complicate their medical care.

In all these situations, the role of the mental health clinician as consultant, liaison, educator, and detective can be crucial in facilitating appropriate care. The mental health clinician practicing in the emergency department setting must be adept at managing hospital systems issues, informed on medical illnesses and their psychiatric manifestations, skilled in conflict resolution, ethically and legally informed about responsibilities for patients' safety, and able to serve as a team leader who can direct staff in a crisis.

A General Approach to the Emergency Psychiatric Patient

While hospital systems and local mental health law and policies may vary by state or even individual hospital settings, an overall approach to the psychiatric emergency patient involves an understanding of systems and a focus on patient and clinician safety.

Understanding Health Care Systems

Psychiatrists and mental health workers, including psychologists, social workers, and psychiatric nurses, work in a variety of different capacities within emergency departments. Delivery of efficient care requires that clinicians in the emergency department know their role within the overall health care system in which they are practicing. Issues that commonly arise include admission privileges, follow-up planning, insurance issues, safety, medical care, available facilities at the emergency department or at affiliate hospitals, and supervision, particularly for trainees or nonphysician consultants. Every hospital has its own method of dividing responsibility and varying levels of support staff. The answer to the question, "Who does what?" is primarily determined by the training of the clinician within the emergency department and the department's overall policy for handling psychiatric cases (Brown 2005).

The settings of emergency psychiatric care delivery exist on a spectrum. In most community hospitals, the volume of psychiatric cases is not high enough to warrant dedicated psychiatric evaluation space or a comprehensive psychiatric evaluation team. Typically, in primary care and community-based centers, the mental health clinician acts as consultant to the emergency department. The facility may not have dedicated space for psychiatric evaluation and assessment, and the nursing and support staff may be less familiar with psychiatric issues (Woo et al. 2007). In facilities with more psychiatric cases, particularly in hospitals with active inpatient psychiatric services, emergency departments may set aside space or have more support services available for psychiatric emergencies, as advocated by the American Psychiatric Association (Allen et al. 2002). A true comprehensive psychiatric emergency department is most common in large, urban settings, where a higher volume of psychiatric cases is common. For example, dedicated social work staff, psychiatrically trained nursing and support staff, a separate locked area, and the possibility of extended observation (up to 72 hours) are features of the Comprehensive Psychiatric Emergency Program in New York State. Variations on this model have developed across the country. Although a comprehensive psychiatric emergency department can be a stressful work environment, the role of each clinician working in such a setting is clearer and more support is available.

Regardless of the system in which the clinician works, the same basic principles apply. The patient should receive as comprehensive an evaluation as possible, followed by a thorough disposition plan—whether admitted or discharged—in a setting that is safe and as therapeutic as possible.

Assuring Safety

Although the idea of emergency department psychiatry commonly brings to mind wildly out-of-control patients, the reality is much more mundane. The vast majority of psychiatric patients are not violent toward others, and self-harm in a supervised setting is not common. However, one must still act to assure the safety of the patient, the doctor, the staff, and other patients in the area.

Hospital systems play a large role in how safety is achieved, so it is important for the clinician to know the particular challenges in his or her emergency department and have a plan in mind for ensuring patient and staff safety when a potentially dangerous situation arises. If contingency plans for safety are already established, the staff can execute them more easily. Emergency departments should establish policies regarding searching patients for weapons and specifying when and how to call for backup support if a patient becomes violent. Ideally, all patients should be searched prior to the interview. If a search is not performed routinely, the clinician should request a search or at least request that the patient change into hospital gowns or pajamas prior to the interview, thereby making it harder to conceal weapons. At the start of a shift, consultants—particularly those who work only occasionally in the emergency department—should introduce themselves to security staff so staff know whom to contact if backup support is needed. Although some facilities have security cameras or panic buttons, it is also helpful to notify staff prior to meeting with a patient so they can be ready to respond if a crisis situation arises.

Approaching Agitated or Violent Patients

Asking staff how the patient has been behaving prior to the clinician's arrival can help the clinician tailor an initial approach. If the patient has been calm and cooperative, then the clinician may elect to interview the patient following the hospital's standard safety protocol. However, if the patient has been agitated, then additional precautions may be warranted prior to interviewing the patient.

Prior to initiating an encounter with an agitated patient, the clinician should first determine some key points about the patient, both through the clinician's own observation and by asking the staff for their input. Who is the patient, including his or her basic physical characteristics and presenting complaint? Is the patient upset about a specific issue or psychotic and disorganized? What is the patient's behavior? Is he or she yelling? Throwing things? Making any specific threats? Finally, are there any indicators as to the etiology of the agitation, such as appearing ill, smell of alcohol on the patient's breath, or obvious head trauma?

Once the nature of the situation is clear, the clinician can determine the environment in which to further assess the patient. For example, the degree of agitation may warrant interviewing the patient in a more public area than usual so that other staff members can monitor the interaction directly. Additionally, the clinician may request that security staff be present on standby in the emergency department to provide assistance rapidly if needed. Finally, the clinician may elect to begin the interaction with the patient by addressing the agitation directly rather than trying to determine the chief complaint, the history of the presenting illness, and so forth. For example, the clinician may start by pointing out the level of agitation to the patient and then offering to help. This may include an offer of a medication to calm the patient. Given that situations may not always be as they appear, the clinician should always err on the side of caution and containment of the patient in the least restrictive method possible.

Maintaining a calm demeanor goes a long way toward preventing escalation of agitation to violence. Many patients will resonate with the nonverbal communication of the clinician, and a clinician who is becoming more agitated may cause the patient to become more agitated as well (Flannery 2007). The clinician should be vigilant for signs of escalating tension, such as clenching fists, increased respiratory rate, threatening postures, or restlessness, and be ready to terminate an interview or interaction before a situation escalates, even if little information has been obtained.

General Rules for Approaching Agitated Patients

When encountering an agitated patient, the following general principles are helpful in maintaining safety and perhaps deescalating the situation.

1. *Take charge and make a plan.* Staff members or other patients, meaning well, may try to intervene in various ways. This is confusing to the patient and can escalate the situation. The team leader should identify himself or herself as such and ask staff to follow his or her directions.
2. *Keep a safe distance.* Crowding someone who is already upset is not generally a soothing tactic, and keeping a safe distance lowers the risk of inadvertent injury by a flailing or agitated patient.
3. *Ask for backup.* Whether security should be present depends on the nature of the situation at hand. If the clinician is concerned that the patient may require a medication or restraints, he or she should ask someone to be preparing those ahead of time.
4. *Provide an easy out.* People who are upset and confused generally want a way to resolve the issue rather than escalating it further. Providing a quick and safe alternative to further escalation allows the patient a way out. For

example, the clinician might say, "I can see you are very upset. Would you be willing to sit down with me and we can figure out a way to resolve this situation?"

5. *Give clear instructions.* Specifically asking the patient to sit down in a certain place, lower his or her voice, put down the chair, and so on, is much more likely to yield a result than general directives to "calm down," "relax," or "take it easy."

Dealing With Escalation

If a patient escalates to violence during an interview, the clinician's priority should always be his or her own safety. Escape is the first priority, followed by alerting other staff and then containment of the patient. A clinician who is injured or incapacitated should leave the situation and get help, because the immediate fear and pain will make being an effective team leader difficult.

Particularly for trainees, who may feel that they are letting other staff down or appearing cowardly if they protect themselves, violent situations can provoke intense feelings of guilt or self-blame. Clinicians who are injured may feel that they provoked the attack or feel intense anger that is unfamiliar and difficult to reconcile with their values and ideals of what constitutes good patient care. Clinicians need to remember that they are also human beings, who exhibit a full range of normal human emotions in response to trauma. Clinicians are advised to seek support from friends, colleagues, or a mental health professional after a frightening incident. There is no one right answer regarding whether the clinician should press charges against an assaulting patient; that decision is best left to the discretion of the clinician.

Etiologies of Agitation

After safety has been assured, the overriding principle in addressing agitation is to rule out life-threatening medical causes. The assumption that a patient is suffering from a psychotic break as the result of schizophrenia could be fatal for a belligerent patient with hypoglycemia and diabetes or a patient experiencing delirium tremens. Table 1–1 covers common causes of agitation and basic approaches to their treatment. Delirium and intoxication/withdrawal syndromes are covered in more detail in later chapters (see Chapter 8, "The Cognitively Impaired Patient," and Chapter 9, "Substance-Related Psychiatric Emergencies").

Treatment

A general progression of options for dealing with agitation starts with verbal/behavioral interventions, then consideration and application of medications, with seclusion/restraints as a final option.

Verbal/Behavioral Interventions

As mentioned previously, speaking with a patient in a calm and rational manner, addressing his or her needs to the extent possible, and giving specific directions for the patient to change behavior may be all that a patient needs to calm down. In a crowded emergency department, moving the patient to a more secluded or quiet area may be helpful. Instituting one-to-one supervision may help by giving the patient someone to talk to, showing that the staff feels that the patient requires supervision, preventing elopement, and providing an early alert for other staff if behavior escalates again. Whenever possible, providing patients with information about how their evaluation is proceeding, why they are at the emergency department, and how long they should expect to remain can prevent further disruption.

Medications

Operating on the principle of using the least restrictive alternative for treatment, offering oral medication to an agitated patient is usually the first option. Most oral medications take effect within 20–30 minutes. Dissolving tablets alleviate the necessity of swallowing but do not take effect any faster than regular oral medications. Dissolving tablets and liquid medication are more difficult to "cheek" or conceal without swallowing. In circumstances where 1) the patient refuses oral medication and safety is a concern, 2) safety is such a concern that oral medication would act too slowly, or 3) the patient might lack the airway control to swallow medication, intramuscular medication is the next best option. The most common protocol is a benzodiazepine plus a neuroleptic (Wilhelm et al. 2008). Table 1–2 lists medications commonly used for agitation, typical dosing ranges for oral and intramuscular routes, and notable benefits and risks of each.

Table 1–1.   Common causes of agitation in the emergency department setting

Cause	Clinical presentation	Treatment approach
Acute cocaine/ stimulant intoxication	Tachycardia, dilated pupils, irritability with or without psychosis, which can present as almost entirely similar to schizophrenia-like symptoms. Cocaine effects usually time limited, as opposed to PCP or amphetamine psychosis, which can persist longer.	Use benzodiazepines for sedation; hold beta-blockers.
Benzodiazepine/ barbiturate withdrawal	Similar to alcohol withdrawal, but may not show vital sign changes, and may present solely as a delirium with or without tremor. High risk of seizure.	Taper benzodiazepine.
Delirium	Waxing and waning level of consciousness, fluctuation in vital signs, confusion. Can be irritable or passive and detached. More common in the elderly or medically frail patient.	Assure safety of the patient, treat the underlying cause, use low-dose neuroleptics to calm the patient so that medical treatment can proceed, provide reorientation cues when possible.
Delirium tremens	All signs of delirium, with or without tremors, with or without hallucinations; intense fluctuation in vital signs. Last drink of alcohol 24–72 hours prior.	If patient has intact airway, aggressively sedate with parenteral benzodiazepines to the point of drowsiness, if possible. Provide ICU-level monitoring, if needed.
Hypoglycemia	Altered mental status with sweating, tachycardia, and weakness.	If patient has patent airway, use oral glucose; otherwise, use dextrose 50% iv.

Table 1–1.   Common causes of agitation in the emergency department setting (*continued*)

Cause	Clinical presentation	Treatment approach
Postictal states	Altered level of consciousness, confusion, ataxia. May have Todd paralysis or other residual neurological signs, such as slurred speech. May have evidence of tongue biting or incontinence from prior seizure.	Assure patient safety, observe for further seizure activity. If agitation requires treatment, use benzodiazepines over neuroleptics because latter may lower seizure threshold. Determine cause of seizure.
Psychosis/mania/ primary psychiatric disorder	Not usually associated with disorientation, no waxing and waning level of consciousness, no vital sign changes. Look for other signs of psychiatric illness or history of same.	Assure safety; offer oral medications or intramuscular medications; or consider restraints if necessary.
Structural brain abnormality	Varies by lesion, but altered mental status with headache, meningeal signs, focal neurological deficit (e.g., agitated patient who wants to leave but cannot walk), or progressive neurological deterioration.	Assure patent airway; use emergent CT scan or other imaging modality.
Toxicologic emergency	Varies by substance, but ingestion of toxic substances can lead to mental status changes. Watch for pupillary changes, sweating, vital sign changes, or other signs of medical illness.	Attempt to identify toxin and contact poison control.

Note.   CT = computed tomographic; ICU = intensive care unit; PCP = phencyclidine.
Source.   Adapted from Moore and Jefferson 2004.

Table 1–2.   Common medications used in management of agitation

Medication	Dosing	Benefits	Risks
Aripiprazole	Only intramuscular administration effective for agitation 9.75 mg im, up to 30 mg/day	Less risk of EPS or dystonia Less sedating	Not in use for long, less experience Akathisia More expensive
Chlorpromazine	25–100 mg po 25–50 mg im	Very sedating Lower risk of EPS/dystonia than other typicals	High risk of orthostatic hypotension
Diazepam	5–10 mg po or im	No EPS or dystonia Also used to treat alcohol or benzodiazepine withdrawal	Respiratory depression Active metabolite resulting in very long half-life and therefore problematic if impaired liver function
Diphenhydramine	25–50 mg po or im	When used with typical antipsychotics, prevents/treats EPS and dystonia Very sedating	Anticholinergic delirium at higher doses or in elderly Paradoxical activating reaction
Fluphenazine	5–10 mg po or im	Sedating Anecdotally less dystonia than haloperidol	EPS Dystonia
Haloperidol	1–5 mg po (liquid or pill) or im; can repeat up to 10–15 mg	Sedating Rapid onset Inexpensive	Dystonic reaction EPS Lower seizure threshold

Table 1–2. Common medications used in management of agitation *(continued)*

Medication	Dosing	Benefits	Risks
Lorazepam	1–4 mg po or im	No EPS or dystonia Also used to treat alcohol or benzodiazepine withdrawal Good for patients with impaired liver function	Paradoxical disinhibition and agitation Respiratory depression
Olanzapine	5–10 mg po (tablet or dissolving wafer) 5–10 mg im, up to 20 mg total/day	Less risk of EPS or dystonia reported Less sedating Wafers excellent for patients with impaired swallowing	Maximum dosing achieved quickly Expensive
Ziprasidone	Only intramuscular administration effective for agitation 10 mg im, maximum 40 mg/day	Less risk of EPS or dystonia reported Less sedating	More expensive Effectiveness unknown

Note. EPS = extrapyramidal symptoms.
Source. Marco and Vaughan 2005; Physicians' Desk Reference 2008; Rocca et al. 2006; Villari et al. 2008.

Seclusion

If available, the option of placing a patient in locked seclusion may be a slightly less restrictive alternative than restraint. Seclusion is safe, however, only if the room is properly designed and the patient is supervised appropriately during the seclusion. Many general emergency departments do not have seclusion rooms.

Restraint

Physical restraint is a last option for assuring safety of an agitated patient and requires training to execute. Careful documentation of the time the patient was restrained, the type of restraint used, and the reasoning behind the decision is essential. Once restrained, the patient should be on one-to-one observation until released, and vital signs should be checked frequently.

More detailed information on restraint and seclusion techniques can be found in Chapter 11, "Seclusion and Restraint in Emergency Settings," but certain principles are important to emphasize here. Restraint or seclusion should always be a last resort and may lead to patient and staff injury. They should never be used punitively and should be used only to contain behavior so unsafe that it cannot be controlled in any other way (Downey et al. 2007; Herzog et al. 2003).

The Emergency Psychiatric Interview

The psychiatric interview of a patient in an emergency setting is unique. Compared with a typical psychiatric interview, the emergency interview is usually shorter and frequently less private, and its primary goals are to assess the patient's safety and determine the appropriate disposition. It can be complicated by the fact that the patient may be unwilling to cooperate and may not have been the person who decided that psychiatric intervention was indicated. Despite the compelling need to uncover complicating medical conditions and sources of collateral information, the interview need not be formulaic. Given that the clinician is trying to establish rapport and ask about intimate issues after only a brief interaction, the clinician should always be flexible enough to switch the topic when necessary, follow the patient's train of thought if indicated, and adapt to the patient's personality style (Manley 2004).

An important part of the assessment occurs before the clinician even enters the room with the patient. Before initiating contact with the patient, the clinician should always find out 1) the reason for seeing the patient, 2) basic available demographic information, and 3) the patient's behavior prior to the clinician's arrival. If possible, brief covert observation of the patient's behavior can also be extremely useful because it may uncover attempts at malingering or reveal behavior that the patient will attempt to hide during the interview itself. Clinicians should always begin an interview by clearly introducing themselves, making the patient aware that they are conducting a psychiatric evaluation, and establishing a safe seating arrangement. It is also helpful to remind the patient that the purpose of the assessment is to figure out how best to help him or her in the given situation.

Components of the Interview

The components of an emergency psychiatric interview (Vergare et al. 2006) are similar to those of a more comprehensive diagnostic interview, but necessarily focus more on immediate medical and safety risk factors and on the events immediately preceding the patient's arrival to the emergency department.

Patient Identification

The clinician first determines who the patient is and how he or she got to the emergency department. A brief sketch of the patient's demographics contextualizes the patient for the rest of the assessment. How the patient arrived (i.e., on his or her own, with family, with police) is helpful for understanding the patient's attitude toward treatment.

Chief Complaint

The clinician should then determine what the patient sees as the presenting problem.

History of Present Illness

A patient who is agitated, intoxicated, or psychotic may have difficulty clearly reconstructing how events unfolded before arriving at the emergency department. The patient may require specific redirection as to times, dates, events, and the chronology of symptoms, and the clinician may require data from collateral informants.

Past Psychiatric History

Information sought about the patient's past psychiatric history should include 1) prior hospitalizations, last hospitalization, and age at first hospitalization; 2) prior suicide attempts or self-harming behaviors; 3) prior episodes of violence or agitation; 4) prior trials of medications or therapies; and 5) history of arrests or incarceration.

Substance Use History

In questioning a patient about his or her history of substance use, the clinician should start by asking about tobacco, which is generally the most socially acceptable. For each substance, a complete history should include the patient's 1) prior use or experimentation, 2) highest level of use, 3) longest sober period, and 4) current level of use. In addition to questioning about alcohol, marijuana, cocaine, and opiates, the clinician should ask about hallucinogens, inhalants, club drugs, and prescription drugs. The clinician should also screen for history of withdrawal symptoms (e.g., delirium tremens and seizures) and prior treatment history (e.g., rehabilitation, outpatient programs, Alcoholics Anonymous).

Medical History

The medical history should include questions about the patient's history of cardiac disease, hypertension, diabetes, epilepsy, head injury, hepatitis, cancer, and surgeries. A general reproductive history for women can also be helpful, specifically asking if the woman is menstruating regularly, is perimenopausal or postmenopausal, might be pregnant, or has undergone any reproductive surgeries. Because the Centers for Disease Control and Prevention (2006) has recommended that all adults be tested for HIV as a routine part of health maintenance, the clinician should routinely ask about HIV status in at-risk individuals. In at-risk populations, history of a positive PPD (purified protein derivative) or tuberculosis diagnosis or treatment is also important in determining whether further evaluation by chest X ray or even respiratory isolation will be necessary.

Social Circumstances

In emergency presentations, instead of taking a detailed developmental history, the clinician should focus on painting a picture of the patient's current social circumstances. The following information is helpful for making disposition determinations: living situation, financial support, employment history, relocation history, social situation and supports, educational background, important developmental events, and legal/immigration status.

Mental Status Examination

The mental status examination in the emergency psychiatric interview is similar to any other mental status examination, except that particular attention must be paid to documenting 1) active psychotic symptoms, 2) thoughts of self-injury or suicide and thoughts of harming others or homicide, 3) evidence of drug or alcohol intoxication, and 4) cognitive functioning.

Safety Alerts

Certain safety-related situations that may present during the emergency psychiatric interview should trigger more immediate action. These include the following:

- Children in the home or other persons for whom the patient is the primary caregiver (The interviewer should ascertain where these individuals are and who is caring for them, document this information carefully, and send authorities to retrieve anyone who is unsupervised while the patient is in the emergency department.)
- Medical conditions requiring immediate treatment
- Active alcohol or benzodiazepine intoxication and withdrawal
- Active suicidal ideation with intent and plan
- Active violent ideation with intent and plan

Collateral Information

Collateral information can be helpful in forming a clear assessment in an emergency situation, and taking steps to obtain this information can be considered a standard of care in certain circumstances. If possible, the clinician should obtain the patient's consent to talk to collateral informants. However, in an emergency situation, the clinician is permitted, even with existing Health Insurance Portability and Accountability Act (HIPAA) regulations, to contact collateral sources of information if demanded by the patient's emergency circumstances. Even though the clinician may obtain collateral information, the physician is still not permitted to unnecessarily share information about the patient without the patient's consent. (This point is discussed further in Chapter 12, "Legal and Ethical Issues in Emergency Psychiatry.") All attempts to gain information via contacting collateral sources should be carefully documented, including why it was deemed necessary to contact the source and whether the contact was made with or without the patient's consent (U.S. Department of Health and Human Services 2003b).

Medical Clearance

The term *medical clearance* has entered into the medical parlance without a consensus about its definition. There is no way to rule out every possible medical illness a patient may have prior to admission to a psychiatric unit (Zun 2005). As such, the goal of the emergency room physician and/or mental health clinician should be to make a reasonable investigation into the possibility that the patient has an illness 1) that would be better treated in a medical setting (e.g., an infection requiring intravenous antibiotics, a stroke, myocardial infarction); 2) that will cause the acute decompensation of the patient in the next few hours and thus require a higher level of care (e.g., active alcohol withdrawal that is not responding to oral medication or a smoldering gastrointestinal bleed); 3) that is causing the behavioral symptoms that brought the patient to the hospital in the first place and should be treated by something other than psychiatric medication (e.g., delirium due to an underlying infection or intracranial hemorrhage); or 4) is worsening the psychiatric process (e.g., untreated pain that is causing agitation). This investigation is accomplished through a careful diagnostic interview, a careful physical examination, and a combination of screening lab tests and imaging studies.

The more that emergency department psychiatrists are able to retain familiarity with routine medical issues and communicate effectively with other services as needed, the more service they will be to their patients. Clinicians without medical training who are working in an emergency department will need to rely more heavily on the emergency department physician to assist with the differentiation of medical and psychiatric issues. However, a familiarity with common medical comorbidities, the medical complications of substance withdrawal, and the differences between delirium and psychiatrically caused psychosis are crucial to a thorough evaluation.

Many hospital systems require that the psychiatrist admitting the patient to a psychiatric unit perform his or her own physical examination as part of the assessment. This examination can be particularly difficult with a patient who is agitated or psychotic, but it may reveal important information that can contribute to treatment decisions. Table 1–3 details the contents of a focused physical examination when seeking medical clearance for psychiatric evaluation, and Table 1–4 details relevant laboratory tests and studies that may be considered.

In summary, the examination of a psychiatric patient in the emergency department should be targeted toward finding occult medical processes that require treatment in a nonpsychiatric setting, are imminently life threatening, or are contributing to the psychiatric process (Guze and Love 2004).

Substance Abuse and Withdrawal Syndromes

Substance abuse accounts for many emergency department visits. Mental health clinicians are frequently called to evaluate patients who are acutely intoxicated or in withdrawal, both to assess their safety and to assist in determining a disposition.

The emergency assessment of substance abuse problems should focus on the immediate issues of safety, which include protecting the acutely intoxicated or withdrawing patient from harming self or others and making a decision about when the patient is safe to leave. Consults can also be called to assess a patient's capacity to refuse medical care when a patient is acutely intoxicated or in withdrawal.

Negative countertransferential feelings may interfere with the appropriate assessment of the substance-abusing patient. Clinicians may be inclined to consider patients who are intoxicated as less deserving of time or attention because they seemingly have brought the problem on themselves. In addition, if these patients are abusive or belligerent and being held against their will, providing appropriate care becomes even more difficult. Despite the difficulties and annoyance that these patients can cause, they require close monitoring and are at greatly increased immediate risk of intentional or unintentional harm to themselves. (For more details on substance abuse in the psychiatric emergency setting, see Chapter 9, "Substance-Related Psychiatric Emergencies," this volume.)

Table 1–3.   Focused physical examination when seeking medical clearance for psychiatric evaluation

Area examined	What to look at	What to look for
General appearance	Weight, stature, grooming, level of distress, skin	Cachexia—suspicion of tuberculosis, cancer, HIV, malnutrition Obvious respiratory distress Obvious physical distress or agitation Grossly disheveled or malodorous patient Rashes—allergic or infectious illnesses
Head, ears, eyes, nose, throat	Mucous membranes, conjunctiva, pupils and eye movements, any discharge or lesions, evidence of trauma, dentition	Dry mucous membranes—dehydration Pupils and eye movements—focal neurological deficits, evidence of drug intoxication or withdrawal Scleral icterus—jaundice Proptosis—hyperthyroidism Bruises, lacerations—evidence of head or facial trauma Poor dentition—nutritional status, occult abscesses
Neck	Thyroid size, neck mobility	Thyromegaly—goiter, hyperthyroidism Neck rigidity—meningitis, encephalitis
Chest	Breath sounds, accessory muscle use, any evidence of trauma	Rales—congestive heart failure Rhonchi—pneumonia Chest trauma—emergent need for treatment of a wound; risk of future pneumonia from decreased chest expansion
Cardiovascular	Heart sounds, peripheral pulses	Rate, rhythm, regularity of heartbeat Any absent peripheral pulses—vascular disease

Table 1–3.   Focused physical examination when seeking medical clearance for psychiatric evaluation (*continued*)

Area examined	What to look at	What to look for
Abdomen	Any palpable masses, liver size, scars, areas of tenderness	Hepatomegaly—undiagnosed liver disease Surgical scars Acute tenderness—acute pathology that needs to be addressed in emergency department
Back and spine	CVA tenderness, spinal curvature	Curvature—scoliosis or osteoporosis CVA tenderness—kidney infection or stones
Extremities	Movement, strength, range of motion	Any deficits, limps, or pain that might indicate occult neurological illness
Neurological	Cranial nerves, strength, sensation, gait, reflexes	Any focal deficits indicating stroke or occult mass Festinating gait, rigidity—parkinsonism Tremors—parkinsonism, EPS Evidence of tardive dyskinesia Broad-based gait—hydrocephalus, tertiary syphilis

Note.   CVA = cerebrovascular accident; EPS = extrapyramidal symptoms.

Table 1–4.   Common laboratory tests and studies when seeking medical clearance for psychiatric evaluation

Test	Abnormal results and their psychiatric implications
CBC	Macrocytic anemia—vitamin B_{12}/folate deficiency, alcohol abuse
	Microcytic anemia—iron deficiency
	Normocytic—acute bleeding or chronic inflammatory disease
	Leukocytosis—acute infection
	Leukopenia—advanced HIV disease, immune suppression, leukemia, carbamazepine
	Low platelets—side effect of valproate or carbamazepine, autoimmune thrombocytopenia
Basic metabolic	Elevated creatinine—renal failure
	Hyponatremia—can be caused by SSRIs, particularly in elderly
	Hypernatremia—dehydration, renal failure
	Low potassium—risk for arrhythmia; may be due to diuretic use, bulimia, diarrhea
	High potassium—risk for arrhythmia; may be due to renal failure
	Low bicarbonate—acidosis; aspirin ingestion
Liver enzymes	Elevated ALT:AST ratio—alcohol abuse
	Elevated ALT and AST—liver failure due to multiple causes (e.g., drugs, acetaminophen ingestion, hepatitis)
Urinalysis	Urinary tract infection in elderly or sick patient can lead to severe delirium
Urine drug screen	Positive—detection of some common drugs of abuse
TSH	Elevated—hypothyroidism leading to depression, cognitive changes
	Low—hyperthyroidism leading to manic-like symptoms, agitation
Vitamin B_{12}/folate	Low B_{12}—neurological changes, memory problems
	Low folate—evidence of general malnutrition; may be associated with depression, thromboembolic events
RPR	Latent syphilis—can lead to dementia, mood changes, neurological deficits
Chest X ray	Considered for all homeless patients, any patients with risk factors for tuberculosis, and elderly patients—look for evidence of tuberculosis, occult masses, pneumonia

Table 1–4. Common laboratory tests and studies when seeking medical clearance for psychiatric evaluation *(continued)*

Test	Abnormal results and their psychiatric implications
Head CT	Occasionally used for screening for gross masses or bleeding in patients with altered mental status or new-onset psychosis Less sensitive than MRI but less expensive, more accessible, and faster
EEG	If available acutely, can be used to look for nonconvulsive status epilepticus, evidence of metabolic encephalopathy (delirium)
Lumbar puncture	Indicated for any patient with new mental status changes, fever, and/or meningeal signs Look for evidence of viral or bacterial meningitis, encephalitis, bleeding, cryptococcal infection

Note. ALT = alanine aminotransferase; AST = aspartate aminotransferase; CBC = complete blood count; CT = computed tomography; EEG = electroencephalography; MRI = magnetic resonance imaging; RPR = rapid plasma reagin; SSRI = selective serotonin reuptake inhibitor; TSH = thyroid-stimulating hormone.

Documentation

Whenever a patient is hospitalized or released, either voluntarily or involuntarily, one of the clinician's most important jobs is to provide clear and thorough documentation. The purpose of emergency department documentation is twofold. First, the report may communicate details to other interested clinicians, such as the patient's outpatient psychiatrist or therapist, admitting doctor, and primary care doctor, when the treating clinician is not available to communicate with them. Second, the report will be used as evidence of what happened and what contributed to the assessment of the patient both by insurance companies and other organizations involved in utilization review activities and by courts if the patient is involved in a legal case (e.g., currently incarcerated, possibly raped) or if a malpractice case is brought against the treating clinician. Clinicians need to be aware not only of the liability involved in releasing a patient who may turn out to be dangerous, but also of the fact that lawsuits have been filed charging doctors with false imprisonment and deprivation of civil rights by patients who feel they were unjustly committed against their will. Therefore, documentation should be thorough regardless of disposition.

Components of Documentation

Documentation for every psychiatric admission or release should include the following:

- The facts on which an assessment is based, including the sources of these facts, such as the patient, collateral informants, and laboratory tests and studies
- A risk assessment of the patient's chronic *and* immediate risk of danger to self and others (Jacobs et al. 2003)
- A reasoned argument for the decision that was made and against the alternative disposition
- In the case of admission, clear documentation of all evidence that proves the patient's dangerousness or inability to care for self and the manner in which this will be addressed by psychiatric admission
- In the case of discharge, clear documentation of the lack of imminent dangerousness (A follow-up plan of some kind—even if it is merely a listing of information given to the patient for use on his or her own—is always warranted.)

It is absolutely essential that the risk assessment be documented in a clear and coherent manner that justifies the decision regarding admission and treatment that has been made by the treating psychiatrist. Readers of the assessment should not be left to deduce or infer the clinician's thought process.

Examples of Documentation

Ms. A is a 34-year-old single white woman, employed, domiciled, and recently divorced, with a history of alcohol dependence and depressive episodes. She was brought to the emergency department by emergency medical services after she called 911 reporting that she had taken an overdose of alcohol, diazepam, and painkillers. After medical stabilization, she was referred for psychiatric evaluation. Ms. A currently denies that she was intending to harm herself and maintains that she accidentally ingested these medications. She does not recall calling 911 for help and denies any current depressive symptoms. Collateral information from her ex-husband reveals that their divorce has resulted in the loss of custody of her children and that she has been absent from work and drinking more heavily since. Despite Ms. A's assertions of her safety, it is evident that she is at high risk for harming herself in the near future, given the potential lethality of her ingestion, her lack of insight into the dangerousness of her behavior, and reports of her decreasing ability to function. In addition, losing custody of her children is likely to have increased her risk of suicidal behavior due to feelings of guilt. She has no support in the community and no current psychiatric care. Due to these risks, she will be admitted for 72-hour observation for improvement in her mood with supportive and group psychotherapy, and plans for aftercare will be made before her release.

Mr. B is a 55-year-old single white man with no formal psychiatric history who was recently released from a brief jail stay for domestic violence. He presented to the emergency room after his mother called 911 stating that he was "acting crazy" and smashing items in her home. The patient was agitated on arrival but has maintained behavioral control since then and has shown no evidence of aggression or agitation. He admits to "having problems with my temper" and using cocaine earlier in the day. He is currently staying with his mother since his arrest for domestic violence. He admits to having angry feelings toward his ex-girlfriend who filed charges, and states that if he knew where she was staying, he would probably "knock some sense into her." However, he evidences no symptoms of mental illness and has a clear and coherent thought process. He is fully aware of the legal implications and risks of assaulting his ex-girlfriend. He declined referral to substance abuse treatment. Despite Mr. B's assertions of violent ideation, he does not demonstrate symptoms of a mental illness at this time and does not warrant psychiatric hospitalization. Prior to his release, the precinct in his ex-girlfriend's neighborhood was warned of his impending release. She has not been notified, according to her family, because she has entered a domestic violence shelter and they do not know her location. In addition, staff spoke with the patient's mother and advised her to call police if her son's behavior escalated and to take steps to assure her own safety.

Special Situations

Telephone Emergencies

Emergency departments frequently receive calls from people in the community seeking medical advice. When these calls are of a psychiatric nature, they may be directed to the consulting mental health clinician or routed to the psychiatric emergency department. Calls cover a wide range of questions, including issues of medications, side effects, and drug use. The clinician should try to help to the degree that he or she can. Patients should always be assured that they can come to the emergency department for further evaluation of their complaint and encouraged to contact their personal physician or mental health clinician for further assistance. When phone calls involve threats of violence or self-harm, the clinician should attempt to remain on the line with the patient, be supportive, and try to obtain as much information as possible about the patient's location. If the patient refuses to reveal his or her identity or location, the clinician should notify other emergency department staff to contact the police so that they can attempt to trace the call, although in the age of cellular phones, tracing can be difficult. If a clinician is concerned about the safety of the caller, notifying police and asking them to visit the caller to check on him or her is the safest option.

Rape

Although many rape victims never seek treatment, some victims may request a psychiatric consultation, emergency department staff may request a psychiatric consultation if they are concerned that a rape victim may be suicidal or otherwise psychiatrically compromised by the event, or a patient may reveal an assault while being evaluated for another psychiatric issue. Clinicians should ensure that all appropriate medical, legal, and counseling services are made available to the patient. The hospital's social work department can be helpful for finding victims services available in the area. Patients who have experienced rape or sexual traumatization should be offered and encouraged to have a full physical examination by a nurse or physician trained in evidence collection, even if they do not want to press charges at that time. Women should be offered prophylactic contraception to prevent pregnancy, and all patients should be counseled about and offered prophylaxis for sexually transmitted diseases and HIV. Patients may not wish to report the incident, but should be offered the opportunity to do so, and whenever possible they should be assisted by a rape crisis counselor or victim's advocate during this process. Patients who are considered "mentally ill" may experience more difficulty in reporting assaults because of the significant stigma attached to psychiatric diagnosis. The mental health clinician may have to assume more of an advocacy role in assisting the patient in making a report if the patient wishes to do so.

Chapter 7, "The Anxious Patient," provides further information about preventing psychiatric sequelae in victims of trauma.

Domestic Violence

As in cases of rape, the psychiatrist may be a part of the evaluation of a patient reporting domestic violence. Counseling or advocacy services, legal services, physical exams if indicated, and psychiatric follow-up should be made available to patients affected by domestic violence. An adult reporting domestic violence is not required to report the events to the police. However, if children in the home are at risk as a result of the violence, the clinician may be mandated by state law to report suspected child abuse. The clinician should avoid giving patients any pamphlets or fliers that are obviously about domestic violence, because these materials can lead to escalation if discovered. Leaving the abuser is not always immediately possible or indicated for victims; however, victims should be encouraged to make a "safety plan" for how to leave the home safely when they are ready. Victims sometimes require multiple tries before they successfully leave a violent situation. Once again, social work services should also be involved.

If the clinician suspects that a patient is unable to make a reasoned decision about his or her own safety due to mental illness, the clinician can arrange for psychiatric admission or make a report to adult protective services. For example, a patient with severe psychosis may not be able to organize herself to get out of an abusive situation and therefore may be deemed unable to care for herself.

Child Abuse

In most states, physicians are mandated to report child abuse. If a clinician has a reasonable suspicion that a child is being abused, neglected, or mistreated by a caregiver, the clinician should inform the appropriate agency of the suspicion. Child abuse can range from obvious episodes of physical abuse and torture, to sexual abuse or exploitation, to neglect of food, shelter, clothing, or even appropriate educational services. In the emergency department setting, suspicion of child abuse or neglect should be triggered when children 1) appear afraid of their parents or unwilling to speak in front of them, 2) have unexplained physical injuries, 3) have evidence of malnutrition or poor hygiene, or 4) are found to have excessive truancy from school. If a patient with dependent children is to be admitted to the hospital, efforts should be made to contact someone who can care for the children during the hospitalization to avoid referral to child protective services.

Elder Abuse

The aging of the population has led to a rise in the number of elderly adults in need of various levels of care. This care frequently falls to their adult children or spouses, who may lack the resources to adequately care for them. Nonjudgmental questioning of caregivers by the clinician is the best route toward discovering information. For example, saying, "It seems like your mom's care can be quite overwhelming. Do you ever feel like you can't handle it?" is more likely than an accusation of maltreatment to elicit a relieved request for assistance. Report of elder abuse is not mandated, but suspicion should increase when certain situations arise, including elderly patients who are dirty, unkempt, or malnourished; who have unexplained injuries; or who repeatedly present to the emergency department with no clear medical pathology or with medical conditions that are a result of noncompliance with treatment that is supposed to be monitored or administered by family members.

The Patient in Legal Custody

Patients in legal custody are brought for psychiatric evaluation to an emergency setting for a variety of reasons, including evaluation for suicidality, behavioral problems, treatment or prevention of withdrawal, or the need for a recommendation for psychiatric observation or treatment while in custody. Prior to interviewing the patient, the clinician should consider several key points that will determine what kind of interview takes place, whether any assessment is even indicated, and what question is being asked by those who are bringing the patient for evaluation. Most important, the clinician needs to remember that *patients do not surrender their right to doctor-patient confidentiality simply because they are under arrest or serving a jail or prison term* (U.S. Department of Health and Human Services 2003a). The clinician should ask the officers escorting the patient to delineate the patient's current legal status; to state the charges against the patient, so that the clinician can determine if the patient understands the charges; and to explain why the patient is being brought for evaluation. If the patient is released from the emergency department, the officers should know where the patient will go next—that is, to court, to jail, or to the community. They can also provide information about the patient's behavior while he or she was in custody. The patient should be interviewed without the police present, but should remain handcuffed to ensure safety.

The nature of the evaluation is determined by the question being asked, but the following general points are helpful when interviewing any patient in custody.

- Clarify to the patient at the outset what the nature of the interview is, what information will be held confidential, and what information, if any, will be disclosed to officers.
- Clarify the evaluator's role and the parameters of the evaluation. Patients in legal custody may be under the impression that the mental health clinician can arrange for charges to be dropped or for provisions to be made for what sort of housing they will have while incarcerated.
- Inform the patient not to make statements during the interview about his or her guilt or innocence regarding the charges because the medical record could be subpoenaed.
- Document the interview thoroughly in the medical record, particularly an assessment of the patient's risk for injury to self or others while in custody and any recommendations to the officers or the court for special precautions while in custody.

The Patient Who Does Not Speak English or Who Requires Sign Language Interpretation

All hospitals are required to make accommodations for patients who do not speak English or who are deaf or hard of hearing. Although the ideal is to provide a trained medical interpreter, this is not always possible. For language interpretation, the best available option may be use of phone interpreter services, which can offer the widest range of languages. If emergency department staff speak the patient's language, they can also be useful, but they should be asked to provide direct translation of what the doctor and patient are saying and to not interject their own opinions or questions. It is *never* acceptable to rely entirely on a family member or friend who is accompanying the patient, because this practice violates patient confidentiality and may prohibit the patient from making a full and honest accounting of his or her situation. If absolutely no other option is available, then it is better to at least get some information from the friend or family member, but more appropriate alternatives should be sought. Hospitals have been and can be sued for not providing appropriate language interpretation services or interpreter services for people who are deaf and hard of hearing.

The Pregnant Patient

Pregnancy should be suspected in women of reproductive age until proven otherwise by laboratory testing. The range of what is considered reproductive age is vast, so liberal use of beta-HCG (human chorionic gonadotropin) testing is advised to avoid missing a pregnancy.

Safety data on the use of psychiatric medication in pregnant patients are limited to case reports and population surveillance, so more data are available about older medications (Menon 2008). According to the American College of Obstetricians and Gynecologists (ACOG Committee on Practice Bulletins— Obstetrics 2008), it is better practice to treat pregnant women for their psychiatric problems with medication if indicated, because the risk of teratogenicity due to psychiatric medication is smaller than the known risk of low birth weight and other complications from having an untreated psychiatric illness during pregnancy. In the emergency department, discovery of a pregnancy can influence multiple areas of the patient's psychiatric care but should not preclude appropriate treatment, including treatment of agitation if indicated (Ladavac et al. 2007).

For many women, discovery of a pregnancy may be an unexpected or unpleasant surprise and thus may complicate whatever crisis brought them into the emergency department in the first place. The following are considerations for the pregnant emergency psychiatric patient:

- *Disposition planning.* Concerns include providing obstetric gynecological care as part of discharge planning, increased risk of suicide after discovery of an unplanned pregnancy, and referral to appropriate services.
- *Pharmacotherapy.* The clinician should make an informed choice of psychotropic medication based on risks and benefits and clearly document the thought process involved in either prescribing or refraining from prescribing medication.

- *Restraint.* Safe restraint becomes more complicated as a pregnancy progresses and should be avoided if possible. Patients in advanced stages of pregnancy should not be restrained on their back due to compromised blood flow through the vena cava.

The legal and ethical issues surrounding pregnancy in psychiatric patients are complicated. Patients with psychosis or severe psychiatric illness do not automatically surrender their right to reproductive choices, including choosing to terminate or continue a pregnancy, choosing to use or not use contraception, and so forth. The most appropriate option for dealing with pregnancy in the psychiatric patient is to treat the patient first, because optimizing her physical and psychiatric health is the best way to optimize the health of her fetus, and to put her in the best position to make decisions regarding her pregnancy and overall health.

Conclusion

Emergency psychiatry is a developing field, providing an opportunity for exposure to a vast array of patients and situations. Clinicians in this practice need to have skills in consultation-liaison psychiatry, crisis management, brief psychotherapy, and risk assessment, as well as a broad knowledge of medicine, hospital and health care systems, and general psychiatry. To best direct the care of patients, the mental health clinician working in the emergency department must view patients as individuals, as part of their social environment, and as part of the health care system.

Key Clinical Points

- Clinicians should consider their personal safety first. Clinicians should be aware of the protocols in the emergency department in which they are working, the environment in which they will be seeing patients, and patient factors that may lead to violent escalation.

- Assessment should focus on the patient's safety. Critical questions to consider are whether the patient's presentation is due to a medical condition better treated by a different clinician and whether the patient can adequately maintain his or her safety and the safety of others in the current outpatient setting.

- All emergency department encounters should be documented in the medical record, with sufficient detail that the reader of the documentation can understand the factors that went into the assessment and disposition of the patient.

References

ACOG Committee on Practice Bulletins—Obstetrics: ACOG practice bulletin: clinical management guidelines for obstetrician-gynecologists number 92, April 2008 (replaces practice bulletin number 87, November 2007). Use of psychiatric medications during pregnancy and lactation. Obstet Gynecol 111:1001–1020, 2008

Allen MA, Forster P, Zealberg J, et al; American Psychiatric Association Task Force on Psychiatric Emergency Services: Report and recommendations regarding psychiatric emergency and crisis services: a review and model program descriptions. August 2002. Available at: http://archive.psych.org/edu/other_res/lib_archives/archives/tfr/tfr200201.pdf. Accessed September 19, 2009.

Baillargeon J, Thomas CR, Williams B, et al: Medical emergency department utilization patterns among uninsured patients with psychiatric disorders. Psychiatr Serv 7:808–811, 2008

Brown JF: Emergency department psychiatric consultation arrangements. Health Care Manage Rev 30:251–261, 2005

Centers for Disease Control and Prevention: Revised Recommendations for HIV Testing of Adults, Adolescents, and Pregnant Women in Health-Care Settings. MMWR Morbidity and Mortality Weekly Report Recommendations and Reports (Vol 55, No RR14), September 26, 2006. Available at: http://www.cdc.gov/mmwr/PDF/rr/rr5514.pdf. Accessed January 20, 2009.

Downey LV, Zun LS, Gonzales SJ: Frequency of alternative to restraints and seclusion and uses of agitation reduction techniques in the emergency department. Gen Hosp Psychiatry 29:470–474, 2007

Flannery RB Jr: Precipitants to psychiatric patient assaults: review of findings, 2004–2006, with implications for EMS and other health care providers. Int J Emerg Ment Health 9:5–11, 2007

Guze BH, Love MJ: Medical assessment and laboratory testing in psychiatry, in Kaplan and Sadock's Comprehensive Textbook of Psychiatry. Edited by Sadock BJ, Sadock VA. Philadelphia, PA, Lippincott Williams & Wilkins, 2004, pp 916–928

Hazlett SB, McCarthy ML, Londner MS, et al: Epidemiology of adult psychiatric visits to U.S. emergency departments. Acad Emerg Med 11:193–195, 2004

Herzog A, Shore MF, Beale RR, et al: Patient safety and psychiatry: recommendations to the Board of Trustees of the American Psychiatric Association from the APA Task Force on Patient Safety. January 2003. Available at: http://archive.psych.org/edu/other_res/lib_archives/archives/tfr/tfr200301.pdf. Accessed September 19, 2009.

Jacobs DG, Baldessarini RJ, Conwell Y, et al; American Psychiatric Association Work Group on Suicidal Behaviors. Practice guideline for the assessment and treatment of patients with suicidal behaviors. Washington, DC, American Psychiatric Association, 2003

Ladavac AS, Dubin WR, Ning A, et al: Emergency management of agitation in pregnancy. Gen Hosp Psychiatry 29:39–41, 2007

Manley M: Interviewing techniques with the difficult patient, in Kaplan and Sadock's Comprehensive Textbook of Psychiatry. Edited by Sadock BJ, Sadock VA. Philadelphia, PA, Lippincott Williams & Wilkins, 2004, pp 904–907

Marco CA, Vaughan J: Emergency management of agitation in schizophrenia. Am J Emerg Med 23:767–776, 2005

Menon SJ: Psychotropic medication during pregnancy and lactation. Arch Gynecol Obstet 277:1–13, 2008

Moore DP, Jefferson JW: Handbook of Medical Psychiatry, 2nd Edition. Philadelphia, PA, Mosby, 2004, Section XVII, Chapters 155–156, pp 281–286

Physicians' Desk Reference, 62nd Edition. Montvale, NJ, Thomson Healthcare, 2008

Rocca P, Villari V, Bogetto F: Managing the aggressive and violent patient in the psychiatric emergency. Prog Neuropsychopharmacol Biol Psychiatry 30:586–598, 2006

U.S. Department of Health and Human Services: Health information privacy: disclosure for law enforcement purposes. May 2003a. Available at: http://www.hhs.gov/ocr/privacy/hipaa/faq/permitted/law/505.html. Accessed September 19, 2009.

U.S. Department of Health and Human Services: Summary of the HIPAA privacy rule, May 2003b. Available at: http://www.hhs.gov/ocr/privacy/hipaa/understanding/summary/privacysummary.pdf. Accessed November 24, 2009.

Vergare M, Binder R, Cook I, et al; Work Group on Psychiatric Evaluation: Practice guideline for the psychiatric evaluation of adults, 2nd edition. June 2006. Available at: http://www.psychiatryonline.com/pracGuide/loadGuidelinePdf.aspx?file=PsychEval2ePG_04-28-06. Accessed September 19, 2009.

Villari V, Rocca P, Fonzo V, et al: Oral risperidone, olanzapine and quetiapine versus haloperidol in psychotic agitation. Prog Neuropsychopharmacol Biol Psychiatry 32:405–413, 2008

Walsh PG, Currier G, Shah MN, et al: Psychiatric emergency services for the U.S. elderly: 2008 and beyond. Am J Geriatr Psychiatry 16:706–717, 2008

Wilhelm S, Schacht A, Wagner T: Use of antipsychotics and benzodiazepines in patients with psychiatric emergencies: results of an observational trial. BMC Psychiatry 8:61, 2008

Woo BK, Chan VT, Ghobrial N, et al: Comparison of two models for delivery of services in psychiatric emergencies. Gen Hosp Psychiatry 29:489–491, 2007

Zun LS: Evidence-based evaluation of psychiatric patients. J Emerg Med 28:35–39, 2005

Suggested Readings

Allen MA, Forster P, Zealberg J, et al; American Psychiatric Association Task Force on Psychiatric Emergency Services: Report and recommendations regarding psychiatric emergency and crisis services: a review and model program descriptions. August 2002. Available at: http://archive.psych.org/edu/other_res/lib_archives/archives/tfr/tfr200201.pdf. Accessed September 19, 2009.

Dubin WR, Lion JR (eds): Clinician Safety (APA Task Force Report 33). Washington, DC, American Psychiatric Association, 1993

Manley M: Interviewing techniques with the difficult patient, in Kaplan and Sadock's Comprehensive Textbook of Psychiatry. Edited by Sadock BJ, Sadock VA. Philadelphia, PA, Lippincott Williams & Wilkins, 2004, pp 904–907

2

The Suicidal Patient

Felicia Kuo Wong, M.D.

Ana Wolanin, M.S., R.N.

Patrick Smallwood, M.D.

Case Example

Mr. J is an 18-year-old single white male who was referred to emergency mental health services (EMHS) by his outpatient provider after Mr. J made threats to kill his coach for cutting him from the basketball team. In addition, he had threatened violence toward his mother and made statements of planning to hang himself. When he presented to the emergency department, he was extremely agitated and upset.

Suicide is a major health problem and one of the most common reasons why people present to psychiatric emergency rooms in crisis. In 2006, it was the eleventh leading cause of death in the United States for all age groups (National Institute of Mental Health [NIMH] 2009). The overall rate for suicide in the United States in 2006 was 11 per 100,000 (Centers for Disease Control and Prevention [CDC] 2009a). More than 33,000 completed suicides occur in the United States each year, which is equivalent to 91 suicides per day or one suicide every 16 minutes (CDC 2009a). It is estimated that there are 8–25 suicide attempts for every completed suicide (Moscicki 2001; NIMH 2009). Although only a small minority of suicide attempts result in death, each attempt increases the risk of death, serious long-term physical injury, and psychological suffering (Borges et al. 2006).

Demographics

Age

The prevalence and lethality of suicide differ across age groups. For example, although suicide attempts are more common for persons ages 15–34 years, the lethality is much higher in the elderly population. Among young adults ages 15–24, suicide is the third leading cause of death, accounting for 12% of all deaths in this group annually, and it is the second leading cause of deaths for adults ages 25–34 years (CDC 2009a). In young adults, there is one suicide for every 100–200 attempts, whereas in the elderly population ages 65 and older, there is one suicide for every four attempts (Goldsmith et al. 2002). The rate of suicide for elderly adults is estimated at 14 per 100,000 (Goldsmith et al. 2002).

Although the teen suicide rate has declined by over 25% since the early 1990s, it still remains a major problem. Adolescence is a difficult and turbulent time for teenagers as they attempt to navigate through a vast array of new experiences, including new relationships, decisions about their future, and physical changes that are taking place in their bodies due to hormonal influences. These changes can affect their mood and ability to adapt and cope, which may lead to an increased risk for suicide (American Psychiatric Association 2005).

The strongest risk factors for attempted suicide in the youth population are the presence of depression, alcohol or drug abuse, aggressive or disruptive behaviors, and a previous suicide attempt (American Psychiatric Association 2005). Other risk factors include frequent episodes of running away, incarceration, family loss or instability, significant problems with parents, expressions of suicidal thoughts or talk of death or the afterlife during moments of sadness or boredom, withdrawal from friends and family, difficulty dealing with sexual orientation, diminished interest in enjoyable activities, and unplanned pregnancy. The presence of depression results in a 14-fold increase in the risk of a first suicide attempt. Over half of the youth who have depression will attempt suicide at least once, and more than 7% will be successful (American Psychiatric Association 2005). Substance abuse or dependence also plays a significant role in youth suicide; 53% of young people who commit suicide have a known history of substance abuse. Firearms, the most common method of suicide completion in this age group, are used in over half of all youth suicides (American Psychiatric Association 2005).

Older Americans are disproportionately likely to die by suicide and have the highest suicide rates of any age group. In 2005, individuals ages 65 years and older accounted for 12.4% of the population but represented 16.6% of all suicide deaths. In 2004 in the United States, 14.3 per 100,000 people ages 65 and older committed suicide, compared with 10.9 per 100,000 in the general population. Among elderly individuals, an average of one suicide occurs every 90 minutes (National Strategy for Suicide Prevention [NSSP] 2009). The rates of suicide in the elderly population generally increase according to age: 13.1 per 100,000 for those ages 65–69 years, 15.2 per 100,000 for those ages 70–74 years, and 21.0 per 100,000 for those ages 85 years and older (NSSP 2009).

Risk factors for suicide among persons older than age 65 years differ from those of the rest of the population. In addition to having a higher prevalence of depression, older persons tend to be more socially isolated, make fewer attempts per completed suicide, and use more lethal methods (Goldsmith et al. 2002; NSSP 2009). The most common methods for suicide by older adults include firearms (71%), overdose (11%), and suffocation (11%) (Goldsmith et al. 2002). Because elderly persons have a higher burden of physical illnesses, they most often visit a health care provider before their suicide. It is estimated that prior to committing suicide, 20% of elderly persons had visited a physician within the preceding 24 hours, 41% within the previous week, and 75% within the previous month (NSSP 2009). Those who are divorced or widowed have the highest suicide rates, and men account for approximately 84% of suicides in this age group (NSSP 2009).

Gender

Suicide manifests differently in men and women. In 2004, suicide was the eighth leading cause of death for males and the sixteenth leading cause of death for females. Although women attempt suicide almost two to three times more often than men during their lifetime (Krug et al. 2002), almost four times as many males as females die from completed suicide (NIMH 2009). Males represented 78% of all suicides in the United States in 2005 (NIMH 2009). Although firearms, suffocation, and poisoning are the three most common methods of suicide for both males and females, males most often use firearms (56%), followed by suffocation (23%) and poisoning (13%), whereas females most often use poisoning (40%), followed by firearms (31%) and suffocation (19%) (NIMH 2009).

Race and Ethnicity

Data show different patterns or rates of suicide across various racial and ethnic groups in the United States. According to the CDC (2009a), for Native Americans ages 15–34 years, suicide is the second leading cause of death, with a rate of 19.7 per 100,000, which is 1.8 times higher than the national average for that age group. A study by Eaton et al. (2006) demonstrated that Hispanic female high school students in grades 9–12 reported a higher percentage of suicide attempts (14.9%) than their non-Hispanic white (9.3%) or non-Hispanic black (9.8%) counterparts. Caucasians have a substantially higher rate of suicide completion than African Americans, Hispanics, or Asians. For example, of every 100,000 people, the highest rates of death by suicide occurred in non-Hispanic whites (12.9) and Native Americans (12.4), whereas the lowest rates were among the non-Hispanic blacks (5.3), Asian Pacific Islanders (5.8), and Hispanics (5.9) (NIMH 2009).

Risk Factors

Research has clearly identified several risk factors related to suicide. The clinician needs to weigh the complex interaction of these factors when assessing a patient's risk for suicide and not simply consider each factor individually, because the cumulative effects of these factors place a patient at greater risk (Moscicki 1999). For example, the acute or immediate risk of suicide in a patient who is experiencing major depression and who may also be struggling with an impending loss increases considerably if he or she also has an alcohol abuse or dependence disorder, because alcohol may increase the patient's impulsivity and behavioral disinhibition (American Psychiatric Association 2003).

Demographics

The major demographic features that are linked to increased risk for suicide are marital status, age, gender, sexual orientation, and race. Men and women who are unmarried (never married, divorced, or widowed) have higher suicide rates than people who are married (American Psychiatric Association 2003). Cutright and Fernquist (2007) found that marital status has a greater protective effect on men than on women. The effect of age on suicide risk should be assessed in conjunction with race and gender. Caucasian males have a higher rate of suicide in late life (over age 65) (American Psychiatric Association 2003; U.S. Public Health Service 1999). Asian females have a dramatically high rate of suicide after age 80 and have the highest suicide rate among all women (American Psychiatric Association 2003; U.S. Public Health Service 1999). Native American males experience higher rates of suicide in adolescence and young adulthood compared with the national average for those age groups (CDC 2009a). Among all youth, 30% of attempted and completed suicides are related to sexual identity issues, especially among gay males (American Psychiatric Association 2003; U.S. Public Health Service 1999). Overall, men have the highest rate of completed suicides, whereas women have the highest lifetime rate of suicide attempts (Moscicki 1997).

Psychiatric History

Approximately 90% of people who have completed suicide have been diagnosed with a major psychiatric disorder (American Psychiatric Association 2003; Arsenault-Lapierre et al. 2004; Harris and Barraclough 1997). People with mood disorders, substance-related disorders, psychotic disorders, and personality disorders were found to have the highest risk for suicide (Arsenault-Lapierre et al. 2004; Moscicki 1999). The majority of completed suicides were by people with mood disorders, especially in the depressive phase. However, suicide risk is increased in those with bipolar disorder experiencing *mixed* episodes (American Psychiatric Association 2003). For people with mood disorders, the risk of suicide increases in those with comorbid alcohol abuse, anxiety and panic attacks, and symptoms of global insomnia and hopelessness (American Psychiatric Association 2003). People with schizophrenia and schizoaffective disorder also have high rates of suicide attempts, with risk increased in those with schizophrenia who had higher premorbid functioning (American Psychiatric Association 2003). The period of time immediately after hospitalization has been shown to increase the risk of suicide for patients with schizophrenia and schizoaffective disorders (American Psychiatric Association 2003). Importantly, suicide attempts by people with schizophrenia and schizoaffective disorder tend to be of greater lethality compared with attempts made by the general population and produce higher mortality and morbidity (American Psychiatric Association 2003).

Psychiatric comorbidity has also been found to increase a person's risk for suicide. Arsenault-Lapierre et al. (2004) found that on average suicide completers had 2.36 diagnoses. Studies show that 70%–80% of completed suicides have been by people with comorbid disorders and that the most important diagnostic comorbidities in increasing a person's risk for suicide are mood disorders combined with substance abuse disorders and personality disorders (American Psychiatric Association 2003).

In people diagnosed with a personality disorder (especially borderline personality disorder and antisocial personality disorder), the incidence of substance abuse and past history of suicide attempts are high, and when these patients have depressive states or experience a particular interpersonal loss, their risk for suicide is augmented (American Psychiatric Association 2003). The premise for increased suicide risk in people with substance abuse disorders and personality disorders is that they have a higher predisposition to aggression and impulsivity (Mann et al. 1999).

Psychological and Cognitive Dimensions

Psychological factors that have been found to potentiate suicide risk are anxiety and hopelessness (Fawcett 1999; Jacobs et al. 1999). Fawcett (1999) defined anxiety in the presence of depression as unremitting psychic pain. Hopelessness has been suggested as the culminating factor that explains why some depressed patients choose suicide whereas other depressed patients do not (Jacobs et al. 1999). Shame, worthlessness, and poor self-esteem in vulnerable individuals can lead to narcissistic injury that can be intolerable and increase the person's suicidal intent (American Psychiatric Association 2003). People who exhibit thought constriction and polarized thinking are unable to consider options when faced with stressful situations and are at higher risk for suicide (American Psychiatric Association 2003).

Psychosocial Dimensions

An important factor to establish when assessing patients for suicide risk is their access to firearms. The availability of firearms in combination with a mood disorder and intoxication is an acutely lethal profile (Moscicki 1999). Stressful life events can also significantly increase suicide risk. Stressors that have been identified as proximal risk factors include interpersonal loss, relationship conflicts, rejection, legal issues (e.g., incarceration), economic difficulties, and lack of social supports (American Psychiatric Association 2003; Moscicki 1999).

Childhood Trauma

Patients with a history of childhood trauma (physical and sexual abuse) may develop complex and incapacitating disorders as adults. These disorders include dissociative disorders, personality disorders, eating disorders, substance abuse disorders, and posttraumatic stress disorder (Chu 1999). In addition, these patients may express symptoms of severe impulsivity, mood lability, and self-injurious behaviors (Mann et al. 1999). The combination of these disabling disorders and complex traits places these patients at significant risk for suicide (American Psychiatric Association 2003; Chu 1999).

Family History

Both environmental and genetic factors have been identified as contributing to the increased risk of suicide. Although specific genetic factors involved in the transmission of suicidal behavior have yet to be identified, the clinician should make an effort to determine if the patient has a family history of suicide, particularly among any first-degree relatives, because this history has been shown to increase the patient's risk for suicide (American Psychiatric Association 2003; Mann et al. 1999). Environmental factors that are most likely to be associated with suicide risk are parental separation or divorce, parental legal problems, child abuse and neglect, and a family history of mental illness and/or substance abuse (Jacobs et al. 1999).

Physical Illness

The following physical illnesses and conditions are associated with an increased risk of suicide: malignant neoplasms, ulcer, lung disorders (especially asthma and chronic obstructive pulmonary disease), HIV/AIDS, Huntington's disease, brain injury, multiple sclerosis, lupus erythematosus, renal hemodialysis, and seizure disorders (Harris and Barraclough 1997; Jacobs et al. 1999). These illnesses have been found to increase suicide risk due to their association with chronic pain, impaired functioning, debilitation, and chronicity (American Psychiatric Association 2003; Jacobs et al. 1999). Likewise, the treatment of these illnesses may precipitate or exacerbate underlying mental illness (American Psychiatric Association 2003; Jacobs et al. 1999).

Assessment

The depth and breadth of information obtained from a psychiatric evaluation will vary with the setting, the patient's ability or willingness to provide information, and the availability of information from collateral sources. In some emergency mental health (EMH) settings, the psychiatrist may work with a team of professionals to gather all pertinent clinical information. In this instance, the psychiatrist should take on the leadership role of ensuring that all necessary information is obtained and then integrated into a final assessment and treatment plan. Because the patient may minimize the severity or even the existence of his or her difficulties, other individuals may serve as valuable resources for the psychiatrist in providing information about the patient's current mental state, activities, and psychosocial stressors. Sources of collateral information that may be helpful include the patient's family members and friends, physicians, other medical or mental health professionals, teachers or school personnel, colleagues or coworkers, and staff from supervised housing programs where the patient may reside (American Psychiatric Association 2003).

A thorough psychiatric evaluation is essential to the suicide assessment process. Information regarding the patient's psychiatric and medical history, current circumstances, and mental state must be obtained during this evaluation and used by the clinician to a) identify specific factors and features that may increase or decrease the risk of suicide or suicidal behaviors and that may be amenable to acute and ongoing interventions, b) address the patient's immediate safety and determine the most appropriate treatment setting, and c) develop a multiaxial differential diagnosis that can help guide the next step of treatment (Jacobs et al. 2003).

Psychiatric Signs and Symptoms

When evaluating a suicidal patient, the clinician should attempt to identify specific psychiatric signs and symptoms that have been correlated with an increased risk of suicide or other suicidal behaviors by asking the patient directly or through collateral information if available. These include aggression and violence toward others, impulsiveness, hopelessness, agitation, anxiety, anhedonia, global insomnia, and panic attacks (Fawcett 2001). Other psychiatric signs and symptoms, such as psychosis or depression, can help inform the clinician as to whether the patient has a psychiatric syndrome that should be addressed in treatment.

Past Suicidal Behavior

One of the most significant risk factors for suicide is a past history of suicide attempts (Moscicki 1997). Because suicide risk can be further increased by more serious, frequent, or recent attempts, the psychiatrist needs to explore in depth any past suicide attempts, aborted suicide attempts, and self-destructive behaviors. Details surrounding the attempts should be elicited, including information about the precipitants, timing, intent, consequences, and medical severity. If the patient was intoxicated with alcohol and/or drugs prior to the attempt, this should be noted, because intoxication can facilitate suicide attempts, as well as be part of a more serious suicide plan. Any interpersonal issues involved in the attempt should also be documented. The patient's thoughts about the attempts, including his or her perception of the lethality, ambivalence toward living, visualization of death, degree of premeditation, persistence of suicidal ideation, and reaction to attempt should be explored. Finally, information about prior self-injurious behaviors, including risk-taking behaviors such as unsafe sexual practices and reckless driving, may be relevant (Jacobs et al. 2003).

Past Psychiatric and Medical History

A patient's past psychiatric treatment history can provide information on co-morbid diagnoses, prior psychiatric hospitalizations, current suicidal ideation, and any previous suicide attempts. Information regarding a history of medical treatment can also help to identify medically serious suicide attempts, as well as any medical conditions that may be associated with increased suicide risk. A study by Druss and Pincus (2000) found that in models controlling for major depression, depressive symptoms, alcohol use, and demographic characteristics, the presence of a general medical condition predicted a 1.3 times greater likelihood of suicidal ideation. They also found that pulmonary diseases (e.g., asthma, bronchitis) were associated with a two-thirds increase in the odds of lifetime suicidal ideation, and cancer and asthma were associated with a more than fourfold increase in the likelihood of a suicide attempt (Druss and Pincus 2000).

Many patients who present with suicidality or after a suicide attempt are already in treatment, either with psychiatrists, mental health professionals, or primary care physicians. Collateral information from these caregivers can provide important insight that may be useful in determining a treatment plan and setting. The strength and stability of the therapeutic alliance should be gauged, because a positive therapeutic alliance is considered protective against suicidal behaviors, whereas a less reliable therapeutic alliance may represent an increased risk of suicide (Jacobs et al. 2003).

Family Psychiatric History

Because a family history of completed suicide and psychiatric illness significantly and independently increases the risk of suicide, the clinician must investigate the family's history of psychiatric hospitalizations, mental illness, substance use, and completed suicides or suicide attempts (Qin et al. 2002). Other information regarding the patient's childhood and current family milieu may also be relevant, because many aspects of family dysfunction, such as a history of family conflict, parental legal trouble, family substance use, domestic violence, and physical and/or sexual abuse, can be linked to self-destructive or suicidal behavior (Moscicki 1997).

Current Psychosocial Stressors and Function

Acute psychosocial crises or chronic psychosocial stressors may augment suicide risk and should be thoroughly assessed. Significant precipitants may include perceived losses or recent or impending humiliation. Understanding the patient's psychosocial situation is essential in helping the patient to mobilize external supports and can also have a protective influence on suicide risk (Jacobs et al. 2003).

Psychological Strengths and Vulnerabilities

A patient's psychological strengths and vulnerabilities should be considered when evaluating suicide risk and formulating a treatment plan. These strengths and vulnerabilities may include coping skills, personality traits, and thinking style, as well as developmental and psychological needs. Determining the patient's tendency to engage in risk-taking behaviors as well as past responses to stress, including capacity for reality testing and ability to tolerate rejection, subjective loneliness, or psychological pain when his or her unique psychological needs are not met, may give clues to the patient's suicide risk (American Psychiatric Association 2003). Factors such as thought constriction or polarized ("either-or") thinking, closed-mindedness, or perfectionism with excessively high self-expectations have also been noted in clinical practice to be possible contributors to suicide risk (American Psychiatric Association 2003).

Suicide Inquiry

Two important predictors of suicide are current suicidal ideation and a history of suicide attempts (American Psychiatric Association 2003; Mann 2002). Careful inquiry into the patient's current and past thinking and behavior in relation to suicide are extremely important in determining proximal risk (American Psychiatric Association 2003; Mann 2002). The essential features of a suicide inquiry are assessment of suicidal ideation, suicidal intent, suicide plan, suicidal behavior, and suicide history.

Suicidal Ideation and Suicidal Intent

When interviewing a suicidal patient, the clinician needs to explore the frequency and intensity of current and recent suicidal ideation as a means of determining the severity. Clinicians must also ask specifically when the thoughts began, how frequently they occur, and whether the patient can control the thoughts or the thoughts are obsessive (Jacobs et al. 1999). Also, clinicians must determine if the patient's thoughts are passive (i.e., a wish to be dead) or if the patient is actively planning to kill himself or herself, because suicidal ideation with a clear, detailed, and well-conceived plan increases proximal risk (American Psychiatric Association 2003; Jacobs et al. 1999). It is also important to determine what patients believe they will accomplish by killing themselves, because such motivations as a wish to reunite with a dead loved one, ending intense psychological pain, escaping shame, and perceiving death as peaceful all increase the severity of intent and proximal risk of suicide (American Psychiatric Association 2003). Not all patients will admit to suicidal ideation, but the clinician can elicit thoughts of suicide by asking the patient to talk about his or her future (American Psychiatric Association 2003).

Suicide Plan and Suicidal Behavior

It is important to determine if a patient has a plan and the lethality of that plan. Plans with high lethality that are irreversible, such as the use of firearms, jumping, hanging, and suicide via motor vehicles, place the patient at higher risk (American Psychiatric Association 2003). The clinician should also investigate if the patient has rehearsed the plan or made preparations, because rehearsal and preparations, such as completing a will or purchasing the means to accomplish the plan, indicate an increased wish to die (American Psychiatric Association 2003). Even if the plan is not one that will likely result in death from an objective medical standpoint, the clinician should still consider the patient's expectation, because the patient's belief that the plan will culminate in death places the patient's risk as high (American Psychiatric Association 2003).

Suicide History

Clinicians should assess the patient's history of suicide attempts and assess the lethality of previous attempts as a means of defining the patient's current risk (American Psychiatric Association 2003; Jacobs et al. 1999; Mann 2002). Attempts that resulted in medical or intensive care unit admission, loss of consciousness, or extensive tissue or organ damage are considered high-risk attempts (Jacobs et al. 1999). Attempts made with low potential for rescue, such as attempts made in locations and at times with low probability of discovery or in locations with poor accessibility for rescue, are also attempts of high lethality (Jacobs et al. 1999).

Estimated Suicide Risk

No body of scientific literature is available to inform the clinician on how to assign suicide risk to a patient. The clinician must integrate the clinical data gathered, evaluate the data in light of the severity and acuity of the patient's symptoms and psychosocial stressors, and apply clinical judgment to formulate risk. Risk factors should be considered cumulative and synergistic and should be weighed against the patient's protective factors, which can attenuate risk (American Psychiatric Association 2003). Protective factors or factors that mitigate risk include a) a positive therapeutic relationship; b) psychosocial supports, such as family and friends; c) evidence of coping skills, such as the ability to tolerate rejection, loss, and humiliation; d) flexibility; e) a sense of responsibility to family; f) children (except in cases of postpartum depression); g) religious prohibition; h) pregnancy; i) full-time employment (especially in persons with substance abuse disorders); and j) the ability to cite reasons for living and optimism (American Psychiatric Association 2003). Finally, the patient's access to means must be determined and restricted if possible. Table 2–1 provides guidelines for determining whether hospital admission is indicated based on a patient's risk factors and psychopathology.

Case Example *(continued)*

Mr. J had just learned that he did not make the varsity basketball team 2 days prior to his referral to EMHS. He reported active suicidal ideation with the aforementioned plan but denied intent to the EMHS clinician. He denied any homicidal ideation but endorsed being "upset" and "frustrated." He had no previous history of psychiatric hospitalizations, suicide attempts, or aggression. He denied any history of trauma or abuse. His family psychiatric history was significant only for schizophrenia. He had been seeing his outpatient psychiatrist for treatment of bipolar disorder and attention-deficit/hyperactivity disorder since age 15. He was clear that he did not like his provider, stating, "I don't think he has helped me at all." Upon medical clearance in EMHS, the toxicology screen was positive for cannabis, which he reported using three times a week. In addition, he acknowledged occasional use of alcohol on the weekends but denied blackouts or alcohol withdrawal symptoms. He described his main support system to be his girlfriend of 2 years and various close friends. He did not get along with his mother but reported a close relationship with his father and grandmother. He was a high school student with a B/C average who enjoyed hanging out with his friends and "playing ball."

Psychiatric Management of Suicidal Behaviors

The management of suicidal patients who present to the emergency department or an EMH unit includes a broad array of therapeutic interventions targeting the suicidal behavior, as well as any comorbid major mental illnesses, personality disorders, psychosocial issues, and interpersonal difficulties that may be present. According to the "Practice Guideline for the Assessment and Treatment of Patients With Suicidal Behaviors" (American Psychiatric Association 2003), "Psychiatric management includes establishing and maintaining a therapeutic alliance; attending to the patient's safety; and determining the patient's psychiatric status, level of functioning, and clinical needs to arrive at a plan and setting for treatment" (p. 29). Once the initial evaluation is complete and the treatment plan has been determined, additional goals of psychiatric management may be applied in the emergency setting; these include crisis intervention, facilitating treatment adherence, and providing education to the patient and family members.

Establishing Therapeutic Alliance

When a suicidal patient presents to an EMH unit, he or she may never have had an encounter with a mental health professional. During this initial encounter, the psychiatrist must work to build trust and develop a therapeutic relationship, with the ultimate goal of reducing the patient's suicide risk. An individual who is determined to commit suicide may be unmotivated to develop a cooperative doctor-patient relationship and may view the emergency intervention as adversarial. In working with a suicidal patient, no matter how brief the intervention, the psychiatrist should practice empathy and demonstrate an understanding of the suicidal individual, as well as provide emotional support and expand the patient's sense of possible choices other than suicide (Jacobs et al. 2003).

Table 2–1. Guidelines for selecting a treatment setting for patients at risk for suicide or suicidal behaviors

Admission generally indicated

After a suicide attempt or aborted suicide attempt if:

Patient is psychotic

Attempt was violent, near-lethal, or premeditated

Precautions were taken to avoid rescue or discovery

Persistent plan and/or intent is present

Distress is increased or patient regrets surviving

Patient is male, older than age 45 years, especially with new onset of psychiatric illness or suicidal thinking

Patient has limited family and/or social support, including lack of stable living situation

Current impulsive behavior, severe agitation, poor judgment, or refusal of help is evident

Patient has change in mental status with a metabolic, toxic, infectious, or other etiology requiring further workup in a structured setting

In the presence of suicidal ideation with:

Specific plan with high lethality

High suicidal intent

Admission may be necessary

After a suicide attempt or aborted suicide attempt, except in circumstances for which admission is generally indicated

In the presence of suicidal ideation with:

Psychosis

Major psychiatric disorder

Past attempts, particularly if medically serious

Possibly contributing medical condition (e.g., acute neurological disorder, cancer, infection)

Lack of response to or inability to cooperate with partial hospital or outpatient treatment

Need for supervised setting for medication trial or electroconvulsive therapy

Source. Reprinted from "Practice Guideline for the Assessment and Treatment of Patients With Suicidal Behaviors." *American Journal of Psychiatry* 160(suppl):31, 2003. Copyright 2003, American Psychiatric Association. Used with permission.

Determining the Appropriate Treatment Setting

Perhaps the most important decision made during the evaluation of a suicidal patient in a psychiatric emergency is the determination of appropriate treatment setting. Jacobs et al. (2003) suggested that patients with suicidal thoughts, plans, or behaviors should be seen and evaluated in the least restrictive safe and effective treatment environment. Treatment settings span a continuum of different levels of care, ranging from the most restrictive, involuntary inpatient hospitalization; through partial hospitalization and intensive outpatient programs; to the least restrictive setting of ambulatory care. The choice of treatment setting should be based on the best estimate of the patient's current suicide risk, risk of harm toward others, and other aspects of the patient's presentation. These factors may include medical and psychiatric comorbidity; strength and availability of a psychosocial support network; and ability to provide adequate self-care, give reliable feedback to the psychiatrist, and cooperate with treatment.

Hospitalization, the most restrictive treatment setting, should always be considered when the patient's safety is in question. Inpatient treatment is usually indicated for individuals who pose a serious threat of harm to themselves or others. Significant factors favoring inpatient hospitalization over alternative treatment settings for suicidal patients include psychosis, past suicide attempts, and persistence of a specific suicidal plan with high lethality or intent (Goldberg et al. 2007). Other considerations for inpatient treatment include factors based on the severity of illness and the intensity of services needed by the patient. For example, severely ill individuals may require inpatient care because they cannot be safe in a less restrictive environment or because they lack structure or social support outside of a hospital setting. In addition, hospitalization is indicated when there is a new, acute presentation that is not part of a repetitive or chronic pattern. Those individuals with a complicated psychiatric or general medical condition that has not responded adequately to outpatient treatment may also need to be hospitalized. Some patients with lesser degrees of suicidality may end up needing more intensive treatment if they lack a strong psychosocial support system, are unable to gain timely access to outpatient care, have limited insight into the need for treatment, or are unable to adhere to recommendations for ambulatory follow-up. In geographic areas where partial hospital or intensive outpatient programs are not readily accessible, inpatient care may be necessary at lower levels of suicide risk to keep certain individuals safe (Jacobs et al. 2003).

It is important to recognize that hospitalization is not a treatment, but rather is a treatment setting that can facilitate continued evaluation and treatment of suicidal persons. In considering an intensive intervention such as inpatient hospitalization, a clinician should weigh the risks and benefits of hospitalization, and balance a person's right to privacy and choice against the issue of potential dangerousness to self or others. The decision to hospitalize should not be taken lightly; although the benefits of treatment seem obvious to a trained professional, hospitalization carries the potential for negative effects for the patient, such as social stigma, financial difficulties, and loss of employment. Some people may feel frightened or humiliated in the hospital, whereas others may feel a sense of emotional relief.

Hospitalization can occur on a voluntary or an involuntary basis. This decision is often made during the EMH evaluation and depends on a variety of factors. These factors include the estimated level of risk to the patient and others, the patient's level of insight and willingness to seek care, and the legal criteria for involuntary hospitalization in the clinician's jurisdiction. Generally, patients who are at imminent risk for suicide will satisfy the criteria for involuntary hospitalization; however, specific commitment criteria vary from state to state, and emergency psychiatrists must know the specific state statutes regarding involuntary hospitalization. Under some circumstances, the decision to hospitalize may be made before additional history is available, based on the high potential of dangerousness to self or others, or the patient's inability or unwillingness to cooperate with a psychiatric evaluation (e.g., in the presence of extreme agitation, psychosis, or catatonia).

For those patients who are not found to be at imminent risk for suicide and who do not require inpatient treatment, outpatient services may be appropriate. A "step-down" level of care from hospitalization includes two options: an intensive outpatient program or partial hospitalization. Less intensive treatment may be more appropriate if suicidal ideation or actual attempts are part of a chronic, repetitive cycle and if the patient is aware of the chronicity. For those patients with a history of suicidal ideation without suicidal intent and a strong ongoing doctor-patient relationship, the benefits of continued treatment outside of the hospital may outweigh the potential negative effects of hospitalization.

Under some circumstances, individuals who are not involved in outpatient treatment may be referred for care after a suicide attempt or emergency psychiatric evaluation. Adherence can often be a problem for those individuals referred for outpatient follow-up after an emergency psychiatric evaluation. Therefore, the clinician should discuss the referral with the patient during the course of the interview and, if possible, arrange a specific appointment time. Related issues are discussed further in Chapter 13, "Disposition and Resource Options."

Providing Treatment

Psychopharmacological interventions that modify risk factors may be helpful in preventing suicide. The following treatment modalities have been studied, and some limited evidence indicates that they may help reduce the risk of suicide in certain populations. In this section, we provide a broad overview of treatment modalities, with an emphasis on those interventions that can take place or begin in the emergency psychiatric setting.

Medications can be lifesaving not only in the long term, but also in the short term, such as in the treatment of severe acute anxiety in a depressed patient. In the emergency setting, medications can provide significant immediate relief, but have time-limited effects that require close supervision of the patient's mental status, because the effects of the medications can wear off and symptoms may reemerge, with subsequent recurrence of suicidal impulses. Even if medications are given for acute treatment, a patient at high risk for suicide must still be monitored closely or hospitalized until the crisis resolves. Research will continue to investigate and delineate the role of different types of psychopharmacological interventions in acute suicide prevention.

Antidepressants

Currently, evidence remains inconclusive that any type of antidepressant or antianxiety treatment is associated with lowering the acute risk for suicidal behavior (Fawcett 2001). However, the American Psychiatric Association's (2003) practice guideline suggests that a strong association exists between clinical depression and suicide, and that the reasonable effectiveness and safety of antidepressants support their use. In the EMH setting, although antidepressants are rarely prescribed on an acute basis without secured outpatient follow-up, nontricyclic, non–monoamine oxidase inhibitor antidepressants should be considered first and dosed in a conservative manner, because they are relatively safe and present minimal risks of lethality on overdose (Jacobs 2003).

Lithium

A recent meta-analysis of studies of suicide rates with versus without long-term lithium maintenance in patients with recurring bipolar disorder and major depressive disorder found an almost 14-fold decrease in suicidal acts. Lithium maintenance treatment was associated with an 80%–90% decrease in risk of suicide and more than a 90% decrease in suicide attempt rates (Jacobs 2003). As with antidepressants, initiation of lithium should not be considered in an emergency department setting unless secured follow-up or inpatient psychiatric hospitalization occurs.

Benzodiazepines

Clinical evidence suggests that aggressive treatment of panic, anxiety, and agitation with benzodiazepines or other anxiolytic agents may reduce suicidal risk. In the EMH setting, the concern for benzodiazepine dependency should be viewed as less important than the risk of suicide. However, benzodiazepines should be used cautiously in patients with borderline personality disorder because behavioral disinhibition may occur (Fawcett 2001).

Anticonvulsants

Anticonvulsant medications, such as divalproex, have been used to reduce agitation in a whole host of psychiatric conditions. However, the long-term effectiveness of anticonvulsant agents in protecting against recurrent mood episodes or reducing risk of suicidal behavior has not been well established (Jacobs 2003). As with all psychotropic medications, initiation of anticonvulsants should be carefully weighed against the risk of potential overdose or misuse.

Atypical Neuroleptics

Atypical neuroleptics, such as olanzapine and quetiapine, seem to produce anxiolytic and antiagitation effects in some patients and may play a role in reducing suicide risk. In patients with schizophrenia and schizoaffective disorders, studies have shown that clozapine substantially reduces suicide attempts. Olanzapine has been found to be more effective than haloperidol in reducing suicide attempts in patients with schizophrenia (Fawcett 2001). In the psychiatric emergency setting, neuroleptics are used primarily to reduce aggression and agitation.

Documentation and Risk Assessment

Case Example *(continued)*

Mr. J allowed the EMHS clinician to contact his father and his school for collateral information. His father reported that Mr. J "has a mighty temper" but had never committed any acts of violence toward others or property. The school reported that he had been suspended for disruptive behaviors in class but was not considered a dangerous student. When evaluated by the clinician, Mr. J was calm and stated he felt he could maintain his safety as an outpatient. Although Mr. J was initially reluctant to allow the clinician to talk to his psychiatrist, he eventually agreed. The EMHS clinician and psychiatrist determined that the most appropriate disposition for him would be to go home and continue psychopharmacological treatment with his psychiatrist, with a strong consideration of a mood stabilizer trial. In addition, the EMHS team felt that Mr. J would benefit from a referral to a psychotherapist who could help him learn techniques aimed at affect modulation. This referral was made, and Mr. J was discharged after agreeing to the plan. He was given phone numbers for a suicide hotline and EMHS, with a recommendation to return to EMHS if he were to feel suicidal or unsafe.

The clinician has a duty of care to the patient and, as such, is expected to act affirmatively to protect the patient from self-injurious behaviors. Also, the clinician is expected to practice within the accepted standard of care, which is defined as the conventional practice undertaken by professionals of similar training under similar clinical circumstances. Negligence is determined by a court of law by establishing that the clinician violated his or her duty of care to the patient through omission or commission and that the clinician did not practice within the established standard of care. Although it is not possible to predict suicidal behavior, the clinician is expected to make a reasonable evaluation of foreseeability based on the interpretation of the data gathered during the assessment (Berman 2006). Furthermore, the data gathered, the interpretation of that data, and the assessment of the patient based on that data should be rooted in scientific evidence and not solely on clinical experience (Berman 2006; Simon 2006). Whether duty of care and standard of care were met and practiced in a reasonable and prudent manner is determined through documentation. Therefore, documentation should include the assessment of suicide risk, the interventions, and the aspects of the assessment that justify the interventions. The clinician must also document the rationale and the decision-making process for the clinical choices made or rejected at each major transition in the patient's care (e.g., discharge, change in observation level, admission) (American Psychiatric Association 2003; Berman 2006).

Clinicians must be mindful to assess and document a patient's *proximal* suicide risk, based on the presence of a suicide note, access to firearms, a history of near-lethal attempts, a recent and severely stressful life event, and incapacitating physical illness (American Psychiatric Association 2003; Moscicki 1997). Restricting the means by which a patient can commit suicide, especially by removal of firearms, must be attempted, and the efforts to restrict means must be documented (American Psychiatric Association 2003).

An integral component of the risk assessment is the collection and documentation of collateral information from family or care providers. In emergency situations, and to protect the patient from self-harm or harm to others, the clinician may breach the patient's confidentiality and contact family and care providers without the patient's consent as long as the clinician does not disclose patient information (American Psychiatric Association 2003). Prior to any breach of confidentiality, the patient's permission to contact family and care providers should be aggressively sought, because in addition to obtaining information from the family, it is also essential to involve and educate the family in the patient's care as a means of attenuating the patient's risk (Berman 2006). Table 2–2 outlines risk management and documentation issues relative to suicide assessment and management.

Suicide Prevention Contracts

The suicide prevention contract, also known as the no-harm contract, was originally developed in 1973 to facilitate the management of the patient at suicide risk (Centre for Suicide Prevention 2002). Even today, clinicians readily report that patients are either able or unable to "contract for their safety." However, despite the widespread use of verbal and written suicide contracts in

Table 2–2. General risk management and documentation considerations in the assessment and management of patients at risk for suicide

Good collaboration, communication, and alliance between clinician and patient

Careful and attentive documentation, including:

    Risk assessments

    Record of decision-making processes

    Descriptions of changes in treatment

    Record of communications with other clinicians

    Record of telephone calls from patients or family members

    Prescription log or copies of actual prescriptions

    Medical records of previous treatment, if available, particularly treatment related to past suicide attempts

Critical junctures for documentation:

    At first psychiatric assessment or admission

    With occurrence of any suicidal behavior or ideation

    Whenever there is any noteworthy clinical change

    For inpatients, before increasing privileges or giving passes and before discharge

Monitoring issues of transference and countertransference in order to optimize clinical judgment

Consultation, a second opinion, or both should be considered when necessary

Careful termination (with appropriate documentation)

Firearms

    If present, document instructions given to the patient and significant others

    If absent, document as a pertinent negative

Planning for coverage

Source. Reprinted from "Practice Guideline for the Assessment and Treatment of Patients With Suicidal Behaviors." *American Journal of Psychiatry* 160(suppl):41, 2003. Copyright 2003, American Psychiatric Association. Used with permission.

clinical practices, no studies have proved their effectiveness in reducing or preventing suicide. Clinicians should be warned that suicide prevention contracts are based on subjective rather than objective evidence, are not legally binding, and should not serve as a substitute for careful clinical assessment. Under no circumstance should a patient's willingness or reluctance to enter into a verbal or written suicide contract be used as an indicator for discharge planning, especially from an emergency department setting (Jacobs et al. 2003).

Conclusion

Suicide is a major health problem and one of the most common reasons why people present to psychiatry emergency rooms in crisis. More than 33,000 completed suicides occur in the United States each year, which is equivalent to 91 suicides per day or 1 suicide every 16 minutes. Although only a small minority of suicide attempts end up in death, each attempt increases the risk of death, serious long-term physical injury, and psychological suffering. The prevalence and lethality of suicide differ across age groups, gender, and race/ethnicity.

Research has clearly identified several risk factors related to suicide. The major demographic features linked to increased risk for suicide are marital state, age, gender, sexual orientation, and race/ethnicity. Approximately 90% of people who have completed suicide have been diagnosed with a major psychiatric disorder. Psychological factors found to potentiate suicide risk are anxiety and hopelessness. Other important risk factors to ask about include access to firearms, childhood trauma, family history, and physical illness.

The depth and breadth of information obtained from a psychiatric evaluation will vary with the setting, the patient's ability or willingness to provide information, and the availability of information from collateral sources. A thorough psychiatric evaluation is essential to the suicide assessment. Information regarding the patient's psychiatric and medical history, current circumstances, and mental state must be obtained during this evaluation. Two important predictors of suicide are current suicidal ideation and history of suicide attempts. A comprehensive suicide inquiry should include assessment of suicidal ideation, suicide intent, a suicide plan, suicidal behavior, and suicide history.

Psychiatric management of suicidal behaviors includes establishing and maintaining therapeutic alliance, attending to the patient's safety, and determining the patient's psychiatric status, level of function, and clinical needs to arrive at a plan and setting for treatment.

Key Clinical Points

- The prevalence and lethality of suicide differ across age, gender, racial, and ethnic groups. Understanding that different risk factors and methods used for self-harm pertain to each group can help with determining the most appropriate assessment and treatment planning for an individual.

- Research has clearly identified several risk factors related to suicide. Demographics, past psychiatric history, psychological and cognitive dimensions, psychosocial dimensions, childhood trauma, family history, and physical illness can all influence an individual's risk of suicide. The cumulative effect of these factors places a patient at greater risk.

- A thorough psychiatric evaluation should include a review of psychiatric signs and symptoms, past suicidal behavior, past psychiatric and medical history, family psychiatric history, current psychosocial stressors and functioning, psychological strengths and vulnerabilities, and a suicide inquiry.

- The essential features of a suicide inquiry are assessment of suicidal ideation, suicidal intent, suicide plan, suicidal behavior, and suicide history.

- The management of suicidal patients who present to the emergency department includes a broad array of therapeutic interventions targeting the suicidal behavior, as well as any comorbid major mental illnesses, personality disorders, psychosocial issues, and interpersonal difficulties that may be present.

- Perhaps the most important decision made during the evaluation of a suicidal patient in an emergency setting is the determination of appropriate treatment setting. Psychopharmacological treatment options should also be considered. In the emergency setting, medications can provide significant immediate relief but have time-limited effects that require close supervision of the patient's mental status, because the effects of the medications can wear off and symptoms may reemerge, with subsequent recurrence of suicidal impulses.

- Those patients at high risk for suicide must be monitored closely or hospitalized until the crisis resolves.

- Documentation should include the assessment of suicide risk, the interventions, and the aspects of the assessment that justify the interventions. The clinician should note the rationale and decision-making process for the choices made or rejected at each major transition in the patient's care (e.g., admission, change in observation level, discharge). Restricting the means by which a patient can commit suicide must be attempted, and the efforts to restrict means must be documented. Collection and documentation of collateral information from family or providers is important.

- Despite the widespread use of suicide contracts in clinical practices, no studies have proved their effectiveness in reducing or preventing suicide. Suicide prevention contracts are based on subjective rather than objective evidence, are not legally binding, and should not serve as a substitute for careful clinical assessment.

References

American Psychiatric Association: Practice guideline for the assessment and treatment of patients with suicidal behaviors. Am J Psychiatry 160(suppl):1–60, 2003

American Psychiatric Association: Let's talk facts about teen suicide. May 2005. Available at: http://www.healthyminds.org/Document-Library/Brochure-Library/Teen-Suicide.aspx. Accessed November 13, 2009.

Arsenault-Lapierre G, Kim C, Turecki G: Psychiatric diagnoses in 3275 suicides: a meta-analysis. BMC Psychiatry 4:37, 2004

Berman AL: Risk management with suicidal patients. J Clin Psychol 62:171–184, 2006

Borges G, Angst J, Nock MK, et al: A risk index for 12-month suicide attempts in the National Comorbidity Survey Replication (NCS-R). Psychol Med 36:1747–1757, 2006

Centers for Disease Control and Prevention: Suicide facts at a glance, Summer 2009. 2009a. Available at: http://www.cdc.gov/ViolencePrevention/pdf/Suicide-DataSheet-a.pdf. Accessed September 20, 2009.

Centers for Disease Control and Prevention: Welcome to WISQARS (Web-based Injury Statistics Query and Reporting System). 2009b. Available at: http://www.cdc.gov/injury/wisqars/index.html. Accessed September 20, 2009.

Centre for Suicide Prevention: No-suicide contracts: a review of the findings from the research. SIEC Alert #49, September 2002. Available at: http://www.suicideinfo.ca/csp/assets/alert49.pdf. Accessed January 21, 2010.

Chu JA: Trauma and suicide, in Harvard Medical School Guide to Suicide Assessment and Intervention. Edited by Jacobs DG. San Francisco, CA, Jossey-Bass, 1999, pp 332–354

Cutright P, Fernquist RM: Three explanations of marital status differences in suicide rates: social integration, marital status integration, and the culture of suicide. Omega 56:175–190, 2007

Druss B, Pincus H: Suicidal ideation and suicide attempts in general medical illnesses. Arch Intern Med 160:1522–1526, 2000

Eaton DK, Kann L, Kinchen S, et al: Youth risk behavior surveillance—United States, 2005. MMWR CDC Surveill Summ 55(5):1–108, 2006

Fawcett J: Profiles of completed suicides, in Harvard Medical School Guide to Suicide Assessment and Intervention. Edited by Jacobs DG. San Francisco, CA, Jossey-Bass, 1999, pp 115–124

Fawcett J: Treating impulsivity and anxiety in the suicidal patient. Ann N Y Acad Sci 932:94–105, 2001

Goldberg J, Ernst C, Bird S: Predicting hospitalization versus discharge of suicidal patients presenting to a psychiatric emergency service. Psychiatr Serv 58:561–565, 2007

Goldsmith SK, Pellmar TC, Kleinman AM, et al. (eds): Reducing Suicide: A National Imperative. Washington, DC, National Academy Press, 2002

Harris EC, Barraclough B: Suicide as an outcome for mental disorders: a meta-analysis. Br J Psychiatry 170:205–228, 1997

Jacobs DG, Brewer M, Klein-Benheim M: Suicide assessment: an overview and recommended protocol, in Harvard Medical School Guide to Suicide Assessment and Intervention. Edited by Jacobs DG. San Francisco, CA, Jossey-Bass, 1999, pp 3–39

Krug EG, Dahlberg LL, Mercy JA, et al. (eds): World Report on Violence and Health. Geneva, World Health Organization, 2002

Mann JJ: A current perspective of suicide and attempted suicide. Ann Intern Med 136:302–311, 2002

Mann JJ, Waternaux C, Hass GL, et al: Toward a clinical model of suicidal behavior in psychiatric patients. Am J Psychiatry 156:181–189, 1999

Moscicki EK: Identification of suicide risk factors using epidemiologic studies. Psychiatr Clin North Am 20:499–517, 1997

Moscicki EK: Epidemiology of suicide, in Harvard Medical School Guide to Suicide Assessment and Intervention. Edited by Jacobs DG. San Francisco, CA, Jossey-Bass, 1999, pp 40–51

Moscicki EK: Epidemiology of completed and attempted suicide: toward a framework for prevention. Clin Neurosci Res 1:310–323, 2001

National Institute of Mental Health: Suicide in the U.S.: statistics and prevention. July 27, 2009. Available at: http://www.nimh.nih.gov/health/publications/suicide-in-the-us-statistics-and-prevention.shtml. Accessed September 20, 2009.

National Strategy for Suicide Prevention: At a glance—suicide among the elderly. Available at: http://mentalhealth.samhsa.gov/suicideprevention/elderly.asp. Accessed September 20, 2009.

Qin P, Agerbo E, Mortensen P: Suicide risk in relation to family history of completed suicide and psychiatric disorders: a nested case-control study based on longitudinal registers. Lancet 360:1126–1130, 2002

Simon RI: Suicide risk assessment: is clinical experience enough? J Am Acad Psychiatry Law 34:276–278, 2006

U.S. Public Health Service: The Surgeon General's call to action to prevent suicide. 1999. Available at: http://www.surgeongeneral.gov/library/calltoaction/default.htm. Accessed September 20, 2009.

Suggested Readings

American Psychiatric Association: Practice guideline for the assessment and treatment of patients with suicidal behaviors. Am J Psychiatry 160(suppl):1–60, 2003

3

Violence Risk Assessment

Vasilis K. Pozios, M.D.

Ernest Poortinga, M.D.

Mr. C is a 34-year-old married white male veteran with a history of bipolar disorder and polysubstance—cocaine and alcohol—dependence. He had been psychiatrically hospitalized twice previously, once while in the military and again shortly after discharge 10 years ago. He was brought to the psychiatric emergency services by his brother, who had become increasingly concerned about Mr. C's paranoid ideation. Per the patient's brother, the patient believed that his wife was having an affair and had become increasingly verbally aggressive with his wife. Through repeated interrogation, Mr. C admitted that he had been making threatening phone calls to his wife's coworker, whom he believed was involved in an extramarital affair with his wife. In the emergency department, the patient admitted to wanting to kill his wife's coworker. He also reported that he had stopped taking his valproic acid and risperidone and had been binging on both alcohol and cocaine. The patient's wife, who was contacted by telephone for corroborating information, stated that she feared for both her coworker's life and her own. She stated that the patient owns a handgun, but when she had attempted to remove it from the home, she discovered it was missing. A search of the patient's vehicle revealed a loaded handgun in the glove compartment.

Psychiatric treatment in an emergency setting is one of the more challenging aspects of the practice of psychiatry. Whether services are provided in standard emergency departments or in designated psychiatric emergency services, the setting is usually complex, with the provider typically managing several emergency situations at one time. Also, clinicians in the emergency setting may face external pressures from various sources; for example, insurance companies may exert pressures to avoid patient hospitalization. Needless to say, even in the best of situations, subtle clues can be overlooked, and mistakes can be made.

Emergency psychiatrists provide an undeniably fundamental service in medicine: maintaining the safety of the patient and protecting the patient from harm (self-inflicted or otherwise). Unlike other emergency medicine practitioners, however, the emergency department psychiatrist is more commonly charged with the responsibility of supporting the safety not only of the patient but, indirectly, of others as well (usually those with whom no doctor-patient relationship exists). This responsibility—exemplified in the case of Mr. C, in which the emergency psychiatric services clinician was asked to assess a patient's dangerousness to others—raises the importance of assessment and management of the potentially violent patient.

Our goal in this chapter is to describe strategies that the busy emergency psychiatrist and resident psychiatrist can use to assess the short-term risk of violence in an orderly and standardized manner. Recognizing the absence of a foolproof method of predicting the perpetration of violent acts upon others, we present accepted clinical methods of assessing risk in the context of landmark legal cases in which such methods have been highlighted. Although generally perceived as superior to clinical assessments of risk of violence in the long term (Monahan 2008), structured risk assessment methods based on the use of actuarial instruments largely fall outside the scope of this text because of our focus on psychiatric emergency situations. Ultimately, it is the duty of the individual clinician to determine what combination of assessment strategies best serves his or her duties in the determination of violence risk assessment.

Violence and Mental Illness

To better understand the potential of patient violence, one needs to study the culture of violence that exists in the United States in the early twenty-first century. Studies have consistently shown that violent acts are directly related to low social class, low IQ and education levels, and employment and residential instability. Statistics have also demonstrated that violent acts in the United States are at an all-time low. Since 1994, the rate of violent crimes (including rape, robbery, aggravated and simple assault, and homicide) has declined, reaching the lowest level ever recorded in 2005 (Bureau of Justice Statistics 2009).

Perceptions with regard to the part played by mental illness in the perpetration of violence on others are similarly misinformed. According to Appelbaum (2008), only 3%–5% of the risk for violence in the United States can be attributed to mental illnesses. Instead, the effects of substance abuse and personality disorders far outweigh the role played by other mental illnesses (e.g., schizophrenia, major depression) alone; individuals with these other mental illnesses are far more likely to be victims than perpetrators of violent crimes.

Why does the popular perception of those with mental illnesses as violent predators persist? According to "Mental Health: A Report of the Surgeon General" (Satcher 1999), one series of surveys found that selective media reporting reinforced the public's stereotypes linking violence and mental illness, and encouraged people to distance themselves from those with mental disorders. The portrayal of persons with mental illness on television and in film may consciously or subconsciously influence the treatment of persons with mental illness who are in the custody of law enforcement (and who oftentimes wind up in psychiatric emergency services). Media portrayals may also influence the decisions of practitioners regarding the clinical treatment of persons with mental illness, especially those who are homeless or are otherwise in situations of compromise; homeless persons with mental illness commit 35 times more crimes than persons with mental illnesses who are not homeless (Martell et al. 1995).

Although the entertainment industry is making more responsible efforts to accurately depict the risk of violence from persons with mental illness, it is the duty of psychiatrists to determine the context in which the potential risk of violence posed by their patients exists, and to make efforts to appropriately assess that risk. Certainly, some mental disorders and symptoms of mental illnesses can contribute more to the risk of violence than others. Command auditory hallucinations are perhaps the most common cause for concern with regard to risk of violence attributable to a specific symptom; disturbing visual hallucinations, irritability secondary to mania, and hopelessness secondary to depression can all contribute to a patient's potentially becoming violent (Appelbaum 2008). Paranoid patients may seek to "preemptively strike" targets who, in the patients' mind, are plotting to do them harm (Resnick 2009). All of these symptoms are exacerbated by the disinhibiting effects of substance abuse, which is more common in people with mental disorders (Appelbaum 2008).

The bottom line is this: persons with mental illness are not violent most of the time, and those with tendencies toward violence are not always violent. Given this understanding, how does one accurately and reliably perform an assessment of risk of violence in an emergency setting?

Clinical Assessment of Risk for Violence

All psychiatrists are intimately familiar with safety evaluations with regard to suicidality. The same thorough approach should be applied to the evaluation of risk of violence toward others.

The clinical assessment of violence risk in the emergency setting is a challenging endeavor. In the best of circumstances, a clear account of the incident leading to the patient's presentation to the emergency room is given, a chart containing the patient's medical and psychiatric history is available for review, and a family member or other third-party source of information is present for corroboration. It is rare that all of these sources of information are available to the clinician evaluating the patient; a clinician's familiarity with the patient is considered icing on the cake. Taking these realities into account, a reliable violence risk assessment can seem daunting for even the most capable clinician. Given the obstacles potentially impeding a reliable emergency department violence risk assessment, it is necessary to perform the assessment in a uniform manner.

Just as universal precautions are taken to prevent infectious disease, some level of a standardized approach should be employed with regard to short-term violence risk assessment. Similar to the assessment of suicidality, the clinical violence risk assessment should comprise an evidence-based survey of the most important risk factors that contribute to an increased risk of violence. A more probing investigation can then be pursued if certain red flags are raised in the initial investigation. An effective violence risk assessment is a marriage of clinical and nonclinical information, which is synthesized to form the complete assessment profile.

Risk factors for violence can be divided into those that may change over time (dynamic) and those that do not change over time (static). Static risk factors include the patient's past use of violence, patterns of past violence, patterns of family violence, substance use history, institutional history, military history, work history, sexual aggression history, and demographics. Changes in internal or environmental circumstances can influence the propensity for an individual to act on violent impulses. Dynamic risk factors include ownership of weapons, social supports, living situation, current psychiatric symptoms, and noncompliance with medication.

Static Risk Factors for Violence

A History of Violence

Courts have emphasized that in addition to obtaining the patient's self-report of previous violence, the emergency mental health practitioner needs to obtain collateral information (*Jablonski by Pahls v. United States* 1983) from family and/or other mental health clinicians. For each reported act of violence, the clinician should ask the patient why it occurred, how he or she felt about the violence, and the degree of physical injury inflicted. Minimization of injury inflicted in prior episodes of violence and lack of empathy are additional risk factors for future violence (Resnick 2009).

Patterns of Past Violence

The clinician should evaluate whether the patient's previous violence occurred during psychotic states, manic states, depressed states, or intoxicated states. Another important question is whether the violence was predatory (i.e., planned, purposeful, and goal directed), which is common in psychopathic individuals. Whether a patient knew prior targets of violence can be important, as well as whether the patient has ever been violent toward a victim outside of the family. This information can be useful when establishing a risk reduction plan (Henning and Feder 2004; Shields et al. 1988).

Violence Within the Family of Origin

The clinician should learn whether the patient experienced early violence in his or her family. Children, especially boys, who have been abused by their parents are more likely to be violent as adults (Fries et al. 2008; Yesavage and Brizer 1989).

Substance Use History

A detailed substance use history, including information regarding recent substance use and intoxication, should be obtained. Swanson et al. (1990) found that substance abuse or dependence is a stronger risk factor for violence than any psychotic or affective diagnosis. A more recent study showed that nonpartner violence was associated with "heavy" drinking, cocaine use, and depressive symptoms (Murray et al. 2008).

Institutional History

The frequency of inpatient hospitalization can be telling. Studies show that once a person exceeds 10 psychiatric hospitalizations, the likelihood of future violence is increased (Klassen and O'Connor 1988).

Military History

Important details about military history include whether the patient was involved in combat and what type of discharge he or she received (Resnick 2009).

Work History

Evaluators should explore reasons for a patient's previous job terminations as well as imminent loss of a current job. Persons who are unemployed after being laid off are six times more likely to be violent than their employed peers (Catalano et al. 1993).

History of Sexual Aggression

Deviant sexual or violent fantasies are related to the commission of sexual and violent offenses (Quinsey et al. 1984; Salfati 2000).

Demographics

The younger the person is at the time of the first known violence, the greater the likelihood of subsequent violent conduct (Harris and Rice 1997; Harris et al. 1993). Men are more likely than women to seriously injure their victims (Resnick 2006).

Dynamic Risk Factors for Violence

Weapons

Clinicians should ask emergency department patients if they own weapons. Another important question is whether they have recently *removed* their weapons from storage (Resnick 2009).

Social Supports

A lack of social support is a significant risk factor for violence. The presence of patient, tolerant, and encouraging family members or peers can be of great assistance in maintaining a risk management plan. A recent decrease in social support is also a risk factor (Estroff and Zimmer 1994).

Housing/Living Situation

Difficulty in achieving basic social needs, such as housing, finances, and food, is a predictor of violence (Bartels et al. 1991).

Current Psychiatric Symptoms

Several groups of researchers have demonstrated that psychotic symptoms that override one's sense of self-control and are threatening to one's safety (e.g., delusions in which patients believe that people are seeking to harm them or that outside forces are controlling their minds) have higher correlations with violence than psychotic symptoms without these characteristics (Link and Stueve 1994; Monahan 1996). Swanson et al. (2006) found that positive symptoms of schizophrenia were associated with a higher risk of violence, whereas negative symptoms were actually associated with a lower risk of violence. Additionally, a lack of insight into one's mental illness and negative attitudes toward other people, social agencies/institutions, and authority have been associated with increased risk for violence (Amador 1993).

Medication Nonadherence

Patients who do not take their medications as prescribed are at higher risk of enacting violence (Resnick 2006). Medication nonadherence is often part of a multidimensional construct of insight that should include assessment of a patient's awareness of his or her violence potential (Amador et al. 1993). As such, fear of exerting violence can be used as a tool to improve medication compliance. Some authors prefer to split the noncompliance issue into 1) a lack of insight into mental illness and 2) negative attitudes toward treatment (Webster et al. 1997). This duality should be kept in mind when addressing noncompliance with the patient.

Actuarial Assessment of Risk for Violence

Structured risk assessments, which use various degrees of actuarial assessment in the determination of violence risk, have become increasingly commonplace and accepted in courts of law. A classification of violence risk assessment has been proposed that places structured assessments on a continuum, with completely unstructured (i.e., clinical) risk assessment at one end and completely structured (i.e., actuarial) risk assessment at the other (Monahan 2008). The goal of completely structured risk assessments is to replace clinical judgment with evidence-based predictions of risk.

Structured assessments, such as the Historical, Clinical, and Risk Management–20 (Webster et al. 1997; see also Douglas et al. 1999), Classification of Violence Risk (Monahan et al. 2006), and Violence Risk Appraisal Guide (Harris and Rice 1997; Harris et al. 1993), were primarily designed to predict recidivism and, therefore, pertain mostly to the assessment of long-term risk of violence of patients being discharged from inpatient units. These instruments were not designed to predict an imminent threat of violence over the course of hours, days, or even weeks. Although Stefan (2006) suggested that a structured assessment tool, such as the Classification of Violence Risk, can be modified for use in an emergency setting due to the relatively short amount of time it takes to administer, no primary research was found pertaining to the application of such an instrument in this manner. McNiel et al. (2003) described the potential utility in applying a structured assessment of acute violence risk in an inpatient setting. Criticisms of actuarial assessments commonly include unequal reliance on static rather than dynamic risk factors and the fact that they do not incorporate the judgment of the clinician; because purely actuarial assessments require no clinical patient encounter, they could potentially be administered by anyone, negating any value of involving a trained mental health professional.

Although applicable evidence-based practices are preferable, the utility of clinical experience should not be discounted. So-called anecdotal experience carries with it a less than preferable connotation: that somehow past experiences should be disregarded in favor of a checklist of criteria to be met. The fact is that no actuarial instrument exists that can predict with 100% accuracy and precision those persons who are about to perpetrate acts of violence toward others.

A comprehensive violence risk assessment performed in an emergency setting should take into account both static and dynamic risk factors; all of the previously listed factors should be considered by the clinician before a final short-term violence risk assessment is generated. If the patient is deemed to pose an imminent threat of violence in the short term, the clinician must take action (including medication adjustment, hospitalization, and warning the target of potential violence). The data collected in this assessment, as well as the treatment plan, should be documented in writing, for both continuity of care and legal purposes.

Legal Precedents for Violence Risk Assessment

Despite efforts to standardize the evaluation process through the development and refinement of actuarial instruments, no psychiatrist can state with certainty that he or she can accurately predict violent acts perpetrated by psychiatric patients. The courts, however, have decided otherwise, and negligence to dutifully determine risk of violence can result in malpractice and liability.

None of the cases identified as landmarks by the American Academy of Psychiatry and the Law involve risk assessment in the emergency department. Legal opinions seldom differentiate between the standard of care expected in a physician's office and the standard of care expected in the emergency department. Therefore, we can glean useful information from legal opinions rendered about hospital and outpatient cases. Applicable landmark cases are often referred to as "duty to protect" cases and are summarized here.

Tarasoff I

Mr. Poddar felt distraught that fellow University of California at Berkeley student, Ms. Tarasoff, had kissed other men. He informed his university psychologist that he intended to get a gun and harm Ms. Tarasoff. The psychologist gave written and oral alerts to campus police, who interviewed Mr. Poddar and decided that he was not dangerous. Mr. Poddar stalked, stabbed, and shot Ms. Tarasoff; the parents of Ms. Tarasoff sued the university and the psychologist. The trial and appeals courts both dismissed the case. In *Tarasoff v. Regents of the University of California* (1974), the California Supreme Court disagreed and ruled that the "doctor bears a duty to use reasonable care to give threatened persons such warnings as are essential to avert foreseeable danger arising from the patient's condition. The protective privilege ends where the public peril begins."

Tarasoff II

The university and the psychologist petitioned for and were granted a new hearing, and so the California Supreme Court heard the case again. The following is a direct quote from the *Tarasoff* (1976) decision:

> When a therapist determines, or pursuant to the standards of the profession, should determine, that his patient presents a serious danger of violence to another, he incurs an obligation to use reasonable care to protect the intended victim against such danger. The discharge of this duty may require the therapist to take one or more of various steps, depending on the nature of the case. Thus, it may call for him to warn the intended victim or others, likely to apprise the victim of the danger, to notify police, or to take whatever steps are reasonably necessary under the circumstances.

Tarasoff holds sway in California, Michigan, New Jersey, Pennsylvania, and Nebraska. It has been rejected or significantly modified in Maryland, West Virginia, Florida, and Connecticut.

Tarasoff Progeny

Lipari v. Sears (1980)

After being an inpatient at a Veterans Administration (VA) hospital, Mr. Cribbs purchased a shotgun from Sears. He quit his outpatient program and 4 weeks later fired the shotgun into a nightclub, killing Mr. Lipari. Mrs. Lipari sued Sears for selling a gun to a person with mental illness. Sears filed a third-party complaint against the VA, alleging that they knew Mr. Cribbs was dangerous but did not properly manage his case.

Jablonski by Pahls v. United States (1983)

Mr. Jablonski threatened his girlfriend's mother with a sharp object and attempted to rape her. He voluntarily went to the Loma Linda VA, where he was evaluated by a psychiatrist as an outpatient. Police gave the VA information about Mr. Jablonski's previous obscene phone calls and malicious property damage; it was unclear whether this information was passed on to the psychiatrist. The interview revealed that Mr. Jablonski had served 5 years in prison for the rape of his then-wife and also discussed the more recent attempted rape. Mr. Jablonski mentioned that he had received psychiatric treatment previously but refused to sign a release of information or even to state where the treatment took place. The psychiatrist diagnosed Mr. Jablonski with antisocial personality disorder and offered voluntary hospitalization for dangerousness. Mr. Jablonski refused, and the psychiatrist planned to see him in 2 weeks. His girlfriend was told to leave Mr. Jablonski alone but was given no other warning.

Four days later, Mr. Jablonski was seen by the psychiatrist and his supervisor; both agreed that Mr. Jablonski was "dangerous, but not committable." He was prescribed diazepam and was asked to come back in 3 days; his girlfriend was again told to stay away from Mr. Jablonski. One day before the scheduled appointment, the girlfriend went to Mr. Jablonski's apartment to get diapers and was murdered. The victim's family sued the VA, and the district court found malpractice based on 1) failure to adequately warn the victim, 2) failure to obtain old medical records, and 3) failure to record or transmit the information from police.

The court of appeals affirmed the decision and suggested that the Loma Linda VA could have called neighboring VA hospitals without Mr. Jablonski's consent. Records would have revealed that Mr. Jablonski had a history of homicidal ideation toward his former wife, multiple murder attempts, and a diagnosis of schizophrenia. The court emphasized the importance of, at minimum, requesting the records and leaving the burden of breaching confidentiality to the party that holds the records.

This case extends the duty to protect to a victim who had not been specifically identified by the patient. Some states (including California) have statutes that limit liability to cases involving an explicit threat.

Notice that neither the district court nor the court of appeals criticized the VA for not committing Mr. Jablonski to inpatient treatment (one clear method of satisfying a Tarasoff duty). One can speculate that the courts viewed Mr. Jablonski as "uncommittable," because antisocial personality disorder does not meet most statutory definitions of "mental illness." To commit a patient to psychiatric treatment, most states require a person to meet statutory definitions for mental illness. Michigan's definition is representative and reads, "a substantial disorder of thought or mood which significantly impairs judgment, behavior, capacity to recognize reality, or ability to cope with the ordinary demands of life" (Michigan Compiled Laws 330.1400a).

Lessons From Tarasoff and Its Progeny

What can we learn from these landmark cases involving psychiatric assessment of risk of violence? What are the "standards of the profession" for predicting violence in the emergency setting? Although predicting violence has no standards, there is a standard for the assessment of dangerousness (Beck 1990). In other words, when faced with a potentially violent patient in the emergency department, psychiatrists can and should perform a careful, thorough assessment of the risk of danger, as outlined in the earlier section "Clinical Assessment of Risk for Violence." Notably, there are no landmark cases involving inappropriate commitment to treatment. Psychiatrists have protection from litigation in commitment issues, because the probate courts screen these cases with due process.

Moreover, the court's suggestions in the Jablonski case can be highly illustrative. Psychiatrists are expected to make a legitimate attempt to obtain previous medical records and to record information from police in the medical record. The first suggestion is difficult, given the time constraints in an emergency setting. The second suggestion may require psychiatrists to overcome their reluctance to place inflammatory material in a medical record.

Conclusion

The evaluation of dangerousness to others is a necessary and vital component of any emergency psychiatric evaluation. Although psychiatrists possess no special powers of prediction, evidence-based principles used in combination with insight gained through experience can prove invaluable in preventing acts of violence perpetrated on innocents by those with mental illness.

The task of the psychiatrist practicing in an emergency setting with regard to violence risk assessment is twofold: 1) the recognition of factors commonly attributed to an increased risk of violence and 2) appropriate intervention once that determination of risk has been made. A responsible psychiatrist should employ evidence-based practices when evaluating patients for dangerousness to others and risk of violence; "shoot-from-the-hip" assessments based purely on hunches or gut feelings are dangerous and potentially destructive, and serve only to fan the flames of stigma. Likewise, although it is inadvisable and foolhardy to practice psychiatry based on unstructured assessments alone, past experience can certainly add color commentary to the play-by-play provided by evidence-based practices.

All mental health practitioners concerned for the equitable treatment of their patients should pay close attention to the effect that acts of violence committed by those with mental illnesses has on the stigma associated with mental illness. In order not to contribute to stigma, a psychiatrist must treat all patients with respect, while paying careful attention to the cues detailed in this chapter.

Psychiatrists can—and in fact should—intervene when they suspect that a patient is at risk of causing physical harm to another person because of factors attributed to the exacerbation or decompensation of a mental illness. Unfortunately, there is no hard-and-fast rule to ensure the foolproof prediction of the violence perpetrated on others by psychiatric patients. There are, however, evidence-based methods that, when used in combination with clinical judgment and experience, form the basis of most accepted approaches to violence risk assessment in an emergency department setting.

Key Clinical Points

- Patients with mental illness do commit violent acts; however, popular media and other sources may exaggerate the risk attributable to mental illness as a category.

- Specific mental illnesses (e.g., antisocial personality disorder, substance dependence) carry more risk than others (e.g., major depression).

- Specific symptoms (e.g., positive symptoms of schizophrenia) carry more risk than others (e.g., negative symptoms of schizophrenia).

- Psychosocial factors can be subdivided into static and dynamic risk factors, which can be diminished to decrease the risk of violence.

- Although there is no perfect way to predict future violence, landmark court cases have established a "duty to protect" potential victims. This obligation may apply to evaluations in the emergency department.

References

Amador XF, Strauss DH, Yale SA, et al: Assessment of insight in psychosis. Am J Psychiatry 150:873–879, 1993

Appelbaum PS: Foreword, in Textbook of Violence Assessment and Management. Edited by Simon R, Tardiff K. Washington, DC, American Psychiatric Publishing, 2008, pp xvii–xxii

Bartels SJ, Drake RE, Wallach MA, et al: Characteristic hostility in schizophrenic outpatients. Schizophr Bull 17:163–171, 1991

Beck JC (ed): Confidentiality and the Duty to Protect: Foreseeable Harm in the Practice of Psychiatry. Washington, DC, American Psychiatric Press, 1990

Bureau of Justice Statistics, U.S. Department of Justice, Office of Justice Programs: Crime characteristics. September 2, 2009. Available at: http://www.ojp.usdoj.gov/bjs/cvict_c.htm#vtrends. Accessed September 24, 2009.

Catalano R, Dooley D, Novaco RW, et al: Using ECA survey data to examine the effects of job layoffs in violent behavior. Hosp Community Psychiatry 44:874–879, 1993

Douglas KS, Ogloff JR, Nicholls TL, et al: Assessing risk factors for violence among psychiatric patients: the HCR-20 violence risk assessment scheme and the Psychopathy Checklist: Screening Version. J Consult Clin Psychol 67:917–930, 1999

Estroff SE, Zimmer C: Social networks, social support, and violence among persons with severe, persistent mental illness, in Violence and Mental Disorder: Developments in Risk Assessment. Edited by Monahan J, Steadman HJ. Chicago, IL, University of Chicago Press, 1994, pp 259–295

Fries AB, Shirtcliff EA, Pollak SD: Neuroendocrine dysregulation following early social deprivation in children. Dev Psychobiol 50:588–599, 2008

Harris GT, Rice ME: Risk appraisal and management of violent behavior. Psychiatr Serv 48:1168–1176, 1997

Harris GT, Rice ME, Quinsey VL: Violent recidivism of mentally disordered offenders: the development of a statistical prediction instrument. Crim Justice Behav 20:315–335, 1993

Henning K, Feder L: A comparison between men and women arrested for domestic violence: who presents the greater threat? J Fam Violence 19:69–81, 2004

Jablonski by Pahls v United States, 712 F.2d 391, 395, 9th Cir. (1983)

Klassen D, O'Connor WA: A prospective study of predictors of violence in adult male mental health admissions. Law Hum Behav 12:148–158, 1988

Link BG, Stueve A: Psychotic symptoms and the violent/illegal behavior of mental patients compared to community controls, in Violence and Mental Disorder: Developments in Risk Assessment. Edited by Monahan J, Steadman HJ. Chicago, IL, University of Chicago Press, 1994, pp 137–159

Lipari v Sears, Roebuck and Co., 497 F.Supp. 185, D.Neb. (1980)

Martell DA, Rosner R, Harmon RB: Base-rate estimates of criminal behavior by homeless mentally ill persons in New York City. Psychiatr Serv 46:596–601, 1995

McNiel DE, Gregory AL, Lam JN, et al: Utility of decision support tools for assessing acute risk of violence. J Consult Clin Psychol 71:945–953, 2003

Michigan Compiled Laws 330.1400a. Available at: http://www.legislature.michigan. gov. Accessed September 24, 2009.

Monahan J: Violence prediction: the last 20 and the next 20 years. Crim Justice Behav 23:107–120, 1996

Monahan J: Structured risk assessment of violence, in Textbook of Violence Assessment and Management. Edited by Simon R, Tardiff K. Washington, DC, American Psychiatric Publishing, 2008, pp 17–31

Monahan J, Steadman HJ, Appelbaum PS, et al: The classification of violence risk. Behav Sci Law 24:721–730, 2006

Murray RL, Chermack ST, Walton MA, et al: Psychological aggression, physical aggression, and injury in nonpartner relationships among men and women in treatment for substance-use disorders. J Stud Alcohol Drugs 69:896–905, 2008

Quinsey VL, Chaplin TC, Upfold D: Sexual arousal to nonsexual violence and sadomasochistic themes among rapists and non sex-offenders. J Consult Clin Psychol 52:651–657, 1984

Resnick P: Risk assessment for violence: course outline (forensic psychiatry review course). Chicago, IL, American Academy of Psychiatry and the Law, 2006, pp 112–114

Salfati CG: Profiling homicide: a multidimensional approach. Homicide Studies 4:265–293, 2000

Satcher D: Mental health: a report of the Surgeon General. 1999. Available at: http://www.surgeongeneral.gov/library/mentalhealth/home.html. Accessed September 25, 2009.

Shields NM, McCall GJ, Hanneke CR: Patterns of family and non-family violence: violent husbands and violent men. Violence Vict 3:83–97, 1988

Stefan S: Emergency Department Treatment of the Psychiatric Patient: Policy Issues and Legal Requirements. New York, Oxford University Press, 2006

Swanson JW, Holzer CE 3rd, Ganju VK, et al: Violence and psychiatric disorder in the community: evidence from the Epidemiologic Catchment Area Surveys. Hosp Community Psychiatry 41:761–770, 1990

Swanson JW, Swartz MS, Van Dorn RA, et al: A national study of violent behavior in persons with schizophrenia. Arch Gen Psychiatry 63:490–499, 2006

Tarasoff v Regents of the University of California, 118 Cal Rptr 129, 529 P2d 553 (1974)

Tarasoff v Regents of the University of California, 17 Cal. 3d 425, 131 Cal Rptr 14, 551 P2d 334 (1976)

Webster CD, Douglas KS, Eaves D, et al: HCR-20: Assessing Risk of Violence, Version 2. Burnaby, British Columbia, Canada, Simon Fraser University Institute of Mental Health, Law, and Policy, 1997

Yesavage JA, Brizer DA: Clinical and historical correlates of dangerous inpatient behavior, in Current Approaches to the Prediction of Violence. Edited by Brizer DA, Crowner M. Washington, DC, American Psychiatric Press, 1989, pp 63–84

Suggested Readings

Appelbaum PS: Legal issues in emergency psychiatry, in Clinical Handbook of Psychiatry and the Law, 4th Edition. Edited by Appelbaum PS, Gutheil T. Philadelphia, PA, Lippincott Williams & Wilkins, 2007, pp 42–79

Felthous A: Personal violence, in American Psychiatric Publishing Textbook of Forensic Psychiatry: The Clinician's Guide. Edited by Simon P, Gold L. Washington, DC, American Psychiatric Publishing, 2004, pp 471–496

Tardiff K: Clinical risk assessment of violence, in Textbook of Violence Assessment and Management. Edited by Simon R, Tardiff K. Washington, DC, American Psychiatric Publishing, 2008, pp 3–14

4

The Catatonic Patient

M. Justin Coffey, M.D.
Michael Alan Taylor, M.D.

Case Example

Mr. N, a 17-year-old male with no past general medical or psychiatric history, develops over 1 week ideas of reference, increased speech output without pressure, a decreased need for sleep, and a sudden interest in mathematical theory. His father, a physician, brought his son to an emergency room when he noticed him speaking robotically (speech mannerism) and repeating words and phrases that his father had just said (echolalia). The father denied that his son used illicit drugs and said that he had given his son 5 mg of haloperidol on two occasions the day prior to presentation "to see if it would straighten him out."

Mr. N did not speak when prompted (mutism) but occasionally uttered strings of numbers or sounds that became progressively slower and unintelligible (prosectic speech). When asked if he was in any pain or discomfort, he began removing his clothes. He then pointed to the ceiling light, maintaining the position rigidly for several minutes (posturing). The posture could easily be changed into different positions with light pressure (automatic obedience). He was not agitated or dangerous, and seclusion and restraints were unnecessary.

Definition of Catatonia

Catatonia is a syndrome of motor dysregulation characterized by fluctuating stupor, mutism, negativism, posturing, stereotypy, automatic obedience, and mannerisms. Two to four features elicit the diagnosis. Motor dysregulation is present when the patient has the capacity to move normally but cannot. Difficulties include trouble starting and stopping movements, frozen posture, and abnormal or inappropriate reaction times. Parkinsonism is another motor dysregulation syndrome.

Recognizing or eliciting the features of catatonia leads to straightforward diagnosis in the emergency setting. Catatonia, however, is a neurotoxic and potentially lethal state associated with many toxic, metabolic, and neuropsychiatric conditions. Its pathophysiology remains unclear, but its many etiologies likely reflect a common final pathway that involves dysregulation of the frontal lobe circuitry and motor regulatory areas of the brain. Psychiatric emergency clinicians must be aware of the etiologies of catatonia, as well as the conditions mistaken for it. When recognized, catatonia can be treated safely and effectively, regardless of the underlying cause.

Presentation

Epidemiology

The clinical key to catatonia is to look for it. The identification of catatonia, however, is often missed, leading to the false conclusion that the syndrome is rare. In a large Dutch study of acutely hospitalized psychotic patients, the treatment team recognized 2% to be catatonic, whereas systematic assessment identified 18% (Van der Heijden et al. 2005). Similarly designed studies have found about 10% of acutely ill psychiatric inpatients to be catatonic (Taylor and Fink 2003). Catatonia is also common among patients with severe general medical and neurological disease and in persons with autistic spectrum disorders, in whom its prevalence approaches 20% (Taylor and Fink 2003). G. Bush, G. Petrides, and A. Francis (personal communication, 1999) reported that of 249 consecutive psychiatric emergency room patients at a university hospital, 7% were catatonic.

The same systematic studies demonstrate that catatonia has several presentations and that patients with catatonia often are neither mute nor immobile.

Excited forms of catatonia (e.g., manic delirium) are characterized by excessive motor activity, disorientation, confusion, and fantastic confabulation. In retarded forms of catatonia (e.g., the Kahlbaum syndrome), patients are in stupor with a decreased level of response to voice and noxious stimuli. They may retain substantial preservation of awareness, but speech and spontaneous movements are absent or reduced to a minimum, and generalized analgesia may be present.

The emergency department patient should be examined for catatonia when he or she exhibits passive uncooperativeness, muscle rigidity not associated with Parkinson's disease, behavior thought to reflect a conversion disorder or malingering, excited delirium, seizure-like behaviors, mutism or odd speech patterns not consistent with aphasia, or any of the classic features described below (see subsection "Examination"). The course of catatonia may be either simple or malignant. When considering prescribing an antipsychotic, the emergency department physician should first assess the patient for catatonia because most cases of malignant catatonia are triggered by antipsychotics and occur in dehydrated patients with unnoticed catatonic features.

Case Example *(continued)*

On exam, Mr. N's vital signs were stable. His general medical health appeared to be good. His cranial nerves were intact, and his strength and reflexes were symmetric. Sensation to painful stimuli (pinching) was decreased over his extremities and trunk. A motor examination elicited gegenhalten, waxy flexibility, and ambitendency. Urine drug screen was negative, and routine screening laboratory tests were all within normal limits. The patient's creatinine phosphokinase was elevated in the 600s.

One milligram of lorazepam was administered intravenously, as was a 1-liter bolus of normal saline. Roughly 20 minutes later, Mr. N's speech mannerisms resolved. He was able to describe fluently his new fascination with the apparent connections between certain numbers and his laptop computer. Without additional lorazepam, his symptoms returned in roughly 2 hours, although his creatinine phosphokinase had normalized.

Examination

Most patients with catatonia speak and move about (Abrams and Taylor 1976). Associated mood, speech, and language disturbances and psychotic features may be so intense that clinicians lose full attention to motor signs. Mutism and stupor are classic signs, but alone they are not pathognomic. The number of features and their duration required for the diagnosis are not experimentally established, but most patients exhibit four or more signs (Abrams and Taylor 1976). Observed features and elicited signs of catatonia are summarized in Tables 4–1 and 4–2, respectively.

Diagnostic Studies

Laboratory and Imaging Data

No specific diagnostic laboratory test is available for catatonia. The main implications of laboratory findings are summarized in Table 4–3.

Lorazepam Challenge

The most helpful test to verify catatonia is an intravenous bolus of 1–2 mg of lorazepam—a test called the lorazepam challenge. Intravenous administration allows for precise dosing, although intramuscular injections have been used in emergency department settings (Hung and Huang 2006). The patient is reexamined for signs of catatonia after 5 minutes. If there is no change, a second dose is given, and the patient is again examined. Partial temporary relief is diagnostic for catatonia in a patient who is not in nonconvulsive status epilepticus. Favorable responses usually occur within 10 minutes, although patients are observed for longer periods. A positive response to the lorazepam challenge supports a trial of high-dose lorazepam. A positive test also predicts an excellent response to bilateral electroconvulsive therapy (ECT).

Differential Diagnosis

Once catatonia is identified, one must determine its cause. Table 4–4 presents a summary of the differential diagnosis. In the emergency department, patients with catatonia must first be evaluated for life-threatening conditions. Inpatients with catatonia most likely have manic-depressive disorder. About 20% of manic episodes are associated with catatonia, and half of the patients with catatonia have manic-depressive illness (Taylor and Abrams 1977). The second most likely condition underlying catatonia in psychiatric inpatients is depressive illness, particularly melancholia. Catatonia is also present in upward of 20% of patients with autism spectrum disorders. About 10% of pa-

Table 4–1.   Observed features of catatonia

Feature	Description
Stupor[a]	State of decreased alertness in which patients are hypoactive and have diminished responses to voice and to painful stimuli. Stupor is similar in appearance to conscious sedation—the patient seems dazed.
Excitement	Patients are impulsive and stereotypic, with sudden outbursts of talking, singing, dancing, and tearing at their clothes. Complex stereotypic movements may be frantic. Patients may be irritable and damage objects or injure themselves or others. This state may suddenly alternate with stupor.
Mutism	Patients are awake but verbally unresponsive. Mutism is not always associated with immobility and may appear elective. Mutism includes lack of spontaneous speech associated with sluggish responding to questions using automatic answers such as "I don't know" (*speech prompt*) and making utterances of progressively less volume until speech is an inaudible mumble (*prosectic speech*).
Stimulus-bound behaviors	*Echolalia* is present when the patient repeats the examiner's utterances. *Echopraxia* is present when the patient spontaneously copies the examiner's movements or is unable to refrain from copying the examiner's test movements despite instructions to the contrary. *Utilization behavior* is present when the patient appears compelled to use objects (e.g., picking up objects, turning light switches on and off, pulling fire alarms, entering other patients' rooms).
Speech mannerisms	Speech mannerisms include robotic speech, foreign accent syndrome, and verbigeration (constant repetition of meaningless words or phrases) or palilalia (automatic repetition of words or phrases uttered with increasing speed).
Stereotypy	Non–goal-directed, repetitive movements that often are awkward or stiff. They may be complex and ritualistic, or simple (grimacing, teeth/tongue clicking, rocking, sniffing, biting, burning, automatically touching/tapping).
Mannerisms	Patient makes odd, purposeful movements, such as holding hands as if they were handguns, saluting passersby, or making exaggerated or stilted caricatures of mundane movements.

[a]A patient's level of alertness exists along a continuum, and a clinical vocabulary corresponds to points along it. A patient is said to be *alert* when he or she responds spontaneously to environmental stimuli. *Somnolence* is a state of decreased alertness in which patients appear sleepy but awaken with and respond to voice. *Stupor* is a state of decreased alertness in which patients are unresponsive to voice but not to painful stimuli. *Coma* is an unresponsive state from which a person cannot be aroused, even with vigorous, repeated attempts. It is important for clinicians to use terminology that is clear so that communication is effective (e.g., a clinician uncertain of the precise definition of *stupor* should document a patient's level of alertness as "responsive to painful stimuli but not to voice").

Table 4–2.   Elicited signs of catatonia

Feature	Description
Ambitendency	The patient appears "stuck" in an indecisive, hesitant movement, resulting from the examiner's verbally contradicting his or her own strong nonverbal signal, such as offering a hand as if to shake hands while stating, "Do not shake my hand; I don't want you to shake it."
Posturing (catalepsy)	The patient maintains a posture for a long time. Common examples include standing in a room or lying in the same position in bed or on a sofa all day. More striking examples are an exaggerated pucker (schnauzkrampf), lying in bed with head and shoulders elevated and unsupported as if on a pillow (psychological pillow), lying in a jackknifed position, sitting with upper and lower portions of the body twisted at right angles, holding arms above the head or raised in a prayer-like manner, and holding fingers and hands in odd positions.
Waxy flexibility	The rigid patient's initial resistance to the examiner's manipulations is gradually overcome, allowing reposturing (as in bending a candle).
Automatic obedience (mitgehen)	Despite instructions to the contrary ("be limp and let me do all the work…don't help me…pretend you're asleep"), the patient moves with the examiner's light pressure into a new position (posture), which may then be maintained by the patient despite instructions to the contrary. Test bilaterally because this sign may result from contralateral brain lesions.
Negativism (gegenhalten)	The patient resists the examiner's manipulations, whether light or vigorous, with strength equal to that applied, as if bound to the stimulus of the examiner's actions. Negativism in patients' interactions with staff that may be misinterpreted as "bad behavior" includes sleeping under the bed, going to the bathroom when asked but soiling themselves there, turning away when addressed, refusing to open eyes, closing mouth when offered food or liquids.
Stimulus-bound speech	In response to the clinician saying, "When I touch my nose, you touch your chest," the patient touches his or her nose in a mirrored behavior despite understanding the instruction.

Table 4–3. Laboratory findings in catatonia

Laboratory finding	Implication
Increased CPK	Nonspecific finding, but very high levels strongly correlate with malignant catatonia
Low serum iron	Indicator of acute disease and seen in 40% of persons with malignant catatonia
Frontal slowing on EEG	Rules out nonconvulsive status epilepticus and encephalopathy by its waveform and circumscribed pattern
Increased lateral ventricle size or cerebellar atrophy on neuroimaging	The former is seen in mood disorders and the latter in autism spectrum disorders
Frontal hypometabolism on SPECT	Seen in mood disorders
Attention and visuospatial problems on neuro-psychological tests	Nonspecific finding, but rules out encephalopathy by its circumscribed pattern

Note.   CPK= creatinine phosphokinase; EEG=electroencephalography; SPECT= single photon emission computed tomography.

tients with catatonia meet the criteria for schizophrenia (Chandrasena 1986). Many neurological conditions are associated with catatonia, including seizure disorder, encephalitis and postencephalitic states, parkinsonism, ischemic stroke, traumatic brain injury, multiple sclerosis, alcoholic degeneration, and Wernicke's encephalopathy. Electroencephalography (EEG) should be performed on catatonic patients with altered states of consciousness to rule out nonconvulsive or petit mal status epilepticus. Because catatonia is also associated with the same conditions that cause delirium, emergency department clinicians must maintain a high index of suspicion for general medical etiologies of catatonia. Metabolic disorders commonly seen in the emergency department that can present with catatonia include diabetic ketoacidosis, hyperthyroidism, hypercalcemia, Addison's disease, Cushing's disease, the syndrome of inappropriate antidiuretic hormone secretion (SIADH), vitamin B_{12} deficiency, and acute intermittent porphyria.

Table 4–4. Differential diagnosis of catatonia

Life-threatening conditions (MUST BE EVALUATED FOR)	Nonconvulsive status epilepticus (NCSE)
	Ischemic stroke
	Intracerebral hemorrhage
	Traumatic brain injury
Neuropsychiatric conditions	Mania
	Major depression
	Frontal circuitry disease (e.g., basal ganglia syndromes)
	Autism spectrum disorders
	Seizure disorders (particularly postictal states and NCSE)
	Nonaffective psychoses
	Drug-induced states (particularly PCP)
	Withdrawal states (e.g., benzodiazepines, disulfiram)
General medical conditions	Conditions associated with delirium
	Metabolic disorders
	Infection
	Autoimmune disorders (e.g., SLE)
	Endocrine disorders
	Burns
Conditions mistaken for catatonia	Parkinson's disease
	Obsessive-compulsive disorder
	Malignant hyperthermia
	Locked-in syndrome

Note. PCP = phencyclidine; SLE = systemic lupus erythematosus.

Management

Case Example *(continued)*

Mr. N was admitted to the child and adolescent inpatient psychiatry service, where he was given lorazepam 1 mg tid on the first day of hospitalization. No antipsychotic agents were prescribed. His posturing resolved, but his sleep disruption, ideas of reference, and speech mannerisms did not. Lorazepam was increased to 2 mg tid, lithium was added, and the patient was evaluated for ECT. The patient's mother then reported that her father had manic-depressive illness. Roughly a week later, the patient was discharged home on lorazepam and lithium, without having received ECT. He was diagnosed as having manic-depressive illness with catatonic and psychotic features.

Once recognized, catatonia can be treated effectively and rapidly. The overall strategy is to avoid antipsychotic agents, maintain fluid and electrolyte balance, use lorazepam for sedation, and consider ECT as definitive treatment. Catatonia responds well to treatment, regardless of the underlying cause. Neither the number nor the pattern of catatonic features predicts the response to treatment. The safest strategy to prevent relapse is to continue as maintenance treatment whatever prescription was effective during the acute illness. Table 4–5 summarizes the diagnosis and management of catatonia.

Ensuring Safety and Stabilization

Although gratifyingly treatable, catatonia can be lethal. Patients with catatonia, especially those with syndromes of acute onset, need protection and care, best done in a hospital. Patients with excited forms of catatonia may require seclusion and restraint to ensure their safety and that of others. A patient's vital signs should be obtained immediately. Patients with malignant forms of catatonia, which can involve hyperthermia, hypertension or hypotension, tachycardia, and tachypnea with poor oxygen saturation, should be managed in general medical emergency settings with hemodynamic support, intensive nursing care, and rapid assessment for other signs of malignant catatonia, including dehydration, renal failure, and electrolyte derangements (e.g., hyperkalemia).

Avoiding Antipsychotic Agents

To avoid precipitating a neurotoxic reaction, treatment with antipsychotic drugs must be discontinued and avoided. High-potency antipsychotic drugs, especially haloperidol, are commonly used to reduce excited and aggressive behavior, but in patients with catatonia, using these agents risks the development of malignant catatonia or neuroleptic malignant syndrome (MC/NMS; described later in chapter). Nearly all dopamine antagonists have been associated with MC/NMS, although high-potency conventional antipsychotics are associated with a greater risk compared with their low-potency and atypical counterparts. Stübner et al. (2004) reported that over a 7-year period, a typical antipsychotic was imputed alone in 57% of MC/NMS cases. Although atypical antipsychotics are presumed safer than their typical counterparts, MC/NMS is reported for each atypical antipsychotic agent, and a significant

Table 4–5.   Key steps to diagnosing and managing catatonia

Look for it

Does the patient have motor dysregulation with ≥2 of the features below present?

  Features observed: stupor, excitement, mutism, echophenomena, stereotypy
    (including speech), mannerisms

  Features elicited: ambitendency, posturing (catalepsy), waxy flexibility, automatic
    obedience, negativism (gegenhalten)

Are fever and autonomic instability present? If yes, then malignant catatonia (e.g.,
NMS or TSS) is present.

Test for it

Lorazepam challenge: Perform a formal examination for signs of catatonia, then inject
lorazepam 1–2 mg iv and repeat the examination after 5–10 minutes. If no change
occurs, inject another 1–2 mg and repeat the examination. Favorable responses
usually occur within 10 minutes.

Manage it

Determine cause (see Table 4–4). If identified, treat the cause.

Avoid antipsychotics (including atypical antipsychotics) and GABA$_B$ agents.

Hydrate patient.

Lorazepam dosing:

  For stupor, start with 1–2 mg tid, increasing by 3 mg daily every 1–2 days as
    tolerated.

  For excitement, consider physical restraints, followed by lorazepam 2–4 mg iv,
    depending on the patient's size, every 20 minutes until the patient is calm but
    awake.

ECT: Begin workup immediately, and use definitively when there has been no
response to lorazepam after 2 days.

Maintenance: To prevent relapse, whatever prescription was effective during the acute
illness should be continued for 3–6 months and then slowly tapered.

Note.   ECT = electroconvulsive therapy; GABA$_B$ = gamma-aminobutyric acid type B.

number of MC/NMS cases occur at therapeutic doses of these agents (Fink
and Taylor 2003).

A toxic reaction is particularly likely if patients are dehydrated, receive the
medication parenterally or at higher titration rates, or are also receiving high
doses of lithium. Patients with mania who are febrile or have had a prior
episode of catatonia are even more susceptible to developing MC/NMS with
haloperidol and other high-potency antipsychotic drugs.

Benzodiazepine Treatment

If a specific cause of catatonia is identified (e.g., nonconvulsive status epilepticus, anticholinergic-induced delirium, an alcohol toxicity syndrome), treatment of the cause takes priority. If no specific cause is quickly recognized, the patient with catatonia is best treated with benzodiazepines. Most experience has been with lorazepam and diazepam. (Because intravenous diazepam comes in a caustic vehicle, resulting in endothelial scarring and risk for embolus, it is avoided.) These drugs are effective. About 70%–80% of patients with malignant catatonia respond to lorazepam monotherapy (Hawkins et al. 1995; Koek and Mervis 1999; Schmider et al. 1999; Ungvari et al. 1994). Benzodiazepines are safe, and cardiac arrhythmia is extremely rare. Because reduced excitement and sleep occur long before respiratory depression (i.e., the sedation threshold is much lower than the threshold for respiratory depression), even high doses given intravenously are well below levels associated with this potential complication. Initial intravenous administration also permits careful dosing.

Dosages of lorazepam larger than ordinarily prescribed must be administered to be effective. In one study, for example, lorazepam 8–24 mg/day led to 70%–80% remission (Petrides and Fink 2000). For *stuporous* patients, dosing starts at 1–2 mg tid and is increased by 3 mg daily every 1–2 days as tolerated. If no substantial relief occurs after a few days, bilateral ECT becomes the treatment of choice and may be lifesaving. For *excited* patients, lorazepam doses need to be high and repeated at frequent intervals. Patients in manic delirium typically require restraints, followed by lorazepam 2–4 mg iv, depending on the patient's size, every 20 minutes until the patient is calm but awake. For patients with fever, hypertension, tachycardia, and tachypnea, lorazepam 2 mg iv should be administered every 8 hours, increasing by 3 mg/day as needed. Further dosing depends on the balance of response with sedation. Failure to respond within 2 days warrants bilateral ECT, scheduled initially on a daily basis. In extreme instances of excited catatonia, general anesthesia has been required. Typically, a successful acute treatment course will take 4–10 days. When catatonia is relieved by benzodiazepines, further treatment of the associated psychopathology modifies standard treatment algorithms to avoid catatonia-inducing antipsychotic agents, selective serotonin reuptake inhibitors (SSRIs), and gamma-aminobutyric acid type B (GABA$_B$) agonists. To maintain remission, the benzodiazepine is continued at the effective dose for 3–6 months and then slowly tapered.

Electroconvulsive Therapy

When a benzodiazepine challenge does not elicit measurable improvement, preparation for ECT begins immediately. A failed challenge test (i.e., after 2–3 mg of lorazepam or equivalent) predicts a prolonged and often failed clinical trial of benzodiazepines. To wait until the treatment is considered failed before obtaining informed consent, laboratory assessments, and examinations for ECT will needlessly prolong the patient's illness and increase mortality risk. ECT is given at a customary frequency with bitemporal electrode placement and brief-pulse currents. About 90% of catatonic patients remit with ECT, even those who have not responded to benzodiazepines. (For a more complete discussion of using ECT to treat catatonia, including dosing and ECT-induced EEG changes, see Fink and Taylor 2003.)

ECT not only will relieve the catatonia but also may improve the underlying psychopathology, particularly manic-depressive illness. ECT is safe and effective in patients with general medical conditions that may be the cause of or comorbid with catatonia. Although general medical conditions may limit the use of benzodiazepines, dantrolene, or dopamine agonists, there are no absolute contraindications to the use of ECT. Whenever a rapid, definitive treatment is needed, ECT is the treatment of choice for catatonia of any severity, in the widest range of patients, and with virtually any comorbidity. This issue should be considered when determining an inpatient disposition for a catatonic patient.

Special Considerations

Malignant Catatonia/Neuroleptic Malignant Syndrome

Malignant catatonia (MC) is a life-threatening condition characterized by the motor features of catatonia combined with fever and autonomic instability. Patients with MC may also have muscle rigidity, posturing, negativism (gegenhalten), tremor, fever, diaphoresis, and tachypnea with inadequate oxygenation (Adland 1947; Fricchione et al. 2000). MC is the severest form of catatonia and warrants intensive care. Without adequate treatment, patients may die from muscle breakdown and resulting renal failure.

MC is clinically identical to neuroleptic malignant syndrome (NMS), and it is likely that NMS and MC reflect the same pathophysiology, differing only in that NMS is precipitated by an antipsychotic agent (Carroll and Taylor 1997; Fricchione 1985). MC was described before the development of antipsychotic drugs, and NMS has clinical characteristics, course, and response to treatment that are indistinguishable from MC. NMS has also been associated with agents outside the antipsychotic class and with several general medical conditions unrelated to exposure to a medication (Caroff and Mann 1993).

The immediate needs in the management of a patient with MC/NMS involve the discontinuation of antipsychotic medicines[1]; protection of the patient when excited and delirious; temperature regulation and hydration; and intensive nursing care to avoid deep vein thrombosis, aspiration, and loss of skin integrity. ECT provides effective treatment of MC, with overall response rates reported in the literature ranging from 63% to 91% (Troller and Sachdev 1999). It needs to be administered early and intensively in febrile patients to contain the illness. When treatments are deferred beyond the first 5 days of hospital care, mortality increases sharply to over 10%.

Toxic Serotonin Syndrome

A toxic serotonin syndrome (TSS) has been associated with treatments that affect brain serotonin systems. TSS has many features of MC/NMS, with the addition of diarrhea, nausea, and vomiting. The principal differences between TSS and MC/NMS are the inciting agents and the prominence of gastrointestinal symptoms. The descriptive characteristics of TSS are poorly defined, but it is sufficiently like MC in its signs and response to treatment to consider it malignant catatonia (Fink 1996; Keck and Arnold 2000). The similarities between TSS and NMS argue for the treatment of TSS as a form of catatonia (Keck and Arnold 2000).

---

[1]The recognition in 1980 of NMS as a defined toxic response to antipsychotic medicines (see Taylor and Fink 2003) elicited two different treatment approaches. One strategy is based on the idea that NMS results from dopaminergic dysfunction with elements of malignant hyperthermia and involves the use of dopamine agonists (e.g., amantadine and bromocriptine) and the muscle relaxant dantrolene. The second strategy considers NMS to be a variant of MC and is described in this chapter because, we believe, it is safer and more effective.

Children and Adolescents

The signs and symptoms of catatonia in children and adolescents are similar to those in other age groups. Catatonia is sufficiently frequent among children and adolescents that any young patient with motor symptoms should be formally assessed for it. When catatonia is found, the differential diagnosis, in order of decreasing frequency, is mood disorder, seizure disorder, developmental disorder and autism, and psychotic disorders. The same treatments for catatonia that are effective in adults have been found useful in children (Fink 1999).

Key Clinical Points

- Catatonia is a syndrome of motor dysregulation, most commonly associated with mood disorder (not schizophrenia).

- Catatonia can be readily identified when two or more classic features (stupor, mutism, negativism, posturing, stereotypy, automatic obedience) are present on exam.

- The most common error in the evaluation of catatonia is not considering it in the differential diagnosis and not performing an examination because of the mistaken belief that all patients with catatonia are mute, immobile, and frozen in a strange posture.

- Patients with catatonia fall into four broad groups, those with 1) mood disorder, 2) neurological illness, 3) exposure to an antipsychotic or serotonergic medication, and 4) metabolic derangement.

- Catatonia is a potentially neurotoxic and lethal state; it is best to consider neuroleptic malignant syndrome and toxic serotonin syndrome as malignant forms of catatonia with similar pathophysiology and treatment.

- Safe and effective management includes avoiding antipsychotic agents, prescribing lorazepam for symptom relief, and moving swiftly to electroconvulsive therapy as definitive treatment.

References

Abrams R, Taylor MA: Catatonia: a prospective clinical study. Arch Gen Psychiatry 33:579–581, 1976

Adland ML: Review, case studies, therapy, and interpretation of acute exhaustive psychoses. Psychiatr Q 21:39–69, 1947

Caroff SN, Mann SC: Neuroleptic malignant syndrome. Med Clin North Am 77:185–202, 1993

Carroll BT, Taylor BE: The nondichotomy between lethal catatonia and neuroleptic malignant syndrome. J Clin Psychopharmacol 17:235–236, 1997

Chandrasena R: Catatonic schizophrenia: an international comparative study. Can J Psychiatry 31:249–252, 1986

Fink M: Toxic serotonin syndrome or neuroleptic malignant syndrome? Pharmacopsychiatry 29:159–161, 1996

Fink M: Electroshock: Restoring the Mind. New York, Oxford University Press, 1999

Fink M, Taylor MA: Catatonia: A Clinician's Guide to Diagnosis and Treatment. Cambridge, UK, Cambridge University Press, 2003

Fricchione GL: Neuroleptic catatonia and its relationship to psychogenic catatonia. Biol Psychiatry 20:304–313, 1985

Fricchione G, Mann SC, Caroff SN: Catatonia, lethal catatonia, and neuroleptic malignant syndrome. Psychiatr Ann 30:347–355, 2000

Hawkins JM, Archer KJ, Strakowski SM, et al: Somatic treatment of catatonia. Intl J Psychiatry Med 25:345–369, 1995

Hung Y, Huang T: Lorazepam and diazepam rapidly relieve catatonic features in major depression. Clin Neuropharmacol 29:144–147, 2006

Keck PE, Arnold LM: The serotonin syndrome. Psychiatr Ann 30:333–343, 2000

Koek RJ, Mervis JR: Treatment-refractory catatonia, ECT, and parenteral lorazepam. Am J Psychiatry 156:160–161, 1999

Petrides G, Fink M: Catatonia, in Advances in Psychiatry. Edited by Andrade C. Oxford, UK, Oxford University Press, 2000, pp 26–44

Schmider J, Standhart H, Deuschle M, et al: A double-blind comparison of lorazepam and oxazepam in psychomotor retardation and mutism. Biol Psychiatry 46:437–441, 1999

Stübner S, Rustenbeck E, Grohmann R, et al: Severe and uncommon involuntary movement disorders due to psychotropic drugs. Pharmacopsychiatry 37 (suppl 1):S54–S64, 2004

Taylor MA, Abrams R: Catatonia: prevalence and importance in the manic phase of manic-depressive illness. Arch Gen Psychiatry 34:1223–1225, 1977

Taylor MA, Fink M: Catatonia in psychiatric classification: a home of its own. Am J Psychiatry 160:1233–1234, 2003

Troller JN, Sachdev PS: Electroconvulsive treatment of neuroleptic malignant syndrome: a review and report of cases. Aust N Z J Psychiatry 33:650–659, 1999

Ungvari GS, Leung CM, Wong MK, et al : Benzodiazepines in the treatment of catatonic syndrome. Acta Psychiatr Scand 89:285–288, 1994

Van der Heijden FM, Tuinier S, Arts NJ, et al: Catatonia: disappeared or under-diagnosed? Psychopathology 38:3–8, 2005

Suggested Readings

Bush G, Fink M, Petrides G, et al: Catatonia, I: Rating scale and standardized examination. Acta Psychiatr Scand 93:129–136, 1996

Caroff SN, Mann SC, Francis A, et al: Catatonia: From Psychopathology to Neurobiology. Washington, DC, American Psychiatric Publishing, 2004

Fink M, Taylor MA: Catatonia: A Clinician's Guide to Diagnosis and Treatment. Cambridge, UK, Cambridge University Press, 2003

5

Depression, Euphoria, and Anger in the Emergency Department

Philippe-Edouard Boursiquot, M.D.

Jennifer S. Brasch, M.D.

General Approach to Mood States

Mood disturbance is a common presenting symptom or complaint for patients in a psychiatric emergency service (PES). When patients are cooperative, the assessment can be straightforward. However, angry, irritable, and euphoric patients may be agitated or potentially violent and unable to tolerate a lengthy interview. Patients with labile affect can be unpredictable and perplexing to an inexperienced interviewer. Patients who are profoundly depressed may be withdrawn and slow to reply, making it difficult to obtain full information within a busy PES. Accurate assessment of patients with abnormal mood is critical, because they are at increased risk for suicide, violence, and significant morbidity. In this chapter, we focus on the challenges of assessing and managing patients with extreme mood disturbances, specifically depression, mania, and anger.

When a depressed, euphoric, or angry patient arrives in the PES, safety must be the first concern. Although it may be obvious within moments that a patient is probably manic, attention must be directed to assessing the patient's level of agitation and need for a safe, low-stimulus environment. A safe environment and close observation are also necessary for profoundly depressed patients, especially those who may try to die by suicide within the PES setting. Careful assessment of risk of harm to others and suicide is critical because risk issues are central in determining disposition. (See Chapter 2, "The Suicidal Patient," and Chapter 3, "Violence Risk Assessment," for more details.)

The assessment of and emergency interventions for a patient with extreme mood disturbance initially occur simultaneously: mood is observed and monitored, while efforts are made to control the situation. Once immediate safety concerns have been addressed, the assessment can proceed. Assessments in the PES need to focus on the current presentation, including the mood disturbance, neurovegetative symptoms, and recent stressors. It is also important to explore past episodes of abnormal mood, medical illnesses, medications, and functional status. All patients with extreme mood states need to be screened for comorbid psychiatric illnesses, including symptoms of psychosis, personality disorders, and anxiety disorders. Substance abuse and dependence are very common within the PES, and it can be a challenge to determine if a patient's mood disturbance is due to intoxication, withdrawal, drug seeking, or history of use, or if the substance use is an attempt to self-treat. Previous medical notes often can be used to trace the longitudinal pattern of a mood disorder. Collateral information is often essential, especially in evaluating risk of harm to self or others.

Depressed Mood States

Case Example 1

Ms. S, a 61-year-old female, was brought to the PES for suicidal ideation and nihilistic thoughts. She had a past history of depression and had previously been treated with electroconvulsive therapy. During the interview, she did not make eye contact. Her clothes and hair were unkempt. She appeared fatigued.

Her affect was restricted. In a flat voice, she stated, "I am so sad I cannot cry." She had no clear and definite plan to end her life, but she did not see any possibility of recovery. Her goal was to end her inner pain. She had been feeling increasingly depressed since she ran out of her medications 3 months earlier.

Depression is the third most common presenting symptom of patients in the PES, after substance use and psychotic disorders (Currier and Allen 2003). Indeed, major depressive disorder is very common and may affect up to 25% of individuals in their lifetime (Goldstein and Levitt 2006), although the majority will never be seen in the PES. Patients who are seen in a PES or general medical emergency department for a psychiatric assessment following a suicide attempt should always be carefully screened for depression and other mood disorders. In turn, suicide risk should be evaluated in all patients presenting with depressed mood.

Assessment

Many patients with depressed mood will readily admit their distress. Rather than asking closed-ended questions, the clinician should ask open-ended questions, which often yield more accurate information. For example, instead of asking, "Would you say you have been sad and tearful more often than not for the past 2 weeks?" you might say, "How has your mood been lately?"

Symptoms of sadness and/or anhedonia are essential for the diagnosis of a major depressive episode. Other symptoms associated with depressive episodes include sleep disturbance, diminished energy, appetite changes, significant guilt or self-blame, impaired concentration, psychomotor retardation, and preoccupation with death or suicide. Additionally, a depressive episode can be diagnosed only if the period of depression includes a significant change in the patient's level of functioning in comparison with the patient's baseline.

The clinician should ask about major stresses and significant losses as part of the history of the presenting illness (see Table 5–1). These stresses and losses may trigger a depressive episode. A diagnosis of an adjustment disorder should also be considered if the mood symptoms begin after a significant stress.

Interviewing patients with psychomotor retardation can be challenging. These patients can be slowed in their responses and provide only limited information. Inexperienced interviewers may empathize with the patient to the

Table 5–1. Categories of stressors to explore in patients with abnormal mood

Financial	Income, debt, gambling losses
Employment	Instability, unemployment, dissatisfaction, retirement
Shelter	Insecurity, homelessness
Relationship	Loss (bereavement), violence, infidelity, sexual orientation, bullying, conflict, abuse
Health	Severe or chronic illness, pregnancy, disability, chronic pain
Other	Cultural, developmental, life transition, spiritual

extent that the interview can slow down and almost grind to a halt. The clinician needs to keep the questions gentle but persistent.

Some patients may minimize their symptoms of depression for cultural reasons or fears of stigma and discrimination. These patients may have decided to die by suicide and may deny depressed mood in order to carry out their plans. The clinician should ask open-ended questions and obtain collateral information to minimize the risk of determining disposition with insufficient information.

Interviewers may feel uncomfortable when a depressed patient begins to cry. The clinician should acknowledge the depth and intensity of the patient's distress, and allow some time and silence before continuing the interview. Offering a tissue demonstrates care and concern. Recognizing and addressing these manifestations of suffering can put the patient at greater ease, and empathic listening can relieve the patient's sense of emotional burden.

Asking about past episodes of mood disturbances is important. Past diagnosis, treatment, and follow-up help put the current presentation in context. A history of hypomania or mania must always be ruled out to minimize the risk of precipitating euphoria with an antidepressant.

Obtaining a substance abuse history, particularly for alcohol, benzodiazepines, cocaine, opioids, and sedatives, is essential. It can be very difficult to determine, for example, if a patient is depressed because he or she drinks alcohol or if the patient drinks because he or she is depressed. Some patients may use cocaine or other substances in an effort to self-treat a depressed mood. A substance-induced mood disorder cannot be ruled out if substance use has occurred within a month of the patient's depressive symptoms. (See Chapter 9, "Substance-Related Psychiatric Emergencies," for further information.)

The mental status examination of a patient with depression will often reflect the depth of his or her distress. Hygiene, eye contact, speech, and thought content are salient elements. With respect to thought content, mood-congruent themes of worthlessness, poverty, or nihilism signal severe depression, and may at times reach delusional intensity. Psychotic symptoms are present in 15% of all depressed patients (Glick 2002). In adolescents, psychotic depression may be the first sign of bipolar disorder (Schatzberg and Rothschild 1992). Agitated depression can be difficult to differentiate from a mixed state. The main distinguishing feature is the absence of grandiosity and pleasure-seeking behavior (Glick 2002). Because depression can be the first sign of a dementia in elderly patients, a brief cognitive evaluation, such as the Mini-Mental State Examination (Folstein et al. 1975), can be useful, although the depressed state can distort cognition..

An assessment of mood disorder should always include consideration of medical conditions that may be associated with depressed mood. A physical examination can point to a medical cause of depression (see Table 5–2).

Table 5–2. Some medical disorders associated with a depressed mood

Vascular	Stroke (especially subcortical)
Infectious/inflammatory/ autoimmune	Multiple sclerosis, HIV/AIDS, hepatitis, influenza, Epstein-Barr virus (mononucleosis), systemic lupus erythematosus
Neoplastic	Primary or metastatic brain cancer, pancreatic carcinoma, lung carcinoma
Drugs/toxins	Barbiturates, benzodiazepines, levodopa, antipsychotics, β-adrenergic blockers, ranitidine, lead, other heavy metal poisoning
Degenerative	Dementia, Parkinson's disease, Huntington's disease
Traumatic	Head injury
Endocrine	Hypoadrenalism (Addison's disease), hyperadrenalism (Cushing's disease), hypothyroidism, hyperthyroidism, diabetes, hyperparathyroidism
Metabolic	Seizure disorder, anemia, electrolyte disturbances, vitamin B_{12} and other nutritional deficiencies, uremia

Source. Adapted from Glick 2002; Milner et al. 1999.

Table 5–3.   Suggested investigations for patients presenting with abnormal mood

Complete blood count (CBC)

Thyroid stimulating hormone (TSH)

Urea, creatinine, electrolytes (Na^+, K^+, Ca^{2+})

Liver function tests: alanine transaminase (ALT), aspartate transaminase (AST), gamma-glutamyltransferase (GGT), bilirubin

Beta-human chorionic gonadotropin (β-HCG) in women of childbearing age

Urine toxicology screen; urinalysis (especially in elderly)

Suggested basic investigations for a patient with abnormal mood are listed in Table 5–3. Pregnancy should be ruled out in women of childbearing age because it may influence choice of treatment.

Diagnosis

A depressed mood can be part of many psychiatric disorders. The most common diagnosis associated with depressed mood is major depressive episode, which should be considered first. If the patient's symptoms do not meet full criteria for major depressive episode, the clinician should consider adjustment disorder or bereavement. If the patient is psychotic and depressed, the clinician should consider a diagnosis of major depressive episode, severe, with psychotic features. Depressive episodes, with or without psychosis, can also occur in patients with bipolar disorder, schizophrenia, schizoaffective disorder, or other psychotic disorders. If the patient is actively using a mood-altering substance, substance-induced mood disorder needs to be high on the differential. Alcohol and opioid misuse are frequently associated with depressed mood. Many patients may have more than one diagnosis. For example, high comorbidity exists between anxiety disorders and depressive symptoms. Patients with borderline personality disorder may complain of depressed or rapidly changing mood, in addition to unstable interpersonal relationships and self-image.

Management and Disposition

Disposition of patients is determined by the risk assessment. Patients with depressed mood and significant suicidal ideation and/or psychosis generally

Table 5–4.   Criteria for admission in patients with abnormal mood

Danger to self or others (risk of suicide, violence, or homicide)

Inability to care for self

Strong possibility of a life-threatening medical condition

Symptoms that cannot be safely evaluated or treated on an outpatient basis

Note.   Local criteria for involuntary admission also apply.
Source.   Adapted from Swann 2003.

require hospital admission. Additional factors that may heighten the need for hospital admission include the presence of a disabling medical condition, social isolation, lack of community supports, a hostile home environment, or no follow-up care (see Table 5–4). In fact, over half of all patients seen in the PES with depressive symptoms may require admission (Harman et al. 2004).

Patients with a major depressive episode who will not be admitted to a hospital can be started on antidepressants in the emergency department (Milner et al. 1999). This practice is somewhat controversial, however, because of concerns with compliance, follow-up, and potential drug overdose (Glick 2004), but current first-line treatments for depression are generally safe. The circumstances in which antidepressants can be initiated in the PES are listed in Table 5–5. When prescribing an antidepressant, the clinician needs to carefully explain the purpose of the medication, describe common adverse reactions, and discuss the expected time course for symptom improvement. Patients must have follow-up with a healthcare provider who can monitor their response to the antidepressant and continue the prescription (Glick 2004; Shea 1998). If possible, the patient's family or support person should be included in the discussion. Encourage patients to call a crisis line or return to the emergency department if they struggle with the treatment plan. The clinician should always document that this information was transmitted (Glick 2004).

The choice of an antidepressant agent rests on past response (of the patient or family members), side effects, and known contraindications. Across the lifespan, the selective serotonin reuptake inhibitors (SSRIs) are commonly used as first-line therapy (Sadock and Sadock 2007). Mood improvement typically occurs after 4–6 weeks of therapy, but neurovegetative symptoms may begin to improve in as little as 1–2 weeks. Patients will need to continue

Table 5–5.   Factors supporting emergency department antidepressant therapy and outpatient treatment

Clear diagnosis

No substance use

Low suicide risk

Available social supports

No psychosis or agitation

Clear follow-up plan

Desire to begin treatment

Ability to pay for (or having health insurance for) medications

Source.   Adapted with permission from Glick RL: "Starting Antidepressant Treatment in the Emergency Setting." *Psychiatric Issues in Emergency Care Settings* 3:6–10, 2004. Copyright 2010, *Psychiatric Issues in Emergency Care Settings,*UMB Medica. All rights reserved.

antidepressants beyond their return to euthymia. Common side effects include gastric discomfort, insomnia, jitteriness (in up to 25% of patients), and sexual disturbance (in 50%–80% of patients) (Sadock and Sadock 2007). The starting dose should be reduced in the elderly and in patients with liver disease. In the child and adolescent population, the clinician should carefully weigh the risks and benefits of SSRIs because they may increase suicidal ideation (Bailly 2008). SSRIs are generally considered safe in pregnancy; studies have shown that the risk of congenital cardiac malformations in fetuses exposed to SSRIs does not exceed 2%, although paroxetine is associated with a higher risk compared with other SSRIs (Greene 2007).

Benzodiazepines or low-dose atypical antipsychotics are often prescribed for the insomnia and anxiety associated with depression. Patients should be cautioned about the risk of tolerance, which can occur quite readily with benzodiazepines (Glick 2002).

For a patient with a history of bipolar disorder, mania, or hypomania, antidepressants should not be prescribed alone. A mood stabilizer should be ordered concurrently (Sadock and Sadock 2007). The first-line mood stabilizers in bipolar depression are lithium and lamotrigine. Quetiapine has also shown significant benefit (El-Mallakh and Karippot 2006). If psychosis is present, typical or atypical antipsychotics can be used in conjunction with antidepressants (Glick 2002).

Evidence supports the use of monoamine oxidase inhibitors in patients with atypical depression (hypersomnia, hyperphagia, increased rejection sensitivity); however, cautions include concurrent use of SSRIs (risk of serotonin syndrome), a high-tyramine diet, hypertension (risk of hypertensive crisis), and use of bronchodilators and analgesics. Although inexpensive, tricyclic antidepressants are generally not more effective antidepressants than SSRIs, and the clinician must consider the patient's cardiac history, age, overdose potential, and heightened sensitivity to anticholinergic side effects (Sadock and Sadock 2007). Because these medications carry a higher risk of side effects than SSRIs and because these medications are not typically considered until the patient has attempted trials of SSRIs, strong consideration should be given to establishing a clear pathway for follow-up from the emergency department visit and deferring initiation of these medications to the outpatient provider.

Patients with both depressive symptoms and substance abuse do best when referred to a concurrent disorders program. Unfortunately, these programs are rare, and patients may need to complete substance abuse treatment before receiving care for their mood disorder. Patients should be offered antidepressant therapy because it is safe and efficacious, may improve compliance with substance abuse treatment, and may reduce the patient's substance use (Minkoff 2005).

For patients with mild to moderate depression, a course of brief, structured psychotherapy can be recommended in combination with pharmacotherapy or as an alternative to antidepressants. Unfortunately, access to cognitive-behavioral or interpersonal therapy may be limited by availability or cost. Patients with bereavement or adjustment disorder may benefit more from supportive counseling than from an antidepressant. In patients with borderline personality disorder, dialectical behavior therapy has been proved effective for reducing self-harm behaviors and attenuating mood lability (Sadock and Sadock 2007). Patients and family members benefit from learning about the symptoms and treatment of depression.

Case Example 1 *(continued)*

Given the high risk for self-harm and her inability to care for herself, Ms. S was certified as an involuntary patient and observed closely in the PES until an inpatient bed became available. Her diagnosis was major depressive disorder, current episode severe.

Elevated Mood States

Case Example 2

"Come in, come in!" Mr. M beckoned. "I am so glad to see you! I need to tell you what is going on. You see, today is not April the first. It is April the truth!" he exclaimed in delight. "I am a security guard for Big Town Mall. Today, I am to be promoted to field commander. You have the power to release me, doctor, so I can meet my boss. It is up to you! Up to now I have kept people's bodies safe. Now, now I know how to keep their souls safe." Mr. M smiled with satisfaction and a sense of purpose. His brother had brought Mr. M, age 28, to the PES. Mr. M had slept only 1 or 2 hours per night for the past week and did not abuse substances.

Interviewing a euphoric patient can be an interesting and difficult experience at times. Mania is defined as a state of grandeur, often associated with an elevated, euphoric mood, although manic patients frequently present with irritability. Bipolar disorder has a lifetime prevalence of about 1% and is associated with a high suicide rate and significant morbidity (Sadock and Sadock 2007).

Assessment

Assessing a patient with an elevated mood draws on an interviewer's flexibility, creativity, and patience. As in interviews with depressed patients, safety concerns are a priority. The clinician should consider having security staff present, because even the most euphoric and elated patient can quickly become irritable and uncooperative. Considerable interviewing skill is necessary to interject questions about symptoms consistent with mania that lead to useful information yet avoid causing irritability or excessively lengthy responses (Levinson and Young 2006). Asking questions that are short, closed ended, and focused will increase the amount of useful information from patients who are very talkative, circumstantial, or disorganized. To obtain the history of presenting illness, the clinician should ask questions to elicit a clear timeline of recent events and explore recent stresses. The interview should end before the patient escalates, regardless of how little factual information has been obtained. Even a short encounter provides plenty of data for the mental status examination. Information about the longitudinal pattern of mood disturbance is necessary to determine the diagnosis. Often, this information is easier to obtain from collateral sources.

Symptoms particular to mania that often emerge spontaneously in the interview include grandiosity, decreased need for sleep, increased talkativeness, indulgence in pleasurable or high-risk activities, increased goal-directed activity, flight of ideas, and distractibility. It is important to explore suicidal and homicidal ideation, because manic patients often feel invincible and may lose all sense of mortality or morals. Also, manic patients often engage in behaviors that will inadvertently put them at risk for trauma or neglect (Swann 2003). These should be assessed as well.

Obtaining a patient's medication and substance use history is essential. The clinician should inquire about antidepressant use as a precipitant of a manic state (Sadock and Sadock 2007). Poor compliance with prescribed medications can also contribute to a patient's presentation. Exploring the recent use of substances is important, because substance misuse can mimic or mask a manic episode.

Many patients with mania have excessive motor activity and may be unable to sit down for more than a few seconds. The mental status examination may also reveal hypervigilance, irritability, labile affect, flight of ideas, circumstantiality, tangentiality, delusions, hallucinations, pressured speech, lack of insight, and impaired judgment.

Although patients may not cooperate with a physical examination, it should be attempted, because a number of medical diagnoses are associated with euphoric or elevated mood (see Table 5–6). Brief observation of the patient can suggest substance intoxication or withdrawal. Basic investigations are recommended (see Table 5–3). Beta-human chorionic gonadotropin testing is warranted in women of childbearing age, because many mood stabilizers are teratogenic (James et al. 2007).

Diagnosis

The key feature of bipolar I disorder is one or more manic or mixed episodes (with or without depressive episodes), whereas bipolar II disorder is associated with hypomanic states. In hypomania, the patient has an elevated, euphoric, or irritable mood but is not psychotic and does not require hospitalization. In mania, the patient has a clear loss of social or occupational functioning, whereas a patient in hypomania usually completes responsibilities despite having a different level of functioning. In a mixed state, features of both depression and mania are present, although a broad range of clinical presentations is seen. Pa-

Table 5–6.   Some medical disorders associated with an elevated mood

Vascular	Primary central nervous system vasculitis, systemic vasculitis
Infectious/inflammatory/ autoimmune	Multiple sclerosis, encephalitis, meningitis, central nervous system syphilis, HIV/AIDS, hepatitis, influenza, Epstein-Barr virus (mononucleosis), systemic lupus erythematosus
Drugs/toxins	Levodopa, methylphenidate, captopril, corticosteroids, lead or other heavy metal poisoning, amphetamine, cocaine
Degenerative	Dementia
Traumatic	History of head injury
Endocrine	Hyperadrenalism (Cushing's disease), hyperthyroidism, sleep deprivation, overstimulation, Wilson's disease, uremia, hemodialysis
Metabolic	Epilepsy, hypoglycemia, electrolyte disturbances, uremia, vitamin B_3 deficiency, vitamin B_{12} deficiency

Source.   Adapted from Milner et al. 1999.

tients with mixed states often demonstrate mood lability and severe agitation, which can make them unpredictable and difficult to manage (Swann 2008).

Manic episodes occur in a smaller number of disorders than depressive episodes. Although most commonly associated with bipolar I disorder, periods of elevated mood also occur in schizoaffective disorder and substance-related disorders. Schizoaffective disorder requires the longitudinal predominance of mood symptoms, as well as a 2-week period of psychotic symptoms in the absence of mood symptoms. Substances associated with a euphoric mood include alcohol, amphetamine, cocaine, hallucinogens, and opioids. The state of mania is associated with disinhibition, which increases the risk of substance use. Mania is also associated with medical conditions (see Table 5–6) and can be induced by an antidepressant.

Management and Disposition

Patients in a manic state or mixed state usually have little or no insight into their potentially harmful ideas and plans. They need to be involuntarily admitted to the hospital (see Table 5–4). Patients with more insight and less severe mood disturbance (e.g., hypomania) may be managed in the community with medication adjustment and close follow-up.

In the emergency setting, patients in a manic state are often irritable, agitated, and intrusive. Staff should try to decrease environmental noise and unpredictability, and offer consistent low-key interpersonal interactions (Swann 2008). Seclusion or restraints may be necessary to contain an agitated patient or prevent harm to others (see Chapter 11, "Seclusion and Restraint in Emergency Settings," for additional information). If a patient will remain in the PES for an extended period, medications should be offered proactively to prevent a reescalation of the manic behaviors.

Atypical antipsychotics are first-line agents to control manic agitation. They have the same antimanic effects as typical antipsychotics and a lower risk of akathisia and extrapyramidal symptoms (Sadock and Sadock 2007; Swann 2003). Risperidone, olanzapine, ziprasidone, quetiapine, and aripiprazole are available in different forms (tablet, soluble, or intramuscular). Benzodiazepines can be used alone or in conjunction with antipsychotics, with the aim of controlling agitation. Caution should be taken when using benzodiazepines in elderly patients due to increased risk of falls. The clinician should keep in mind that the patient may be too agitated and/or incapable of consenting to treatment, and that initially such interventions constitute chemical restraint.

If hospitalization is not required, once the patient is calm, informed consent can be obtained from the patient or a substitute decision maker regarding maintenance therapy. Mood stabilizers are not typically initiated in the PES, unless noncompliance has been identified and the objective of the emergency department visit is simply to reinitiate the patient's usual mood stabilizer. Valproate loading can be attempted (Swann 2003, 2008). Antipsychotics are preferable to mood stabilizers if there are concerns about teratogenicity, although the several risks, such as extrapyramidal symptoms, must be carefully weighed against the benefits (Patton et al. 2002).

Case Example 2 *(continued)*

Mr. M did not see the need for hospitalization. Before transfer to the ward, he became irritable and demanded to be released, but with his brother's support and encouragement, he took soluble olanzapine 10 mg orally and calmed down. He remained calm until transfer to the ward could be arranged.

Angry and Irritable Mood States

Case Example 3

Mr. W, a 17-year-old male, was brought to the emergency department by police for causing a disturbance downtown. He was resistant to the assessment, angry, and verbally abusive with staff. He refused oral sedatives, was uncooperative, and did not interact with his parents. He had a 1-year history of daily cannabis use, corresponding to an escalation of his anger reactions. His parents were unwilling to have him in their home. He was taking bupropion for attention-deficit/hyperactivity disorder (ADHD).

Anger and irritability are the most trying of the extreme moods presented in this chapter. Interviews with angry and irritable patients can be difficult because of pressures on clinicians to accurately predict risk of violence and because nobody likes to deliberately expose themselves to verbal tirades or worse. The threat of aggression is unsettling. Determining the most appropriate diagnosis can be a challenge, because angry and irritable behavior can be the presenting problem for many different diagnostic categories. In addition, many crisis situations may develop from nonpathological angry behavior. In those situations, it is necessary for the clinician to identify the absence of a diagnosis and the limited role of the emergency department.

Assessment

Interviews in the PES to assess angry and irritable patients usually fall into one of two categories: the assessment of a reasonably calm person who was brought in because of angry and irritable behavior in the community or the assessment of a person who is angry at the time of the interview. (See Chapter 1, "Approach to Psychiatric Emergencies," and Chapter 3, "Violence Risk Assessment," for discussion of the assessment and management of agitation and assessment of the risk of violent behavior, respectively.)

As with all other patients in the PES, the assessment of a patient who has a history of angry episodes or is currently angry begins with ensuring everyone's safety and is initially guided by the patient's ability to cooperate. With patients who are reasonably calm and can describe their episodes of anger and irritability, the interviewer can gather specific details about the incident that precipitated the visit as well as about previous episodes of anger. The interviewer should ask open-ended and unbiased questions—for example, "How many times did you hit John?" rather than "Did you hit him a lot of times?" (the latter question allows patients to minimize their aggressive behavior, especially if facing arrest for their actions). Once the history of the presenting illness has been explored, the interviewer can direct questions to ruling in or out specific diagnoses (see Table 5–7).

Assessment of patients who are angry and irritable during the interview presents special challenges. Clinicians need to be aware of their own discomfort with angry patients and avoid revealing any irritability of their own. Setting firm limits may be necessary. It is far better for a clinician to leave the interview room to end a patient's verbal tirade than to become confrontational and thereby escalate the situation. If a patient is not psychotic or delirious and does not settle quickly, it may be safest to terminate the interview until the patient is calmer and more cooperative.

Trying to empathize with the patient can help to establish an alliance and enable the patient to feel understood. This does not mean that the clinician must agree with the patient's ideas or beliefs, but initially offering a rational response to a patient who is angry is unlikely to be helpful. The clinician should allow the angry patient to feel heard, to be supported, and to have his or her feelings validated. Validation can lead to a joining and partnering that can support later problem solving (Shea 1998). It is important to keep in mind that patients can be angry because of long waits in the PES or from having been brought to the emergency room against their will. It is important for the clinician, when assessing an angry patient, to debrief with a colleague and/ or superior and to not take the anger personally.

Diagnosis

Angry and irritable behaviors are associated with many diagnostic categories (see Table 5–7), including mood disorders. People experiencing a depressive episode may present with irritability. This tends to be more common in males,

Table 5–7. Conditions that may present with angry or irritable mood

Major depressive episode; manic episode; mixed episode

Psychotic disorders

Substance intoxication or withdrawal (alcohol, amphetamines, cocaine, "crystal meth," "Ecstasy," hallucinogens)

Drug-seeking behavior (especially benzodiazepines, alcohol)

Impulse-control disorders (especially intermittent explosive disorder)

Personality disorders (especially antisocial and borderline)

Conduct disorder; oppositional defiant disorder

Attention-deficit/hyperactivity disorder; Tourette's syndrome; pervasive developmental disorders

Partner relational problem; parent-child relational problem; adjustment disorder (with disturbance of conduct)

Dementia; delirium; head injury; seizure disorder

Source. American Psychiatric Association 2000.

possibly because the culture discourages men from admitting to depression. Some authors have described a "male depressive syndrome," characterized by low impulse control, episodes of anger, and high irritability (Rutz et al. 1995; Winkler et al. 2005). Patients experiencing a manic or mixed episode can often be angry and irritable, rather than euphoric. Table 5–8 can assist in determining if irritability is due to depression or mania.

Patients with paranoid ideation and other psychotic symptoms can become very angry because they perceive that no one understands their fears of danger. Also, because of the high prevalence rates of substance abuse and dependence seen in patients in a PES, it is important to consider that patients may be intoxicated with alcohol or stimulants. Patients who are in withdrawal may become very irritable and may present to the PES seeking benzodiazepines, opioids, or other prescription medications.

Many other diagnostic categories can also be associated with anger and irritability. The family and friends of patients with borderline or antisocial personality disorders may be more concerned with their outbursts of extreme and inappropriate anger than are the patients themselves. Borderline personality disorder should be suspected in patients with a pattern of instability in interpersonal relationships and self-image, rapidly fluctuating moods, and self-

Table 5–8.   Irritability in depression and mania

	Depression	Mania
To whom the irritability is directed	Irritability is much more likely to be expressed toward loved ones and people who live in close proximity.	Expressed with less selectivity. Therefore, coworkers, strangers, other drivers, etc. receive the wrath of the irritability, although simply as a virtue of time spent together, family is more likely to receive the brunt.
Triggered or not	There is often a "hook to hang the hat" of irritability on. The "infraction" may be small or insignificant, but there is usually a trigger for the irritable outburst.	The irritability is expressed virtually spontaneously. Some patients talk about walking on their own and feeling rage, and yelling, when there is no particular precipitant.
Remorseful?	People with depression most often feel awful about how they are acting and hate the fact that they are irritable.	People experiencing mania are usually remorseful only once the episode is over. During the episode, they do not recognize their behavior as irritable or feel justified in behaving that way.
Associated behavior	The irritability of depression is often associated with distress and expression of other negative emotions such as tearfulness and anguish.	The irritability of mania is often associated with rage and aggression, either verbal or physical.

Source.   Reprinted from Goldstein BI, Levitt AJ: "Assessment of Patients With Depression," in *Psychiatric Clinical Skills.* Edited by Goldbloom DS. Philadelphia, PA, Elsevier Mosby, 2006, p. 350. Copyright 2006, Elsevier. Used with permission.

harm behaviors. Core features in conduct disorder and antisocial personality disorder are verbal and physical aggression, as well as a disregard for the rights of others.

In children and adolescents, oppositional defiant disorder is associated with hostile, disobedient, and defiant behavior but not with a disregard for the rights of others. Poor impulse control is a core symptom in ADHD. In up to 50% of patients, this disorder can persist into adulthood (Sadock and Sadock 2007). ADHD is frequently comorbid with Tourette's syndrome, a condition characterized by motor and vocal tics and episodic rage attacks.

Medical causes for angry outbursts should also be considered. These include dementia, delirium, a history of head injury, and seizure disorders. Any concerns about cognitive impairment should be thoroughly assessed with a standardized instrument such as Folstein et al.'s (1975) Mini-Mental State Examination. These etiologies are discussed further in Chapter 8, "The Cognitively Impaired Patient."

It is important to remember that anger is a normal reaction to many circumstances. Anger is common in sudden losses, unexpected death of a loved one, theft, devastating medical diagnosis, discovery of betrayal, or other crisis. Anger can also be experienced during a disaster. If the anger is situational, interviewing family members may quickly reveal their role in contributing to a patient's angry outbursts.

Intermittent explosive disorder is diagnosed in the absence of other disorders. It is more common in men. Key features include extreme expressions of anger, often to the point of uncontrollable rage, that are disproportionate to the situation at hand. The patient also exhibits genuine remorse afterward and a pleasant demeanor between outbursts.

Management and Disposition

Management of the angry patient depends on the diagnosis. For guidance in assessment and interventions for patients whose anger is not under voluntary control (e.g., in patients with mania or intoxication), see section "Elevated Mood States" earlier in this chapter and also Chapter 1, "Approach to Psychiatric Emergencies." Medication may have a role in the management of angry outbursts if a psychiatric disorder is present. However, any medication needs to be prescribed with a clear plan for follow-up to ensure careful evaluation of any benefit (Sadock and Sadock 2007). Hospitalization should be considered for those patients with a psychiatric disorder whose anger presents a risk of injury to the patient or to others.

Some patients who are in control of their mood state may benefit from anger management training. This training is usually delivered in a group setting and helps patients learn strategies to modulate their angry outbursts, appropriately assert their needs, and develop constructive conflict resolution strategies. The clinician must carefully document the risk assessment of a nonpsychotic angry patient. It is imperative to remind patients that they are responsible for their actions and the consequences of their actions when angry. This should be documented carefully.

Hospitalization or other psychiatric treatment for anger in the absence of a psychiatric disorder is generally not indicated. The most appropriate action may be to release these angry individuals to the custody of law enforcement. Careful documentation of the decision-making process in determining disposition for an angry patient is important for medicolegal purposes.

Case Example 3 *(continued)*

An interview with Mr. W and his family reveals a 6-year history of tantrums and disputes. His mother admitted that she had insulted him about his cannabis use, social isolation, and poor academic performance. Mr. W refused to apologize for his angry outbursts. His parents wanted us to keep him in the hospital. However, Mr. W did not carry psychiatric diagnoses other than his ADHD and cannabis abuse. Moreover, the ADHD appeared well controlled with his bupropion. Hospitalization was not warranted because Mr. W's anger appeared to be independent of his preexisting psychiatric diagnoses, and it would not have been appropriate to use these diagnoses to excuse his behavior. Instead, the diagnosis of parent-child relational problem was given. Reluctantly, his parents took him home. A referral for family counseling was completed.

Key Clinical Points

- In assessing patients with extreme moods, the interviewer should always address safety and risk issues first.

- Angry and depressed mood states occur in a wide range of psychiatric disorders.

- Obtaining a longitudinal history of mood states is important in establishing a mood disorder diagnosis.

- The clinician should screen a patient for a history of hypomania or mania before initiating an antidepressant.

- Depression and mania can present with irritability.

- For patients with depression who do not require admission, the clinician should initiate treatment in the PES and focus on maximizing adherence and follow-up.

- For patients with angry or irritable mood, the clinician should determine if a psychiatric disorder is present and be firm about the limited role of the PES in anger not due to a psychiatric or other medical condition.

References

American Psychiatric Association: Diagnostic and Statistical Manual of Mental Disorders, 4th Edition, Text Revision. Washington, DC, American Psychiatric Association, 2000

Bailly D: Benefits and risks of using antidepressants in children and adolescents. Expert Opin Drug Saf 7:9–27, 2008

Currier GW, Allen M: Organization and function of academic psychiatric emergency services. Gen Hosp Psychiatry 25:124–129, 2003

El-Mallakh RS, Karippot A: Chronic depression in bipolar disorder. Am J Psychiatry 163:1337–1341, 2006

Folstein MF, Folstein SE, McHugh PR: "Mini-mental state": a practical method for grading the cognitive state of patients for the clinician. J Psychiatr Res 12:189–198, 1975

Glick RL: Emergency management of depression and depression complicated by agitation or psychosis. Psychiatric Issues in Emergency Care Settings 1 (winter):11–16, 2002

Glick RL: Starting antidepressant treatment in the emergency setting. Psychiatric Issues in Emergency Care Settings 3:6–10, 2004

Goldstein BI, Levitt AJ: Assessment of patients with depression, in Psychiatric Clinical Skills. Edited by Goldbloom DS. Philadelphia, PA, Elsevier Mosby, 2006, pp 339–359

Greene MF: Teratogenicity of SSRIs: serious concern or much ado about little? N Engl J Med 356:2732–2733, 2007

Harman JS, Scholle SH, Edlund MJ: Emergency department visits for depression in the United States. Psychiatr Serv 55:937–939, 2004

James L, Barnes TR, Lelliott P, et al: Informing patients of the teratogenic potential of mood stabilizing drugs: a case note review of the practice of psychiatrists. J Psychopharmacol 21:815–819, 2007

Levinson AJ, Young LT: Assessment of patients with bipolar disorder, in Psychiatric Clinical Skills. Edited by Goldbloom DS. Philadelphia, Elsevier Mosby, 2006, pp 51–70

Milner KK, Florence T, Glick RL: Mood and anxiety syndromes in emergency psychiatry. Psychiatr Clin North Am 22:755–777, 1999

Minkoff K: Psychopharmacology practice guidelines for individuals with co-occurring psychiatric and substance use disorders (COD). Comprehensive Continuous Integrated System of Care (CCISC). January 2005. Available at: http://www.kenminkoff.com/article1.doc. Accessed September 28, 2009.

Patton SW, Misri S, Corral MR, et al: Antipsychotic medication during pregnancy and lactation in women with schizophrenia: evaluating the risk. Can J Psychiatry 47:959–965, 2002

Rutz W, von Knorring L, Pihlgren H, et al: Prevention of male suicides: lessons from Gotland study. Lancet 345:524, 1995

Sadock BJ, Sadock VA: Kaplan and Sadock's Synopsis of Psychiatry, 10th Edition. Philadelphia, PA, Lippincott Williams & Wilkins, 2007

Schatzberg AF, Rothschild AJ: Psychotic (delusional) major depression: should it be included as a distinct syndrome in DSM-IV? (abstract). Am J Psychiatry 149:733–745, 1992

Shea SC: Psychiatric Interviewing: The Art of Understanding, 2nd Edition. Philadelphia, PA, WB Saunders, 1998, pp 575–621

Swann AC: Psychiatric emergencies in bipolar disorder. Psychiatric Issues in Emergency Care Settings 2 (summer):4–13, 2003

Swann AC: Mania and mixed states, in Emergency Psychiatry: Principles and Practice. Edited by Glick RL, Berlin JS, Fishkind A, et al. Philadelphia, PA, Lippincott Williams & Wilkins, 2008, pp 189–200

Winkler D, Pjrek E, Kasper S: Anger attacks in depression: evidence for a male depressive syndrome. Psychother Psychosom 74:303–307, 2005

Suggested Readings

Edwards CD, Glick RL: Depression, in Emergency Psychiatry: Principles and Practice. Edited by Glick RL, Berlin JS, Fishkind A, et al. Philadelphia, PA, Lippincott Williams & Wilkins, 2008, pp 175–188

Swann AC: Mania and mixed states, in Emergency Psychiatry: Principles and Practice. Edited by Glick RL, Berlin JS, Fishkind A, et al. Philadelphia, PA, Lippincott Williams & Wilkins, 2008, pp 189–200

6

The Psychotic Patient

Patricia Schwartz, M.D.
Mary Weathers, M.D.

Case Example

Mr. S is a 57-year-old undomiciled African American veteran with unknown past psychiatric history, who arrived by ambulance after he was found naked under the highway in the rain, stating that he needed to take a shower. He used military language, asking for a "debriefing" and demanding to see a "medic." He reported that he was a "three-star general" and demanded that staff call the Pentagon.

Definitions

Psychosis refers to "delusions, any prominent hallucinations, disorganized speech, or disorganized or catatonic behavior" (American Psychiatric Association [APA] 2000, p. 297) and is a common reason for patients to present to the psychiatric emergency room. *Delusions* are "erroneous beliefs that usually involve a misinterpretation of perceptions or experiences" (APA 2000, p. 299). *Hallucinations* are sensory perceptions not based in reality, and can be olfactory, visual, tactile, auditory, and even gustatory. *Disorganized speech* occurs when the patient no longer expresses himself or herself coherently in structured sentences. *Disorganized behaviors* can include sudden, unprovoked acts of violence; sexually inappropriate behavior; or even the inability to put on clothing correctly. *Catatonic behaviors* include immobility, posturing, and mutism.

Initial Survey of the Patient

The evaluation of the psychotic patient in the emergency setting begins the moment the patient arrives at the hospital, if not before. The clinician should carefully note the circumstances of the patient's arrival at the hospital and the patient's appearance upon arrival in order to determine how to safely proceed with the assessment.

Mode of Presentation

Psychotic patients present by a number of means and under a variety of circumstances, all of which are relevant to evaluation and treatment. A patient can come to the emergency room by ambulance, arrive under his or her own volition, or be brought to the emergency room by family, friends, strangers, or law enforcement personnel. Whatever the circumstances surrounding patients' arrival to the emergency room, much information can be gleaned from the events leading up to arrival at the hospital, including the manner of their arrival (Dhossche and Ghani 1998).

Patients who self-present to the emergency room for psychosis fall generally into one of three major categories: 1) those who present with medical/somatic complaints, 2) those who present with social complaints, and 3) those who present with psychiatric complaints. Of those patients who have psychiatric complaints, the subjective chief complaint of the psychotic patient often is unrelated to psychosis. Common reasons for such a patient to request help are hallucinations, feelings of persecution or paranoid ideation, mood symptoms, or social stressors. Patients often present complaining of homelessness, financial difficulties, or other social issues, only to reveal themselves to be flagrantly psychotic as well; a patient who requests a social intervention or appears to have secondary motives for presenting to the emergency room requires a full evaluation.

Psychotic patients are often referred to the emergency room by someone else. Behavior intolerable to the community, such as violence, aggression, agitation, and disorganized or inappropriate behavior, will commonly result in the involvement of either law enforcement or emergency medical services. Patients with persecutory delusions may make frequent complaints about others to law enforcement agencies and end up being referred for evaluation, thanks usually to a concerned law enforcement officer. Families of psychotic individuals may bring their loved ones to emergency services for aggressive behaviors, or they may report that the patients have stopped eating, are not sleeping, are behaving oddly, or are otherwise unable to care for themselves. After some change in their baseline behavior occurs, patients already connected within the mental health system may be referred for evaluation by health care providers, case managers, counselors, social workers, staff in shelters or prison systems, or other public agencies.

Choosing a Setting for Initial Patient Evaluation

Having considered the psychotic patient's mode of presentation, a clinician needs to determine the appropriate setting for patient evaluation. In many hospitals, patients are seen in the medical emergency department, and psychiatric consultation is available at the request of emergency department staff. Larger tertiary care centers may have a designated psychiatric emergency room that is separate from the medical emergency room. In such cases, staff must decide whether to evaluate a patient in the psychiatric or medical emergency room.

The initial contact is often a triage nurse, who briefly interviews the patient, obtains a set of vital signs, and determines whether the chief complaint is primarily medical or psychiatric. This is a juncture at which mistakes commonly occur, because this cursory physical assessment may overlook significant medical signs and symptoms (Allen 2002). Vital sign abnormalities, somatic complaints, physical signs, marked intoxication, disorientation, rapid onset of psychotic symptoms, or a waxing and waning mental status are all strong indications for evaluation in the medical emergency department, at least until the patient is determined to be medically stable. Kishi et al. (2007) found that 1) almost half of cases ultimately determined to be delirium that are referred for psychiatric consultation are initially mistaken for psychiatric illness by the referring doctor and 2) delirium is more likely to be missed in those patients with preexisting psychiatric illness. Current or past diagnoses of psychiatric disorders should not influence clinicians in assessing patients for the presence of medical illness (Duwe and Turetsky 2002). Even when no clear physical abnormality is present, patients who are experiencing psychotic symptoms for the first time, elderly patients, and patients with a history of trauma, falls, or significant medical comorbidities warrant a thorough workup in a medical emergency department to rule out a life-threatening medical condition (Marco and Vaughan 2005).

The clinician in the psychiatric emergency department plays a critical role in the medical management of psychiatric patients. The ability to generate a differential diagnosis that takes into account possible medical etiologies for psychosis and to effectively communicate specific concerns about a patient's presentation to other physicians, nurses, and hospital staff can save lives. In tertiary care centers with designated psychiatric emergency departments, a high index of suspicion that a general medical condition may be causing a patient's psychosis will often prompt referral of psychiatric patients to the medical emergency department for further evaluation. In such cases, the psychiatric clinician's role is to assist the medical team in building a differential diagnosis, and therefore he or she should be prepared to address specific concerns and ask specific questions tailored to the individual patient's presentation. Under no circumstances should a potentially medically ill patient be simply referred to the emergency room for "medical clearance" without a conversation between psychiatrist and emergency room physician that addresses the exact nature of the concern.

Two other points bear mentioning about the initial decision regarding the appropriate setting for evaluating a psychotic patient. First, patients with a clear psychiatric history and etiology for their symptoms often present with or develop medical comorbidities significant enough to warrant deferring a thorough psychiatric evaluation until more serious medical concerns are addressed. In fact, a growing body of evidence supports the contention that people with primary psychotic disorders such as schizophrenia have a much higher rate of medical comorbidity (e.g., cancer, heart disease, diabetes) than the general population (Newcomer 2006). When such medical conditions exist, their mortality is also well above the average. Second, when a patient is seen in the psychiatric emergency room, if there is any concern that he or she may have a condition that warrants urgent imaging or lab work, the psychiatrist treating the patient has a responsibility to communicate with the appropriate departments, to ensure that the workup is done in a timely manner, and to follow up the results.

Initial Assessment and Management

The next decision to be made is whether the patient can wait to be fully evaluated or must be seen immediately. If the patient is being evaluated in a medical emergency department, either because the patient is medically unstable or because the facility does not have a designated psychiatric emergency room, the patient should be seen as quickly as possible.

The initial psychiatric assessment is separate from the full interview that will follow, and it has one primary purpose: to assess danger and maintain a safe environment. Any patient who is physically violent on arrival to the emergency room requires immediate assessment and may require urgent behavioral and/or pharmacological intervention. Conversely, a patient who arrives in the psychiatric emergency room in some form of restraint may no longer require it. Patients brought in by emergency medical services, for example, who may have been agitated and dangerous at the time of their initial point of contact, may have calmed sufficiently in transit. For this reason, any patient arriving in physical restraints should be assessed immediately, and a decision needs to be made as to whether physical restraint is absolutely necessary to avoid imminent danger; almost always a less restrictive intervention is available. Other patients who require immediate assessment include those who appear frightened or paranoid, those verbally responding to internal stimuli, those who are verbally aggressive or threatening, those with psychomotor agitation (e.g., pacing or shadowboxing), and those attempting to leave the area without being evaluated.

Special care must be taken in the initial assessment of psychotic patients who present to the emergency room setting involuntarily. A safe and well-run psychiatric emergency department will have adequate staff available to rapidly and effectively deal with any sudden violent outburst with a certain amount of sensitivity to the special needs of this patient population. The psychiatrist should not approach an agitated patient to perform an initial assessment without support staff in the room. On the other hand, the psychiatrist should not leave the initial assessment to the support staff; a team approach works best, and an adequate "show of force" will often be enough to defuse a potentially dangerous situation. The psychiatrist should approach the patient and introduce himself or herself as the doctor who will be performing the evaluation. Patients should be given information about what to expect in language they can understand. It may be appropriate to explain the emergency room procedures, such as performing a search, holding personal valuables in a safe place, or changing into hospital clothes, with emphasis on the fact that these are standard procedures. Any reasonable wants or needs of the patient, such as hunger or thirst or the need for a bathroom, should be addressed. Often, offering food or drink even when the patient has not asked for it may have a calming effect. Patients who want to contact their family or legal services should be given the opportunity to do so.

Unfortunately, some acutely psychotic patients will not respond to verbal interventions or show of force. In such cases, the next step to ensure the safety of both patients and staff and to deescalate potentially dangerous situations generally involves the use of pharmacological interventions, physical restraints, or both. The subject of seclusion and restraint is covered more fully in Chapter 11, "Seclusion and Restraint in Emergency Settings."

The treating physician has several choices to make in determining the best pharmacological intervention for the acutely agitated psychotic patient: which medications to use, what doses to give, and by what route. Most emergency departments use either the intramuscular or oral form of medications to manage psychosis. Unless a patient is physically violent or in imminent danger of becoming so, a good practice, which may assist in establishing a better rapport with the patient, is to offer even the most seemingly agitated patient the option of taking medications by mouth (Currier et al. 2004). When intramuscular medication is required, it is advisable to first have the necessary staff on hand to restrain the patient physically, if necessary, because attempting to give an injection to an unwilling agitated patient without at least temporary restraint poses a significant risk of needlestick or other injury to all involved. In our experience, a *show* of force is typically enough to encourage the patient to cooperate without the *use* of force.

Traditional treatment of agitation and psychosis in emergent settings involved high doses of typical antipsychotics such as haloperidol (Hillard 1998). Over time, these doses were reduced due to the risks of side effects such as acute dystonia. Antipsychotics remain the mainstay of treatment for acute agitation and psychosis in many emergency departments. Benzodiazepines, such as lorazepam, are also frequently used. More recently, atypical antipsychotics have been used to treat psychosis in the emergency department; olanzapine, ziprasidone, and aripiprazole are available in a short-acting intramuscular form. If a patient's agitation or acutely psychotic state can be managed with oral medications, clinicians have a larger field to choose from.

The choice of which medications to use for agitation, and in what doses, should be tailored to the individual. Patients already maintained on an antipsychotic medication as outpatients, and who have tolerated and responded to that particular medication, can be treated accordingly (Hillard 1998). In the absence of any further clinical information, a psychotic but otherwise healthy patient with no known allergies may be given a combination of haloperidol and lorazepam, although olanzapine is increasingly popular in the emergency setting. Patients who are naïve to antipsychotics are likely to be more quickly and heavily sedated, and may require less medication. As with all medications, doses used in elderly patients are typically much less than the dose for a typical adult. It is often best to avoid the use of benzodiazepines in elderly patients because of the potential for falls, respiratory compromise if the patient is medically ill, and paradoxical reactions such as disinhibition particularly in patients with underlying dementia. If a patient has been agitated and required medication shortly after arrival at the emergency room, it is of vital importance that the physician try to garner as much information from the patient as possible, because he or she may soon be too sedated to answer questions, sometimes for a number of hours. If nothing else, information about medical history, substances used, allergies, current medications, any recent trauma, and family to contact in case of an emergency are all important to obtain.

All antipsychotic medications have the potential to cause side effects. The patient in the emergency setting is at particular risk for two reasons: patients may at times need to be medicated without sufficient knowledge of medical comorbidities or previous reactions to medications, and patients treated in the emergency department and subsequently discharged are often lost to follow-up. Patients treated with typical antipsychotics in the emergency room should be observed for signs of acute dystonia, such as muscle spasm or stiffness. Acute dystonia is treated with intramuscular injection of anticholinergic drugs, such as diphenhydramine or benztropine. Patients treated in the emergency department with an atypical antipsychotic, such as olanzapine, should have a fingerstick performed to assess blood sugar levels. Other potential side effects are akathisia (i.e., the subjective sense of being unable to sit still or stop moving) and tardive dyskinesia (i.e., abnormal choreiform movements than can often be observed in patients with a history of treatment with typical antipsychotics; these are unlikely to be caused or significantly worsened by a single antipsychotic dose in the setting of agitation.)

Case Example *(continued)*

Mr. S arrived on a stretcher to the psychiatric emergency room. A cursory examination of his property revealed a veteran's identification card. He was agitated and paranoid during the interview, refusing to answer the majority of questions. He reported that he was in a car with President Bush just 2 weeks ago but said that it would be too dangerous to say why. He asked the medical students present during the interview, "Which one of you jokers grabbed me this morning?" When asked what war he is a veteran of, Mr. S replied, "I'm at war now!" He was malodorous, disheveled, and continually scratching his skin. Mental status examination revealed that he was disoriented to place and time. Because of his agitation, he received prn medications.

Evaluation of the Psychotic Patient

Following the initial triage and assessment of the psychotic patient, the patient should be searched and placed in a safe environment. The full psychiatric evaluation can then begin. During the interview, the same basic safety precautions that apply to all psychiatric patients should be closely followed.

Foreign-Language or Hearing-Impaired Psychotic Patients

As with any psychiatric interview, a thorough examination must be conducted in a language the patient can understand. Patients for whom English is not their preferred language should be offered the opportunity to conduct the interview with a translator or using a translator phone, even if they appear to speak English adequately (Sabin 1975). Conducting an interview with a psychotic patient via translator can be a very challenging process. Live translators, if available, are always preferable to translation by phone. Translators should be informed at the outset that they are being called on to help in a psychiatric evaluation. Translators inexperienced in interviewing psychotic patients should be encouraged prior to the interview to translate *verbatim*, and to resist the temptation to interpret the patient's statements or to try to synthesize them into a cohesive form; disorganized speech is an important psychotic symptom that may go overlooked under such circumstances (Marcos 1979). Often, translators assisting with evaluation of a psychotic patient will report that they are having some trouble with the translation or that something about the patient's speech or vocabulary is difficult to understand. This may be an important clue that the patient is communicating in an unusual way; the clinician should ask the translator to be as specific as possible about what the patient is saying. As is true in any psychiatric evaluation, the clinician intent on making a determination of psychosis should not neglect to assess affective symptoms (Sabin 1975).

Patients who are deaf or hard of hearing should be asked what their preferred means of communication is and should be accommodated. There is a difference, not only in mode of communication but in culture, history, presentation, and sense of identity, between the patient who is deaf, particularly one who has been deaf since childhood, and the patient who is hard of hearing. When using a sign language interpreter, the clinician should always look and speak directly to the patient, not to the interpreter. American Sign Language uses a different syntax and grammar than spoken English, which makes the evaluation of psychosis in the deaf patient a particular challenge, because a literal translation of a deaf person's statements can sound concrete to a hearing person, when in fact the statement is perfectly normal. Unlike a foreign language translator, a proficient and experienced sign language interpreter must interpret some of the patient's statements for the clinician, and likewise must interpret for the patient the many words that do not exist in American Sign Language into their nearest comprehensible meaning. Writing, although on occasion unavoidable in an emergency, is not an appropriate substitute for signing with a deaf person (Iezzoni et al. 2004). In either foreign language or sign language interpretation, it is not appropriate to use a patient's family member or friend as interpreter; such interpretation is apt to be less accurate than that provided by an uninterested third party and is a violation of patient privacy.

The Interview

The evaluation of the psychotic patient should include, as much as the patient will tolerate, a complete history and mental status examination. Within the mental status examination, more time should be spent eliciting psychotic symptoms from the patient. Wording of questions to obtain the necessary information in a nonthreatening manner that is validating to the patient is critical to establishing the therapeutic alliance. Important areas of focus in the mental status examination of the psychotic patient include abstraction, characterization of thought process and content, and characterizing internal preoccupation.

Patients should be asked about hallucinations in the least stigmatizing manner possible, especially patients experiencing a first psychotic episode. When hallucinations are present, it is important to ask whether the patient hears one or more than one voice, whether voices talk to the patient or about the patient, and what the content of the hallucinations is. Patients should be questioned about command auditory hallucinations. If a patient reports command auditory hallucinations, it is of critical importance to obtain a detailed history of the nature of the commands and assess whether the patient has ever acted on commands from auditory hallucinations.

Questions about delusions should cover the range of common delusional types: persecutory, somatic, religious, and grandiose. When inquiring about delusional thoughts, the interviewer should tread carefully, because any fragile rapport he or she has managed to build with a paranoid or frankly delusional patient may be negated if the clinician appears to doubt or challenge a patient's firmly held belief; on the other hand, it is never acceptable practice to collude with a patient's delusions. In the case of somatic delusions, a patient presenting with a somatic complaint must receive a thorough and appropriate medical workup, even if the patient has a primary psychotic disorder, and particularly if there is no documentation of such a workup having been done in the past.

Collateral Sources of Information

The importance of collateral information from other sources, such as friends, family, providers, and outside observers, in the evaluation of the psychotic patient in the emergency setting cannot be overestimated. Patients presenting with psychotic symptoms may be paranoid and refuse to give correct or complete information, or may be too disorganized to give such information. Health Insurance Portability and Accountability Act (HIPAA; U.S. Department of Health and Human Services 2003) regulations allow a clinician to contact outside sources of information in the case of an emergency, so that the patient who lacks capacity to give consent can receive emergency care. Other potential sources of (or clues to) collateral information include the patient's own property and medical records. If the patient will permit a search, his or her cellular phone, wallet, and other items might provide important information that the patient may not be able to recall.

Case Example *(continued)*

Collateral information obtained from a nearby Veterans Hospital revealed that Mr. S was human immunodeficiency virus (HIV) positive, his last CD4 lymphocyte count was 232, and he had been treated with atovaquone and the combination drug Atripla. When asked about this, Mr. S reported noncompliance with his medications. The hospital's records also indicated a history of a parotid mass that had not yet been fully worked up. Although their notes indicated that Mr. S had a history of alcohol dependence, there was no record of any previous psychiatric treatment. Vital signs on arrival to the hospital were within normal limits, and Mr. S was not noted to have any alcohol on his breath.

Differential Diagnosis

After completing the psychiatric evaluation, the clinician must form a differential diagnosis. For all patients presenting to the psychiatric emergency department, it is generally helpful to think about differential diagnosis in terms of several broad categories into which symptoms might fit: 1) medical conditions, 2) substance-induced conditions, 3) psychotic disorders, 4) mood disorders, 5) anxiety disorders, and 6) other miscellaneous conditions.

Medical Conditions

Although medical issues are often the least frequent cause of symptoms in patients who have already been triaged to psychiatry, patients should be examined for medical conditions first both because a medical issue presents a potentially quickly reversible cause of symptoms and because missing a medical condition can cause dire consequences. This situation is clearly illustrated by the clinical case of Mr. S. The clinician should not rush to conclude that a patient who appears psychotic has a primary psychiatric condition.

Table 6–1 presents a list, albeit not exhaustive, of medical conditions that can present with psychotic symptoms, along with the symptoms that they can commonly cause and accompanying signs. Often these symptoms include delirium, a syndrome characterized by waxing and waning mental status that can also be accompanied by psychotic symptoms, including disorganization, hallucinations (particularly visual hallucinations), and false beliefs that are usually not fixed.

Given all the possible medical causes of psychotic symptoms, it is difficult to determine the appropriate medical workup for the psychotic patient (particularly given that most of these conditions are rare and tests will likely be low yield). Regardless of psychiatric history, every patient who presents with psychotic symptoms should at minimum have a complete blood count, a comprehensive metabolic profile, thyroid-stimulating hormone test, and syphilis screening. Given its prevalence and the added benefit as a public health measure, HIV testing should also be encouraged. A more extensive workup should be considered for patients with new-onset psychotic symptoms: imaging, preferably magnetic resonance imaging, should strongly be considered to rule out tumors and other intracranial lesions as the cause of psychotic symptoms, and electroencephalography should be considered to rule out seizures (particularly temporal lobe epilepsy). Further tests should be ordered if history or the results of initial testing are suspicious for a rare medical cause. For instance, a psychotic patient who is found to have elevated liver function tests might warrant further workup for Wilson's disease, including an ophthalmological exam looking for Kayser-Fleischer rings and serum ceruloplasmin. Similarly, a patient with a history of brief psychotic episodes associated with neuropathy and abdominal pain should have urine sent during an episode (checking for uroporphyrin, porphobilinogen, and aminolevulinic acid) to rule out acute intermittent porphyria. Treatment for psychosis secondary to a general medical condition should be directed toward addressing the underlying medical condition and is usually best accomplished on a medical unit with psychiatric consultation.

Substance-Induced Conditions

A variety of substances can cause psychotic symptoms, during either the intoxication phase or the withdrawal phase. Table 6–2 lists some of the substances commonly encountered in the emergency setting and their accompanying symptoms. Substance use can also predispose patients to falls and other accidents with consequent head trauma, which can then present with psychiatric symptoms. It is important not to fall into the trap of incorrectly attributing these symptoms to the substance use, because missing a head injury can lead to dire consequences for the patient. Patients with substance abuse who present with new-onset psychotic symptoms should be examined for evidence of head trauma and, if present, head imaging should be obtained.

All patients presenting with psychotic symptoms in the emergency department should be screened for substance use with urine or serum toxicology. Treatment for substance-induced psychosis usually involves maintaining the patient's safety in a psychiatric setting with supportive interventions until the symptoms resolve. An exception to this is delirium tremens, which requires aggressive medical management (often in an intensive care unit) to prevent seizures, aspiration, and death. Despite the fact that patients with substance-induced psychoses often do not have an underlying psychotic illness, they can benefit from antipsychotics and benzodiazepines on an as-needed basis during the episode to address their symptoms, particularly if agitation is prominent.

Psychotic Disorders

Perhaps the most obvious diagnoses to consider when a patient presents with psychotic symptoms in the psychiatric emergency setting are the primary psychotic disorders. These include schizophrenia, schizoaffective disorder, schizophreniform disorder, and brief psychotic episode. These diagnoses are distinguished from one another by history obtained from the patient and collateral information about time course, presence or absence of mood symptoms, and presence or absence of stressors. The following is a brief review of the criteria for each diagnosis (APA 2000):

- *Schizophrenia.* At least 6 months of symptoms, and at least 1 month of meeting two of the following symptoms: delusions, hallucinations, disor-

Table 6–1. Medical conditions that can present with psychosis

Condition	Signs and symptoms
Electrolyte imbalances *Causes:* primary medical conditions (e.g., renal failure) or related to psychiatric conditions (e.g., eating disorders, psychogenic polydipsia)	Delirium; physical stigmata of underlying cause of electrolyte imbalance (e.g., enlarged parotid glands, dental disease in bulimia)
Hepatic encephalopathy *Causes:* acute or chronic liver failure	Delirium; asterixis; jaundice
Brain tumors	Hallucinations and/or delusions accompanied by headache; disorganization not usually present if tumor is focal
Infections (both systemic and CNS)	Delirium; elevated temperature; elevated WBC; focal signs of infection (e.g., nuchal rigidity)
HIV	Mania; dementia (featuring prominent psychomotor retardation); opportunistic infections can cause delirium or focal symptoms
Wilson's disease	Bizarre behavior; psychosis; motor symptoms; liver and kidney function abnormalities
Huntington's disease	Personality changes; depression; psychosis; choreiform movements; family history usually present
Acute intermittent porphyria	Psychosis; abdominal pain; neuropathy; autonomic dysfunction
Tertiary syphilis	Psychosis; dementia; ataxia; Argyll Robertson pupils
Hyperthyroidism or hypothyroidism	Mood and psychotic symptoms; physical symptoms of each syndrome (e.g., heat or cold intolerance, hair loss, weight loss/gain)
Seizures	Interictal or postictal psychosis; hyperreligiosity; "viscous" or "sticky" style of interaction; auditory hallucinations in temporal lobe epilepsy
Dementia	Visual hallucinations (particularly in Lewy body dementia); paranoid ideation (most typically that people are stealing from them)

Table 6–1. Medical conditions that can present with psychosis *(continued)*

Condition	Signs and symptoms
Medications *Examples:* steroids, interferon, levetiracetam (Keppra), dopamine agonists	Psychosis is usually temporally related to when the patient began taking the medication; would be classified as substance-induced psychosis by DSM-IV-TR

Note. CNS = central nervous system; DSM-IV-TR = *Diagnostic and Statistical Manual of Mental Disorders*, 4th Edition, Text Revision (American Psychiatric Association 2000); WBC = white blood count.

ganized speech, grossly disorganized or catatonic behavior, or negative symptoms.

- *Schizoaffective disorder.* At least 6 months of symptoms, including both mood and psychotic symptoms, with psychotic symptoms present for at least 2 weeks in the absence of mood symptoms at some point during the illness.

- *Schizophreniform disorder.* At least 1 month but less than 6 months of psychotic symptoms.

- *Brief psychotic episode.* Psychotic symptoms appear and resolve fully in less than 1 month; symptoms are often caused by (and it is prognostically better if there is) the presence of an acute stressor.

Treatment for primary psychotic disorders usually involves the use of antipsychotic agents combined with supportive psychotherapy.

Mood Disorders

Both manic and major depressive episodes can present with psychotic features. Given that mood disorders are much more common than primary psychotic disorders, and that the treatment and prognosis are different for patients with mood disorders with psychotic features than for patients with primary psychotic disorders, all patients presenting with psychotic symptoms should be evaluated closely, both during the interview and in the gathering of collateral information, for the presence of mood symptoms. Psychotic symptoms that are present during mood episodes are usually mood congruent (e.g., the manic patient may have grandiose delusions, whereas the depressed patient

Table 6–2.   Substances that can cause psychosis

Substance	Signs and symptoms
Alcohol	*Intoxication:* agitation may appear psychotic *Withdrawal:* hallucinations with alcoholic hallucinosis; hallucinations and delirium with delirium tremens
Amphetamines	*Intoxication:* psychosis similar to that seen with cocaine but often prolonged (3–5 days), dilated pupils; often accompanied by stigmata of chronic amphetamine use (e.g., anorexia, poor dentition)
Cannabis	*Intoxication:* paranoid ideation; if severe, drug may have been laced with other substances (e.g., PCP)
Cocaine	*Intoxication:* disorganization, manic symptoms, delusions, hallucinations (including tactile), dilated pupils; lasts for hours after use *Withdrawal:* depressed mood, hallucinations, somnolence and social withdrawal; beginning hours after use and lasting 24–72 hours
Hallucinogens (LSD, psilocybin mushrooms)	*Intoxication:* vivid visual hallucinations, dissociative symptoms; occasions of recurrence of symptoms of intoxication ("flashbacks") can occur months or years after use
PCP	*Intoxication:* hallucinations, delusions, unpredictable violence; symptoms wax and wane and can last 3–5 days; associated with hyperacusis and nystagmus

Note.   LSD = lysergic acid diethylamide; PCP = phencyclidine.

may have negativistic delusions, such as that his or her organs are rotting). Treatment for mood disorders with psychotic features involves pharmacological treatment, both for the mood symptoms and for the psychotic symptoms, as well as psychotherapy.

Anxiety Disorders

Severe presentations of some anxiety disorders may appear to be psychosis, and this possibility should be considered in patients presenting to the emergency department. Some patients with obsessive-compulsive disorder can hold their obsessive thoughts so rigidly or engage in such bizarre rituals as to appear psychotic. Patients who are in the midst of reexperiencing episodes of posttraumatic stress disorder (particularly when intoxication is also involved) can also appear psychotic. This phenomenon highlights the importance of obtaining a full psychiatric review of symptoms during the interview, because the treatment for these disorders will be very different than for primary psychotic disorders.

Miscellaneous Conditions

Several other conditions should be considered in the differential diagnosis for patients presenting to the emergency department with psychotic symptoms. Patients with borderline personality disorder, as well as other cluster B personality disorders, can develop micropsychotic episodes, particularly in the context of acute stressors. Patients with dissociative disorder can appear disorganized and psychotic.

Although it should always be a diagnosis of exclusion, malingered psychosis is unfortunately not at all uncommon in the psychiatric emergency setting. In general, malingering should be considered in patients who have clear motives for doing so (as in patients under arrest) and exhibit inconsistencies in their history and mental status examination, or are very vague in their descriptions of their symptoms. Patients who report dangerous symptoms that are inconsistent with their affect, behavior, and thought process are suspect (e.g., a patient who appears cheerful in the waiting area but subsequently reports to the doctor, "I'm hearing voices telling me to kill myself and others"). The more detail the psychiatrist presses for during the interview, the more difficult it will become for a malingering patient to keep his or her story straight (Resnick 1999). When available, medical records from within the same institution should be examined; a patient with a history of malingering or with a pattern of brief inpatient admissions from which the patient frequently signs out against medical advice, would be added evidence against a patient suspected of malingering.

Risk Assessment: Important Risk Factors in the Psychotic Patient

The risk assessments of patients who are judged, after careful consideration of the differential diagnoses, to most likely have a disorder other than a primary psychotic disorder are addressed in the chapters appropriate to their underlying diagnoses. In this section, we focus on the evidence-based risk assessment of patients who are thought to have a primary psychotic disorder, although many of the risk factors for this population can be extrapolated to other populations who experience psychotic symptoms in the context of other disorders. This is certainly not an exhaustive listing of all of the risk factors for suicide and violence; this discussion is meant to highlight those factors that are most relevant to the emergency psychiatric assessment.

Risk Factors for Violence

The public perception that patients with psychosis are at elevated risk of violence has sparked a debate in the psychiatric literature that is still far from being resolved, despite the existence of several large-scale studies on the topic (Torrey et al. 2008). Although the jury is still out on this larger question, it is clear from the literature that several factors can predict violence in this population. As might be expected, *past history of violence and criminal behavior* is one of the strongest predictors of future violence and, if present, should be weighted heavily in the risk assessment of any patient. The risk assessment cannot, however, rely exclusively on past behavior as a predictor of future violent behavior, because doing so ends up being both overinclusive and underinclusive. On the one hand, if past behavior were the only factor considered, the risk assessment would fail to identify patients with no such history who go on to become first-time perpetrators of violence (Buchanan 2008). On the other hand, a history of violence is always present in patients who have engaged in that behavior, and so a focus on history fails to consider the patient's acute risks and current symptoms.

Comorbid substance abuse may be one of the largest contributors to violence among patients with a primary psychotic illness (Monahan et al. 2001). However, some authors have found that it is not the substance abuse itself but other factors associated with substance abuse (e.g., childhood conduct disorder and current psychotic symptoms) that are most predictive of violence (Swanson et al. 2006). *Intoxication* certainly raises the risk of violence due to its disinhibiting effects, but it is an easily modifiable risk factor in that the patient's risk can be significantly reduced just by retaining the patient until he or she is no longer intoxicated. *Akathisia* can similarly increase risk of violent acting-out due to the physical discomfort that it causes, and it can be easily modified by changing the psychopharmacological regimen to address this symptom.

Positive psychotic symptoms, including hallucinations and delusions (particularly hallucinations of a command nature and delusions of a persecutory nature), are associated with higher rates of violence, whereas negative symptoms may actually lower the risk of serious violence (Swanson et al. 2006). Command auditory hallucinations to harm others are particularly concerning if the patient has any history of acting on command auditory hallucinations in the past. Given the important role of antipsychotics in preventing positive symptoms, *noncompliance with antipsychotics* increases the risk of violence.

Recent violent threats and behavior leading up to presentation in the psychiatric emergency setting must be given significant weight in the risk assessment, particularly if the patient has a past history of violence or arrest. *Homicidal ideation*, even if it has been communicated as violent fantasies shared only with the assessing clinician, rather than as threats toward a target, will also increase the acute risk of violence. Even when violent ideation or behavior is absent from the current presentation, the risk of repeated violence if the patient has a history of violent behavior when experiencing similar symptoms can be serious enough to justify the classification of the patient as at elevated acute risk.

Risk Factors for Suicide

As with violence, past history is strongly predictive of future behavior when assessing suicide risk, and a history of *past suicide attempts* will chronically elevate a patient's risk for future suicide attempts. Unlike with violence, patients with schizophrenia and other psychotic illnesses are at elevated lifetime risk for completed suicide, with estimates ranging between 5% and 15%. The risk is generally thought to be highest early in the course of the illness, highlighting the importance of engaging psychotic patients early in the course of their symptoms (Melle et al. 2006). *Comorbidities with depressive symptoms and with substance abuse* are thought to increase the risk of suicide attempts among psychotic patients, as is the presence of *command auditory hallucinations to harm oneself* (particularly when the patient has a history of acting on command auditory hallucinations). *Current suicidal ideation*, particularly if there is evidence of planning, should be weighed seriously in the risk assessment. However, the presence of contingency to this suicidal ideation (e.g., "If you don't admit me, I will kill myself") is less predictive than noncontingent suicidal ideation (Lambert 2002). *Social isolation* likely also contributes to suicide risk, whereas the presence of good social and treatment supports may serve as a protective factor. *Akathisia* may also worsen suicide risk and should be given particular attention because this is a modifiable risk factor. As with all psychiatric patients, *access to weapons* will elevate concern about suicide risk.

Other Risk Factors for Harm to Self

A risk assessment also must include a consideration of the potential danger to a patient from inability to care for self. Much of this assessment can be ascertained from the first contact with the patient: if the patient is disheveled, suffering from parasite infestation, or suffering from visible consequences of untreated medical illness that on evaluation appear to be related to the patient's psychotic symptoms, then the patient clearly is unable to care for himself or herself. For example, diabetes-related leg ulcers may turn out to have been caused by the patient not taking prescribed insulin, under the delusion that he or she is cured of diabetes.

If the individual's inability to care for self is not obvious, the clinician must ask questions—often subtle questions—to assess a patient's ability to care for self. For instance, a patient who is afraid to stay in her apartment due to persecutory delusions might choose instead to stay in a shelter. Does this indicate the patient's inability to care for self? The answer to that question hinges on several subsidiary questions about whether the behavior (staying in the shelter) results in adverse consequences for the patient that can lead to potential worsening of her physical or mental health. Appropriate questions might include the following: Does she have access to her psychiatric medications in the shelter? Is she still able to attend her outpatient treatment? Does she still have access to her family and social supports? Has similar behavior led to harm in the past? The availability of support services may alter decisions about whether such a patient needs inpatient psychiatric hospitalization or can be maintained in the community with greater oversight.

Making a Decision About Appropriate Treatment

Having made a thorough risk assessment, the clinician will usually have a good impression of what he or she believes is the appropriate setting for treatment. If the psychotic patient is motivated to follow the clinician's recommendations, the decision about what to do at this point is easier. If the clinician believes that the patient would benefit from inpatient stabilization (either because of the degree of risk or because inpatient treatment would facilitate a more rapid workup and treatment of the patient's symptoms), then the patient can be admitted on a voluntary basis. Alternatively, if the clinician feels that the patient can be safely discharged with a higher level of outpatient care, he or she can feel reassured that the patient is likely to comply with such interventions. The degree of community services that can be accessed from the emergency setting varies in different locations, and will be discussed further in Chapter 13, "Disposition and Resource Options."

If a psychotic patient is not motivated for treatment, or if the patient actively opposes treatment, then the choice of an appropriate treatment setting is far more difficult. A lack of motivation for treatment is often associated with a greater severity of symptoms, increased clinical impression of dangerousness to others, high suspiciousness, and grandiosity (Mulder et al. 2005). Often, such situations require involuntary hospitalization. The clinician faces difficulties when the patient does not meet the legal standards for involuntary commitment but is unlikely to follow up with outpatient treatment. In such cases, the clinician can try to build a therapeutic alliance and to increase the patient's motivation (possibly by using techniques such as motivational interviewing) in the emergency setting. The clinician can also attempt to mobilize the patient's social supports (including family, friends, and treatment providers such as case managers) to encourage the patient's compliance with outpatient follow-up and to monitor closely for any worsening of symptoms that might warrant the patient's return to the emergency room.

Once a decision has been made to hospitalize a patient on either a voluntary or an involuntary basis, the clinician in the emergency department is also charged with initiating a plan for treatment until the patient is reassessed by the inpatient team. At that point, the medical workup should have already been initiated, and the clinician should communicate to the inpatient team what tests or medical issues need to be further pursued. The emergency clinician is also responsible for sending the patient to the inpatient unit on the appropriate levels of observation and for communicating to the inpatient team the patient's level of risk for violence or suicidality. The emergency clinician should also alert the inpatient team to any other management issues that he or she believes the patient may pose (e.g., if the patient is at risk for sexual acting-out based on history or clinical presentation).

A task that often falls to the emergency clinician is to initiate or make changes in the patient's pharmacological regimen. Pharmacological modifications are often required to reduce the patient's level of risk on the inpatient unit, for instance, if he or she has already demonstrated agitation in the emergency setting. However, in this era of managed care and brief hospitalizations, it is often necessary, even if agitation has not been present, to make medication changes immediately—rather than waiting for the inpatient team to make a decision the next day—to facilitate the rapid management of symptoms. What follows is a brief list of factors that should be considered in the choice of neuroleptic agents for the psychotic patient:

- *Side effects.* Atypical (second-generation) antipsychotics pose a greater risk of metabolic syndrome, whereas typical (first-generation) antipsychotics pose an increased risk of extrapyramidal symptoms, tardive dyskinesia, and neuroleptic malignant syndrome. Each patient's situation should be considered individually based on the tolerability of these side effects and any personal or family history (e.g., diabetes) that might put the patient at greater risk of these side effects.
- *Personal history* (or family history) of response to a particular agent.
- *Potential for noncompliance.* The patient considered at high risk for "cheeking" while in the hospital may require an antipsychotic available in liquid or dissolving tablet form. The patient who may require a court order for medications over objection may benefit from an antipsychotic that is also available in a short-acting injectable form. The patient who is at chronic

risk for noncompliance in the outpatient setting, even after being stabilized in the inpatient setting, might be best served by being started on the oral form of an antipsychotic that is also available as a long-acting injectable preparation, onto which the patient may later be titrated.

- *Cost and access issues.* It is important to ensure that after discharge, the patient will still be able to obtain the medication started; otherwise, the patient is more likely to become noncompliant in the future. If uninsured, the patient should be started on a medication that he or she will be able to afford when discharged, or the clinician should initiate efforts to get the patient insured. If the patient is insured but the insurance plan restricts the formulary of available agents, he or she should be started on a formulary agent if possible, or a request to the insurance company for the nonformulary agent needs to be made.

- *Frequency of dosing.* Patients tend to have greater rates of compliance with medications that have once-daily dosing as opposed to more frequent dosing.

Case Example *(continued)*

Suspicion for a medical or substance-induced cause for Mr. S's psychosis was high given the absence of a history of psychosis, the presence of a history of alcohol dependence and multiple medical problems that could present with brain involvement, and the presence of disorientation on mental status examination. Nevertheless, the decision was made that Mr. S could be treated on the psychiatric service (rather than a medical service) because his vital signs were normal and he did not otherwise appear medically unstable, and because he would benefit from being treated in a secure, locked area given his agitation. A medical workup, including blood work, urine toxicology, chest X ray, and head computed tomography (CT), was initiated promptly. Preliminary read of a head CT without contrast revealed a large acute right parietal subdural hematoma, extending from the vertex to the level of the body of the lateral ventricles. A second extra-axial collection along the right frontoparietal convexity, with a more heterogeneous appearance, suggested acute on chronic subdural hematomas. There also appeared a 1.3 cm leftward midline shift and right uncal herniation. The etiology of these injuries was presumably multiple prior falls while intoxicated.

At this time, Mr. S was transferred to the medical emergency department, and neurosurgery was called. By this point, he had become more obtunded, either from the prn medications or from the uncal herniation. Mannitol was administered, but the patient continued to deteriorate, so the decision was made to take him to surgery. Patient went to surgery, where his subdural hematoma was successfully evacuated and a drain was left in place. Follow-up after he was transferred to a rehabilitation unit revealed that Mr. S was organized and able to give a coherent history, with no residual psychotic symptoms. Although he had some residual left-sided weakness, he was able to walk and move independently.

Role of the Emergency Psychiatrist as Psychoeducator

The emergency psychiatrist plays a vital role in providing psychoeducation to patients and their families. Often, the emergency clinician is the first mental health contact for patients who have first-break psychosis and who may have no knowledge about their diagnosis or the way that the mental health system works. Frequently, patients with psychosis present to the psychiatric emergency room in a paranoid state, and the clinician's failure to disclose information about why the decision to admit or discharge has been made or why certain treatments have been ordered only serves to enhance this paranoia, leaving the patient needing to guess at why the clinician is doing what he or she is doing, and often ultimately ascribing a malevolent motive to the clinician. The same can often be true for families, who see that their loved one is ill but, knowing the person in a healthy state, consider him or her as more capable of caring for himself or herself than the patient actually is. The family then perceives coercive measures, such as prn medications and involuntary admission, as victimizing rather than as caring for their loved one. Psychoeducation serves to reverse these misconceptions and helps to build an alliance in which the patient and family are active participants in the treatment plan. This alliance is well worth the time necessary to provide psychoeducation even in the busiest of emergency settings.

Key Clinical Points

- Psychosis is characterized by delusions, hallucinations, and disorganization of speech and behavior.

- Although primary psychotic disorders such as schizophrenia are the most obvious cause, patients presenting with psychosis need to be carefully evaluated for the presence of medical conditions, substance use, and other psychiatric conditions that could be causing their symptoms.

- Care must be taken in evaluating the psychotic patient to maintain safety while obtaining a history from the patient and collateral sources.

- Examining the history for risk factors for violence and self-harm will inform the clinician's decision regarding the need for hospitalization and further treatment.

- Antipsychotic medications play a key role both in controlling agitation and addressing psychotic symptoms, but nonpharmacological interventions such as psychoeducation also are vital in the treatment of psychotic patients in the emergency setting.

References

Allen MH (ed): Emergency Psychiatry (Review of Psychiatry Series; Oldham JM and Riba MB, series eds). Washington, DC, American Psychiatric Publishing, 2002

American Psychiatric Association: Diagnostic and Statistical Manual of Mental Disorders, 4th Edition, Text Revision. Washington, DC, American Psychiatric Association, 2000

Buchanan A: Risk of violence by psychiatric patients: beyond the "actuarial versus clinical" assessment debate. Psychiatr Serv 59:184–190, 2008

Currier GW, Chou JC, Feifel D, et al: Acute treatment of psychotic agitation: a randomized comparison of oral treatment with risperidone and lorazepam versus intramuscular treatment with haloperidol and lorazepam. J Clin Psychiatry 65:386–394, 2004

Dhossche DM, Ghani SO: Who brings patients to the psychiatric emergency room? Psychosocial and psychiatric correlates. Gen Hosp Psychiatry 20:235–240, 1998

Duwe BV, Turetsky BI: Misdiagnosis of schizophrenia in a patient with psychotic symptoms. NeuropsychiatryNeuropsychol Behav Neurol 15:252–260, 2002

Hillard JR: Emergency treatment of acute psychosis. J Clin Psychiatry 59 (suppl 1):57–60, 1998

Iezzoni LI, O'Day BL, Killeen M, et al: Communicating about health care: observations from persons who are deaf or hard of hearing. Ann Intern Med 140:356–362, 2004

Kishi YK, Kato M, Okuyama T, et al: Delirium: patient characteristics that predict a missed diagnosis at psychiatric consultation. Gen Hosp Psychiatry 29:442–445, 2007

Lambert M: Seven-year outcomes of patients evaluated for suicidality. Psychiatr Serv 53:92–94, 2002

Marco CA, Vaughan J: Emergency management of agitation in schizophrenia. Am J Emerg Med 23:767–776, 2005

Marcos LR: Effects of interpreters on the evaluation of psychopathology in non-English-speaking patients. Am J Psychiatry 136:171–174, 1979

Melle I, Johannesen JO, Friis S, et al: Early detection of the first episode of schizophrenia and suicidal behavior. Am J Psychiatry 163:800–804, 2006

Monahan J, Steadman HJ, Silver E, et al: Rethinking Risk Assessment: The MacArthur Study of Mental Disorders and Violence. New York, Oxford University Press, 2001

Mulder CL, Koopmans GT, Hengeveld MW: Lack of motivation for treatment in emergency psychiatry patients. Soc Psychiatry Psychiatr Epidemiol 40:484–488, 2005

Newcomer JW: Medical risk in patients with bipolar disorder and schizophrenia. J Clin Psychiatry 67 (suppl 9):25–30, 2006

Resnick PJ: The detection of malingered psychosis. Psychiatr Clin North Am 22:159–172, 1999

Sabin JE: Translating despair. Am J Psychiatry 132:197–199, 1975

Swanson JW, Swartz MS, Van Dorn RA, et al: A national study of violent behavior in persons with schizophrenia. Arch Gen Psychiatry 63:490–499, 2006

Torrey EF, Stanley J, Monahan J, et al: The MacArthur Violence Risk Assessment Study revisited: two views ten years after its initial publication. Psychiatr Serv 59:147–152, 2008

U.S. Department of Health and Human Services: Summary of the HIPAA privacy rule, May 2003. Available at: http://www.hhs.gov/ocr/privacy/hipaa/understanding/summary/privacysummary.pdf. Accessed November 24, 2009.

Suggested Readings

Allen MH (ed): Emergency Psychiatry (Review of Psychiatry Series; Oldham JM and Riba MB, series eds). Washington, DC, American Psychiatric Publishing, 2002

Monahan J, Steadman HJ, Silver E, et al: Rethinking Risk Assessment: The MacArthur Study of Mental Disorders and Violence. New York, Oxford University Press, 2001

Resnick PJ: The detection of malingered psychosis. Psychiatr Clin North Am 22:159–172, 1999

The Anxious Patient

Divy Ravindranath, M.D., M.S.

James Abelson, M.D., Ph.D.

Case Example

Ms. D, a 35-year-old female graduate student with no prior psychiatric history, was referred to psychiatric emergency services from the medical emergency department for further evaluation after a negative workup for chest pain. The referring doctor's diagnosis was "anxiety." Ms. D characterizes herself as having been an anxious person for the majority of her life. She states that her mind often jumps from worry to worry, leaving her distracted and keeping her up at night. Her tension tends to embody itself in her muscles. She frequently experiences abdominal distress and heartburn but has never been diagnosed with an ulcer. She also says that she cannot think about going

The authors would like to acknowledge the thoughtful comments of Dr. Brian Martis in the preparation of this chapter.

out with friends without developing a panic attack. At the suggestion of going out, she develops a sense of dread, hyperventilates, and feels as if her heart is racing. She gets preoccupied with these physical symptoms, and her panic worsens. She calms herself by slow breathing and counting, and uses alcohol if she goes out, but usually chooses to stay home. She had a fight with her fiancé a few days ago over "something insignificant." She subsequently tried to call him, but he responded only with a one-word text message: "Later." She began to worry about the stability of the relationship, the years she had invested in it, and her future in general. She found the distress intolerable, decided she was better off without him, and went to his house to break off the engagement. He was speechless. She departed abruptly, worrying about what she had done. Since that time, the panic attacks have occurred more frequently and without clear triggers. It has become harder to talk herself out of the panic. She spoke with her ex-fiancé and thinks they will be able to reconcile, but she thinks she needs something to help herself cope better. She doesn't want to become an alcoholic.

Ms. D is a clearly anxious woman with a classic emergency room presentation—featuring elements of multiple DSM-IV-TR (American Psychiatric Association 2000) anxiety disorder diagnoses and a broad anxious predisposition that likely has both biological and psychosocial roots. She demonstrates behavioral tendencies that amplify anxiety (e.g., focusing on physical symptoms) and some reasonable coping efforts to alleviate her anxiety (e.g., taking slow breaths). She also demonstrates one highly dysfunctional but common consequence of anxiety: a vulnerability to impulsive action.

Everyone experiences anxiety. Its complete absence is probably extremely rare, highly pathological, and perhaps incompatible with a long life. Anyone under acute threat should experience some elements of anxiety, both psychologically/emotionally and physically. Activation of the sympathetic nervous system is a normal aspect of the response to threat and is a normal component of physical preparations needed to respond to or cope with threat. However, anxiety also can occur in the absence of genuine threat or in gross excess relative to the magnitude of the threat. In some people, it seems to be present at all times. When it occurs inappropriately, excessively, or uncontrollably and produces impairment in critical life functions, as seen in the case of Ms. D, anxiety is considered pathological, and an anxiety disorder is likely present.

The first challenge in assessing patients who present to the emergency department is differentiating true medical emergencies, which require specific interventions to preserve life or minimize tissue damage, from acute situations that entail less immediate risks. The presence of extreme anxiety does not by itself mean that real risk is low, because serious medical threats, such as chest pain from an impending myocardial infarction, can generate very intense fear. Therefore, the first rule in managing anxiety in the emergency department is to not let it get in the way of careful assessment for medical emergencies requiring immediate intervention.

Once immediate medical risks are ruled out and a likely psychosocial or psychiatric problem is identified, safety is still not assured, so the next step is careful assessment of psychiatric risk. The primary concerns at this point are risk of suicide or self-harm behaviors and risk of violence against others. Patients with only anxiety disorders are rarely violent, but anxiety does increase the risk for suicide, and highly anxious patients may well have other disorders (e.g., paranoid psychosis, borderline personality disorder) in which risks for injurious behavior toward self or others is elevated. (For guidance in assessing these types of risks, see Chapter 2, "The Suicidal Patient," and Chapter 3, "Violence Risk Assessment.")

Anxiety disorders are very common; as many as one in four people may be affected by at least one of the six anxiety disorders. These disorders occur more frequently in women than men and are more common in people at lower socioeconomic levels. Panic disorder has a lifetime prevalence of 1.5%– 5% and is highly comorbid with other disorders. Ninety-one percent of patients with panic disorder have at least one other psychiatric diagnosis. A similar level of comorbidity is reported for generalized anxiety disorder, which has a reported lifetime prevalence of 5%. Up to 25% of the population may have a specific phobia. Lifetime prevalence of social anxiety disorder is variously estimated as between 3% and 13%. Lifetime prevalence of posttraumatic stress disorder (PTSD) is approximately 8%, although the prevalence is much higher in specific populations, such as combat veterans. The lifetime prevalence of obsessive-compulsive disorder is 2%–3% (Sadock and Sadock 2003).

Clearly, many people have anxiety disorders, and anxious people use health care systems much more frequently than other people, increasing their likelihood of presenting to emergency departments and adding to health care costs. Of 171 consecutive patients referred to an anxiety disorders specialty clinic, those with anxiety had visited nonpsychiatric medical providers six times, on average, in the prior year. Patients with panic disorder were the most frequent medical care users, followed by patients with phobias, generalized anxiety disorder, social anxiety disorder, and obsessive-compulsive disorder. The majority of these visits were to the emergency room, cardiology clinic, and primary care clinic (Deacon et al. 2008).

Given the high rates at which anxious patients present to emergency rooms, it is clearly important for emergency department staff to be well acquainted with their presentations and management. In this chapter, we present material related to the chief complaint of "anxiety" in the emergency department. Given that panic attacks are a primary manifestation of this chief complaint and represent a paradigm for understanding acute exacerbation in any anxiety disorder, we focus in the first two sections of this chapter on panic attacks and panic disorder. Trauma is the triggering event for many psychiatric disorders, and trauma patients often first present for medical care in the emergency department. Emergency department intervention could potentially reduce risks for psychiatric sequelae of trauma, so our focus in the third section is on psychiatric aspects of trauma care. In the final section, we discuss other anxiety and anxiety-related conditions.

Panic Attacks

Panic Attacks and Associated Conditions

Anxiety can be a chronic or subchronic condition, but it is also experienced acutely. Sudden onset of acute anxiety is most commonly experienced as fear. A sudden rise in fear may well be an appropriate response to a real threat, but it can also occur in the absence of threat in the form of a panic attack. Sudden-onset fear is often accompanied by activation of the sympathetic nervous system, which may lead to increased heart rate, dilated pupils, and other physiological changes that prepare the organism to respond to threat. It triggers a heightened vigilance to both external cues and internal (bodily) states as the organism scans for sources of risk that may require immediate responses. This vigilance is associated with heightened awareness of physical sensations. In a panic attack, especially when real environmental threats are not present, these physical sensations are interpreted as a source of threat themselves, causing attention to be focused on them and leading to escalating sensations that might include palpitations, shortness of breath, lightheadedness, derealization, paresthesias, and/or nausea. These sensations in turn further heighten vigilance and the sense of threat, and generate catastrophic cognitions (e.g., "I am having a heart attack"), thereby creating an escalating "fear-of-fear" cycle that culminates in a full-blown attack. The subjective sensation of altered bodily states usually far exceeds any real changes in physiological parameters.

Whereas a panic attack may reflect an abnormal activation of fear systems, having a panic attack does not necessarily mean that a person has panic disorder. Over one-third of the population will have a panic attack sometime in their life, but less than 5% will develop panic disorder (Sadock and Sadock 2003). All humans carry the capacity to panic in response to perceived threat. A single attack, whether in response to an identified cue or not, does not constitute a disorder. Some people even have recurrent attacks but manage them effectively and suffer no impairment, and therefore do not qualify for a diagnosis. However, if at least one attack has been spontaneous, fear of further attacks develops, and functioning is impaired, then panic disorder is likely present. Many patients with panic also develop agoraphobia, which involves fear and avoidance of places from which escape might be difficult, with particular fear of having a panic attack and being unable to flee. Not all panic attacks that lead to behavioral avoidance are due to panic disorder. When attacks never occur spontaneously but are consistently triggered by specific, feared cues, specific phobia may be a more appropriate diagnosis. Typical phobic cues can range from small animals (e.g., spiders, snakes, dogs) to particular situational cues (e.g., heights, closed places, airplanes, storms). If the triggers focus on social scrutiny and fear of public embarrassment, the diagnosis might be social anxiety disorder.

People with panic attacks that are always triggered by specific cues can often successfully manage the attacks through careful avoidance of their triggers, although the ability to do this depends on how readily avoidable the triggers are and the "costs" incurred by avoidance behavior. For example, avoiding spiders is much easier than avoiding social situations or all forms of public transportation. When attacks occur spontaneously, as they do in panic disorder, use of avoidance to cope is more challenging and less effective; because the triggers are not circumscribed, the avoidance can become pervasive and disabling. Patients can become housebound, only leaving home to seek medical care for their perceived symptoms.

These differences have bearing on treatment decisions. Panic and avoidance linked to specific, circumscribed triggers can be treated nonpharmacologically, with exposure and desensitization. This treatment is based on the simple principle that fear-based avoidance usually involves automatic, cued triggering of alarm signals at subcortical levels of the brain, and the best way to decouple the triggering cues from the automatic responses is through systematic, graded exposure to the cues in a controlled setting, which allows desensitization of the automatic alarm response system to those cues. Although patients with panic attacks may have avoidance behaviors for which this type of exposure therapy may be useful, patients with panic disorder are much more likely to also require pharmacological intervention. The differential thus becomes important even in the emergency department, because initiation of pharmacological treatment for well-diagnosed panic disorder might well be appropriate, but evaluation by an anxiety specialist might be important before medication is started for a phobia or social anxiety, for which exposure therapy might be the first-line treatment.

Management of a Panic Attack

Panic attacks are obviously frightening and uncomfortable. Patients with panic attacks will present to the emergency department with intense anxious distress, and the anxiety can be "contagious," especially when a threat eliciting this strong response cannot be located. When interacting with a panicking patient, a clinician needs to avoid being pulled into the whirlwind of anxiety. False assurance, such as insisting that nothing threatening is happening even before any data that can support that impression have been collected, is not likely to be helpful. However, the patient may be calmed by assurance that appropriate steps will be taken to identify and address any threats, and that the expressed distress will be taken seriously and reduced. This calm approach will be critical in building the rapport needed to fully evaluate the presenting symptom, to obtain the history and testing needed to ensure that the patient does not have a more emergent medical condition, and to build a foundation for productively addressing the acute anxiety.

In addition to maintaining a calm and confident demeanor, but without false or condescending reassurance, the clinician can take additional steps to help calm the patient. Panic attacks are sometimes associated with hyperventilation, which can trigger and intensify physical symptoms. Helping the patient to slow his or her breathing through attention and control can be helpful, emphasizing that the key is slow breathing, not deep breathing, with enough tidal volume for adequate oxygenation but not with huge breaths that will keep pCO_2 (partial pressure of carbon dioxide) low. Progressive muscle relaxation, with systematic tensing and then relaxing of the various muscle groups of the body, is useful for some patients. Reassurance, as data are obtained, that the patient does not appear to be in acute medical danger can also help. Initiation of education—informing the patient that this could be a panic attack; that panic attacks are overwhelming and frightening but not truly threatening; and that if a panic attack, it will likely pass reasonably quickly if the patient just lets it run its course—can both calm and lay groundwork for subsequent treatment efforts. This education provides foundation for the cognitive component of cognitive-behavioral therapy, which has proved effective for treating panic, and can begin in the emergency department. The behavioral component involves exposure and desensitization to cues that trigger fear, but the acute setting is not likely to be an appropriate context for initiation of this part of the work.

Another cognitive tool used in cognitive-behavioral therapy for panic might also be useful for some patients in the emergency department. This involves directly addressing the catastrophic interpretations that patients with panic often attach to their symptoms with an exploration of past evidence relevant to their interpretations. For example, a patient who interprets chest pain as evidence that he or she is having a heart attack can be asked to review cardiac risk factors with the doctor and can usually be helped to see that he or she has many factors that make a heart attack unlikely; the patient may be young, lack a family history of cardiac disease, have favorable metabolic profiles, have normal blood pressure, and so on. If the patient has had previous episodes like this one that did not prove to be a heart attack, this can be discussed. The provider can also share his or her own experience with other patients with identical symptoms who have come to the emergency room and were proved not to be having heart attacks.

If the patient is preoccupied with fearful beliefs that can be directly addressed with behavioral tests, this can have a strong, beneficial impact. For example, some patients may be convinced that if they stand up, their blood pressure will drop and they will faint. With appropriate support, they may be willing to test this belief, by trying to stand with an automatic blood pressure monitor in place, and seeing exactly what happens to their heart rate and blood pressure, with education provided so they understand the changes. Activating these kinds of cognitive processes can help reduce the emotional focus and intensity.

If the patient's attack cannot be managed with reassurance and the types of techniques described above, use of a benzodiazepine can be considered. A relatively short-acting agent, such as lorazepam in a dose of 0.5–1 mg, is usually sufficient in a benzodiazepine-naïve individual. Lorazepam can be used intramuscularly if the patient is unable to take an oral medication.

Use of medication is presented as a secondary technique because benzodiazepines, even fast-acting ones like alprazolam, take time to enter the bloodstream and exert their effect on the brain. Panic attacks often abate naturally before the medication takes effect, but patients will falsely attribute their recovery to the drug and can rapidly develop psychological reliance on access to it. Even when a benzodiazepine does provide relief, its use can suggest to the patient that the anxiety symptoms cannot be controlled or endured without external assistance, diminishing the patient's self-efficacy and undermining the kind of cognitive and psychological work that is important in optimizing long-term recovery.

Differential Diagnosis and Further Evaluation

As discussed in the previous section, panic attacks can be associated with a number of anxiety disorders. Panic attacks can also occur with nonanxiety psychiatric conditions and medical conditions. Table 7–1 presents a differential of psychiatric and nonpsychiatric conditions that may produce anxiety, panic attacks, or panic-like attacks.

Once the patient is sufficiently calm to participate in his or her care, then evaluation for the etiology of the panic attack should proceed. As with all psychiatric emergencies, the patient should be "cleared" of any medical conditions that may present with psychiatric symptoms forming the chief complaint. A complete discussion of the evaluation and management for these medical conditions is beyond the scope of this chapter.

For the associated psychiatric conditions, indications for hospitalization (e.g., acute suicidal or homicidal ideation) should be assessed. If there are no indications for hospitalization, then the patient should be discharged with re-assurance that the panic attack, though frightening, is not life threatening and with advice that outpatient psychiatric treatment could reduce the patient's chances for experiencing future panic attacks. (For details regarding outpatient follow-up, see Chapter 13, "Disposition and Resource Options.")

One psychiatric condition, panic disorder, merits additional discussion because the anxiety in panic disorder influences emergency room utilization and increases the chances that the patient presents to the emergency department with "physical" complaints. The next section focuses on panic disorder.

Panic Disorder

Why Focus on Panic Disorder?

Panic disorder is a particularly important anxiety disorder for emergency department personnel to understand. The heightened sensitivity to bodily sensations and their catastrophic misinterpretation as serious medical threats that is typical of panic lead to frequent emergency room visits and hospital admissions to rule out myocardial infarctions, manage dyspnea, and evaluate presyncope. Repeated emergency department visits from patients with panic disorder cost the medical system a substantial amount of money; these costs could be significantly reduced with early recognition and effective management of the panic disorder (Coley et al. 2009).

One characteristic of panic disorder that can help differentiate it from other types of anxiety problems is an extreme sensitivity to bodily sensations. Panic patients pay considerable attention to the normal "sounds of the bodily machinery" and are quite frightened by them, whereas most people have habituated and learned to screen out these "sounds" unless something clearly changes or goes awry. Panic attacks are often triggered in panic patients when what should be a "silent" event is attended to and interpreted as a danger signal (D. W. Austin and Richards 2001). Instead of thinking about a perceived palpitation as a normal sensation, a panic patient is prone to catastrophic interpretation (i.e., jumping to the conclusion that a heart attack might be imminent). This reactivity to bodily sensations has been labeled anxiety sensitivity. It can be measured using the Anxiety Sensitivity Index (Reiss et al. 1986) and can be helpful in predicting the appearance of spontaneous panic

Table 7–1. Disorders associated with anxiety syndromes

Psychiatric
    Cognitive disorders
    Depressive episodes with anxiety
    Generalized anxiety disorder
    Obsessive-compulsive disorder
    Panic disorder
    Personality disorders (especially clusters B and C)
    Posttraumatic stress disorder
    Psychotic disorders
    Social anxiety disorder
    Specific phobia
Cardiovascular
    Angina pectoris
    Arrhythmias
    Congestive heart failure
    Hypertension
    Hyperventilation
    Hypovolemia
    Myocardial infarction
    Shock
    Syncope
    Valvular disease
Endocrine
    Cushing's syndrome
    Hyperkalemia
    Hyperthermia
    Hyperthyroidism
    Hypocalcemia
    Hypoglycemia
    Hyponatremia
    Hypoparathyroidism
    Hypothyroidism
    Menopause

Neurological
    Cerebral syphilis
    Cerebrovascular insufficiency
    Encephalopathies (infectious, metabolic, and toxic)
    Essential tremor
    Huntington's chorea
    Intracranial mass lesions
    Migraine headaches
    Multiple sclerosis
    Postconcussive syndrome
    Posterolateral sclerosis
    Polyneuritis
    Seizure disorders (especially temporal lobe seizures)
    Vasculitis
    Vertigo
    Wilson's disease
Respiratory
    Asthma
    Chronic obstructive pulmonary disease
    Pneumonia
    Pneumothorax
    Pulmonary edema
    Pulmonary embolus
Drug related
    Stimulant, marijuana, or hallucinogen abuse
    Alcohol or sedative-hypnotic withdrawal
    Akathisia (secondary to antipsychotic medications or SSRIs)
    Anticholinergic, digitalis, or theophylline toxicity
    Abuse of over-the-counter diet pills

Table 7–1. Disorders associated with anxiety syndromes *(continued)*

Dietary	Neoplastic
Caffeinism	Carcinoid tumor
Monosodium glutamate	Insulinoma
Tyramine-containing foods in those	Pheochromocytoma
taking MAOIs	Infectious/Inflammatory
Vitamin deficiency	Anaphylaxis
Hematologic	Systemic lupus erythematosus
Acute intermittent porphyria	Acute or chronic infection
Anemias	

Note. MAOI = monoamine oxidase inhibitor; SSRI = selective serotonin reuptake inhibitor.
Source. Milner et al. 1999.

attacks as are seen in panic disorder (Schmidt et al. 2006). This trait also contributes to the frequent appearance of panic disorder patients in emergency departments.

Numerous studies have examined presentation of patients with panic disorder to the medical emergency room, and multiple factors that make symptoms such as chest pain more likely to be due to panic disorder have been distilled. If a patient is younger, female, without known coronary artery disease, presenting with atypical chest pain, and reporting high levels of anxiety, the probability of panic disorder is higher than in the absence of these factors (Huffman and Pollack 2003). All of these factors should be readily identified in the initial evaluation of the chest pain complaint. In patients with low risk for cardiac-related chest pain, a simple set of screening questions can then provide data that correlates well with gold-standard techniques for diagnosing panic disorder. Wulsin et al. (2002) have shown that emergency department physicians with no additional training in psychiatric assessment can diagnose panic disorder in patients with low to moderate risk for acute coronary syndrome, with fairly good agreement with psychiatric experts ($\kappa = 0.53$; 95% confidence interval, 0.26–0.80), by asking whether a sudden attack of fear or anxiety has occurred in the 4 weeks prior to the emergency department presentation; whether similar attacks have occurred previously; and whether these attacks come out of the blue, cause worry about having another attack, and feature any cardinal symptoms of panic attacks (shortness of breath, chest pain, heart racing or pounding, sweating, chills or flushing, dizziness, nausea, or tingling or numbness). In this study, diagnosis and initiation of selective serotonin reuptake inhibitor (SSRI) treatment in the emergency department correlated with a significant enhancement of continued treatment at 1-month and 3-month follow-ups.

It can be critically important to screen for and make the diagnosis of panic disorder in the emergency department. Patients come to the emergency room disturbed or distressed by their symptoms and wanting to know what is wrong with them. Simple reassurance that nothing serious can be identified, that tests have "ruled out" the heart attack or other "catastrophic" diagnosis that they feared, often falls on unhearing ears when those ears are attached to a panic-prone brain. The fear associated with a panic attack amplifies the personal importance of the symptoms being experienced, so a provider's assertion that "nothing is wrong" does not match the patient's experience.

Receiving a clear diagnosis of a fairly easily treatable brain-based pathology, based on a carefully done screening approach with proven efficacy, may be far more satisfying to the patient. This diagnosis, however, must be delivered with an appropriate amount of compassion and recognition of the potential need to reduce the stigma attached to psychiatric disorders. It may also help to assure the patient that he or she is not being told that the symptoms are "all in the head," even if those symptoms are generated by misfiring neurons in the brain. Simply ruling out a heart attack, for example, leaves open the possibility of innumerable other interpretations of the symptoms. A panic-prone patient may well go home, do some Internet research, and become convinced the problem was an arrhythmia or something wrong with the lungs. The patient will return to the emergency room for further rule-outs each time symptoms recur, inconveniencing the patient and increasing medical costs. When a careful diagnosis of panic disorder is made during an emergency department visit, on the other hand, it usually proves to be stable 2 years later; and patients with panic disorder who do not receive a panic diagnosis and appropriate panic treatment do worse over that 2-year period, both psychiatrically and medically (Fleet et al. 2003).

Initial Treatment of Panic Disorder

If panic is accurately diagnosed, appropriate treatment can be initiated in the emergency department, using both medications and nonpharmacological treatments. SSRI antidepressants are the drugs of choice; they can reduce both the frequency and intensity of panic attacks, and can be initiated in the emergency department (Wulsin et al. 2002). SSRIs have the advantage of also being useful for treating many of the comorbidities that are common in panic patients, including social anxiety, generalized anxiety disorder, PTSD, and depression.

When prescribing SSRIs, the clinician should keep in mind that these patients have heightened interoceptive sensitivity and a propensity for catastrophic thinking around bodily sensations. Because SSRIs can cause bodily sensations in the first days to weeks of treatment, the risk of having a panic attack and abruptly discontinuing the medication in the titration phase is high. SSRIs can be somewhat activating on first exposure, and panic patients are particularly susceptible to this effect. If started at too high a dose or without adequate preparation, this early activation effect can lead some panic patients to refuse all future efforts to prescribe an SSRI for them, even though this early activation can in fact be a positive prognostic sign that their panic disorder will ultimately prove responsive to this same drug. This early sensitivity risk should be managed with clear instructions to the patient about what to anticipate and very gradual titration of the medication from the lowest possible initiation dose. Sertraline or citalopram are good first-choice drugs for panic patients. Sertraline has a very broad dosing range, so it can be started at very low levels (12.5 mg/day) and titrated slowly to a goal dose of 100–200 mg/day. Citalopram is a good alternative, because it tends to be minimally activating, with fewer bodily sensations for the patient to misinterpret during titration. It can be started at 2.5 mg/day and titrated to a goal dose of 20–40 mg/day. With either drug, the titration pace can be adjusted to individual sensitivities and should be done under supervision, so close follow-up is important. A very slow titration pace should be used while the patient is awaiting follow-up. If the process has been properly explained, sophisticated patients may be capable of learning how to adjust the titration pace themselves, according to their activation sensitivity. Long-acting benzodiazepines, such as clonazepam, can be prescribed in a scheduled fashion to reduce the patient's interoceptive sensitivity during the titration of an SSRI antidepressant. Rapid follow-up and active management of the medication titration is key to successful treatment.

Cognitive management of panic attacks is a cornerstone of treatment for panic disorder and this, too, can and should be initiated from the emergency department. Educating patients about how the amygdala and limbic brain process threats and generate normal fear and anxiety, with associated physiological activation that is adaptive when real threat is present, can lead to an increased sense of comfort that the physical sensations experienced during a panic attack are actually brain based, even if driven by a brain-generated "false alarm." Appropriate education and coaching in how to use this information as a cognitive coping tool may help reduce the pressure felt by these patients to pursue further medical workup through additional emergency department visits. As discussed above, patients can be helped to search for evidence in their own experience and that of others to support the notion that their symptoms do have an explanation based in real biology and modern neuroscience, that their fear does not reflect weakness or psychological problems, and that the alarms ringing in their brains do not reflect real dangers. The simple act of labeling a physical sensation as related to anxiety can lead to increased mastery of the sensation and can directly reduce activity within the fear circuitry (Lieberman et al. 2007). Turning on cognitive processors and engaging in self-talk about one's inner physical and emotional experiences can actually reduce the amygdala outputs that generate or sustain the panic cycle. Knowing that labeling and thinking are, in a way, directly attacking the source of the problem can enhance a patient's motivation to pursue this methodology for coping with their symptoms.

Relaxation techniques—slow breathing and progressive muscle relaxation—were discussed earlier in the chapter (see "Management of a Panic Attack") as useful approaches to managing acute anxiety within the emergency room. Evidence is mixed as to whether these techniques add meaningfully to the standard cognitive-behavioral therapy package used to treat panic, but they definitely will have some value to some patients during initial efforts to manage overwhelming anxiety and initiate a fuller treatment. Slow abdominal breathing can be taught in the emergency department and prescribed for 5–20 minutes at a time, one to three times per day. If the person is already trained in this technique, it can sometimes be helpful in an acute attack as well. Progressive muscle relaxation can also be easily taught in the emergency department. In this technique, patients are asked to scan their muscle groups from head to toe sequentially, contracting each muscle group for a few seconds, then relaxing the group for an equivalent amount of time, focusing on the general sensation of relaxation that occurs and spreads as a tensed muscle is relaxed. This technique can sometimes reduce the muscular tension that accumulates in anxiety disorders. Both techniques may directly reduce emotional arousal, perhaps by activating cognitive processors in the brain that inhibit amygdala output and by focusing attention on relaxation-related physical sensations instead of the fear-generating sensations. Patients can also be advised to engage in other types of meditative practices, although this is clearly more difficult to do in the emergency department setting if they do not have prior training. If the patient already has a meditative practice, its use and application to the panic situation can be reinforced.

As discussed in the earlier section on managing panic attacks, full treatment of anxiety disorders often includes an exposure-based component in the cognitive-behavioral therapy package. This component is always important if the symptom picture includes significant anxiety-based avoidance behavior. In exposure therapy, the goal is to reduce automatic anxiety responses to conditioned cues through a process of repeated exposure and desensitization. In panic disorder, both internal and external cues have become triggers for anxiety or fear, and therapy for panic often includes exposure to both types of cues. Exposure targets may therefore include both interoceptive cues (e.g., heart racing, shortness of breath, dizziness) and exteroceptive cues (e.g., feared places or activities). As discussed previously, the patient in an acute crisis may be too unstable to begin this form of treatment, and the emergency room does not lend itself to the type of support and instruction needed to initiate it. However, it can be valuable to introduce the patient to the idea that anxiety makes people want to avoid the things that trigger it but that this avoidance is the source of the most overwhelming disability imposed by the disorder. Everything patients can do to sustain functioning, to push through fear, to keep doing things that are in reality safe to do, will protect them from the worst consequences of panic. This introduces them to the notion that there is a definitive nondrug treatment for their condition, which can help them reclaim their ability to feel safe in the world, thereby helping to sustain hope and optimism. Rapid follow-up with a skilled clinician experienced with these techniques can then really have an impact and enhance outcomes.

Acute Trauma

Case Example *(continued)*

Two weeks after her previous appearance in the emergency room, Ms. D returns to the emergency department after a car accident. She was the lead driver in a three-car pileup on the local highway. Although she is not seriously injured, a passenger in her car dislocated a shoulder and fractured a leg. Ms. D recalls fearing for her life in the accident and feeling quite distressed afterward, but she was unable to actually describe what happened until she arrived at the hospital. She reports extreme guilt about "causing the accident." On a positive note, she says that she and her fiancé have reconciled and that he is on the way to the emergency department to support her. She has also curtailed her alcohol use, and alcohol was not involved in this accident. Psychiatric input is sought due to recognized risk factors for PTSD.

Acute Stress Disorder and Posttraumatic Stress Disorder

Acute trauma creates risk for psychiatric sequelae, whether the nature of the trauma is interpersonal violence, accident, or natural disaster. After a patient is medically cleared, the clinician can assess the patient for psychiatric sequelae and recommend treatment and/or prevention.

As previously noted, increased anxiety and central nervous system activation are normal responses to threat, but when they are particularly intense, prolonged, or disruptive of functioning, diagnosis and treatment of a stress disorder may be appropriate. The American Psychiatric Association (2000) defines two posttrauma disorders: acute stress disorder (ASD) and PTSD. Both require exposure to events that pose threats of death or serious injury and that elicit reactions of intense fear, helplessness, or horror. Additional symptoms can include dissociation or emotional numbing, reexperiencing of the trauma, avoidance, and hyperarousal. ASD must occur within 4 weeks of the trauma and last less then 4 weeks in total. It often evolves into PTSD, which requires symptoms for at least a month, although it can also resolve on its own.

Given that ASD is a time-limited condition, treatment may not be needed or can itself be time limited. Insofar as the presence of ASD may predict risk for PTSD, early detection and treatment within emergency settings may be able to prevent subsequent complications that can be quite severe.

Evaluation of the Traumatized Patient

Although this is an evolving area of research, a number of risk factors for development of PTSD from ASD have been identified. A prospective study of 200 assault survivors showed that 17% of participants met criteria for ASD at 2 weeks and 24% of participants met criteria for PTSD at 6 months. Statistically significant predictors at 2 weeks of meeting criteria for PTSD at 6 months included prior psychological problems, low posttrauma social support, greater perceived threat to life, peritrauma emotional responses and dissociation, rumination about the trauma, and negative self-appraisals. Elevated resting heart rate at 2 weeks also was found to predict PTSD at 6 months (Kleim et al. 2007).

The nature of the trauma is also salient when assessing risk for progression to PTSD. Interpersonal trauma, such as rape or assault, carries higher risk than other types, such as natural disasters. This is especially true in women. The relative risk of PTSD from nonassaultive trauma fades with time, but the relative risk from interpersonal trauma does not. History of early-life interpersonal trauma increases risk of PTSD from recent trauma (Breslau 2001).

In evaluating trauma patients, therefore, the clinician needs to clarify the nature of the trauma; unearth past history of depression, anxiety, other psychiatric disorders, or early abuse; and explore trauma-related psychological experiences, such as a feeling of mental defeat and a propensity toward rumination or dissociation. It is critical to ensure rapid follow-up to evaluate for additional risk factors, such as ongoing somatic arousal, and to monitor the recovery process.

Aside from serving as a risk factor for development of PTSD, the nature of the trauma is also relevant insofar as patient behavior may contribute to increased risk of repeated exposure to trauma. Alcohol use, failure to use safety restraints, reckless driving, and impulses to harm self or others all contribute to a patient's emergency department presentation and create risk for future visits. For some patients, the emergency room visit may represent an "intervenable moment" in which behavior contributing to traumatic exposure can be addressed with heightened impact.

It is important to note that ASD and PTSD are not the only psychiatric consequences of trauma. Reactivation or new onset of depression, substance abuse, and even psychosis can occur following trauma exposure. This may be especially true after a natural disaster, which can traumatize an entire community and eliminate system-level supports for patients with mental illness (S. L. Austin and Godleski 1999). We have focused on ASD and PTSD, but a prudent emergency department provider will also be vigilant for other psychopathology when treating trauma patients.

Digging too deeply into the details of the trauma with the patient is not without risks, especially for those patients who cannot remember critical details. Pushing too hard when a patient seems frightened by recollections or cannot recall details might intensify traumatic arousal and thus increase risk for PTSD. A form of critical incident debriefing that pushed the immediate recounting of trauma details was once widely used to help first responders to "debrief" after trauma exposure. However, available evidence does not support the effectiveness of this approach in reducing PTSD risk. Emphasis has shifted toward "psychological first aid," which focuses on immediate physical needs, social support, provision of safety, education, and normalization of acute psychological reactions (Litz and Maguen 2007).

Prevention of Posttraumatic Stress Disorder

As mentioned above, longer-term treatment of anxiety often involves reducing avoidance of feared stimuli and increasing engagement with one's usual life events. One of the best proven treatments for established PTSD is prolonged exposure therapy (Foa et al. 2007). In many cases of trauma-related anxiety, core fears include memory of the trauma and the possibility that the trauma will repeat. Bisson et al. (2004) prospectively tested a four-session early psychotherapeutic intervention that included elements of exposure therapy and cognitive restructuring, intended to educate the participants about stress response, minimize avoidance of painful memories, and maximize reintegration into life routines. Enrolled subjects had positive scores at 1 week after trauma on the Posttraumatic Stress Diagnostic Scale, the anxiety or depression subscale of the Hospital Anxiety and Depression Scale, or the Impact of Event Scale. The intervention produced modest improvement in scores on these scales at 13 months when compared with a "repeated assessments only" control group (Bisson et al. 2004). In a study of motor vehicle accident survivors, Ehlers et al. (2003) assessed improvement of PTSD symptoms in a group receiving early cognitive therapy against a group of survivors using a self-help booklet as well as a "repeated assessments" control group. These authors found statistically significant improvement in the cognitive therapy cohort only. A retrospective study of Israeli veterans of the 1982 Lebanon War also suggested that obtaining early treatment and reintegration helped prevent appearance of PTSD, even 20 years after the trauma (Solomon et al. 2005). In a large study in Israel, Shalev et al. (2007) compared a purely cognitive therapy to a purely exposure-based therapy initiated through emergency room–based trauma case finding, and found that both approaches were more effective than medication (escitalopram) or a medication placebo in reducing subsequent PTSD risk.

Findings from these studies suggest that careful, data-based construction of a systematic assessment and treatment approach that identifies and treats high-risk trauma patients may meaningfully reduce PTSD rates, and thus reduce some of the most costly and devastating consequence of trauma exposure. The evolving interventions educate patients about normal and abnormal emotional reactions, support a return to normal life routines and use of social supports, and emphasize a minimization of anxiety-related avoidance after the traumatic event. Although much research is still needed to shape optimal programs, enough evidence is available to suggest that all trauma patients with sustained autonomic arousal (e.g., elevated heart rates) following trauma exposure, prior histories of anxiety or depressive disorders, significant earlier traumas, and particularly intense emotional reactions to the current trauma should be considered for psychotherapeutic PTSD prevention interventions. The probability of patient acceptance of these interventions is much greater if they can be initiated through the emergency department, because most patients have limited interest in prevention and if simply referred to a psychiatric clinic without adequate education will most likely decide to follow through only if severe PTSD actually develops.

If somatic arousal is a risk factor for development of PTSD, it is possible that initiating arousal-reducing intervention in the emergency department could prevent its persistence and reduce PTSD risk. Disintegration of sleep may be a particularly destructive manifestation of arousal, and efforts to normalize sleep may be of considerable value. Sedative-hypnotic agents can be used and clearly have a place in this context; however, risks of tolerance and dependence must be considered, including psychological dependence that can interfere with more definitive psychotherapeutic efforts. Although sedative-hypnotic agents, such as zolpidem and zaleplon, comprise the bulk of agents approved by the U.S. Food and Drug Administration for induction of sleep, many other agents are used off-label for their capacity to induce sleep. These medications include trazodone, gabapentin, and low-dose quetiapine. All may have particular value in specific circumstances for trauma-related sleep disruption. More traditional benzodiazepines, such as lorazepam or clonazepam, should be used with caution. These medications are indeed effective at inducing sleep and may reduce general anxious arousal as well; however, they do not address core symptoms of PTSD and they can actually undermine the effectiveness of prolonged exposure, which may be the most definitive treatment for the disorder. Their use should therefore be restricted to circumstances in which their sedative and rapid anxiolytic properties are clearly needed and are more important than the potential negative impact on subsequent treatment and their traditional risks of tolerance, dependence, and abuse. Also, standard behavioral attention to sleep hygiene should not be ignored.

SSRIs are commonly used in the long-term pharmacotherapy for PTSD, and studies in rats support the notion that these medications may be used to prevent development of PTSD after a traumatic event (Matar et al. 2006). However, early reports from a recent study concluded that SSRIs did not prevent development of PTSD (Shalev et al. 2007). Therefore, it should probably remain standard of care for now to defer initiation of SSRI treatment until and unless a case of ASD turns into PTSD. An exception might be made if the patient has a prior history of anxiety disorders or major depression and has discontinued previously effective SSRI treatment, given that trauma can reactivate these conditions and their prior presence substantially increases the risk of PTSD. In these patients, reinitiation of the SSRI should be considered.

Other Anxiety and Anxiety-Related Conditions

Although panic and trauma have particular salience in the emergency department context, other types of anxiety-related conditions impact the likelihood and nature of patient presentations to the emergency room. All of the anxiety disorders can contribute to heightened fear or worry in the face of physical symptoms and can increase the odds that a patient will appear for emergent care instead of pursuing help through less urgent avenues. Patients with obsessive-compulsive disorder may demonstrate a near-delusional level of concern about germs or infection. Patients with a blood-injection-injury phobia may faint when in the emergency department for another reason. Patients with generalized anxiety disorder may have a somatic focus for their worry, causing them to present to the emergency room for an evaluation that could wait for a primary care appointment. Similarly, somatoform disorders such as hypochondriasis and somatization also involve intense anxiety about physical symptoms, and even though they are not classified as anxiety disorders, they will bring highly anxious patients into the emergency department. A full discussion of these conditions is beyond the scope of this chapter.

Key Clinical Points

- Anxiety is a common complaint in the emergency department, and anxiety disorders pose a significant burden to the medical system if they are not adequately recognized and treated.

- Panic attacks can be managed without medications, using cognitive and behavioral techniques.

- SSRIs provide relief from most anxiety disorders, although a slow titration to the goal dose may be needed given the propensity of SSRIs to cause anxiety-provoking physical symptoms as these medications are initiated.

- Trauma patients with severe distress or dissociation in the aftermath of trauma exposure, a pretrauma history of mental illness, difficulty returning to normal functioning after the trauma, and signs of autonomic arousal are at highest risk of developing PTSD.

- PTSD risk may be reduced with rapid introduction to cognitive-behavioral techniques and normalization of life rhythms (e.g., sleep) after the traumatic event. There is insufficient evidence at this point to support efforts to prevent PTSD pharmacologically.

- High anxiety does not reduce the likelihood of major medical problems requiring urgent attention and should not divert attention from necessary medical evaluation. High risk may remain even if life-threatening medical illness is ruled out, because anxiety may reflect an underlying psychiatric disturbance that carries high risk for self-harm or harm to others.

References

American Psychiatric Association: Diagnostic and Statistical Manual of Mental Disorders, 4th Edition, Text Revision. Washington, DC, American Psychiatric Association, 2000

Austin DW, Richards JC: The catastrophic misinterpretation model of panic disorder. Behav Res Ther 39:1277–1291, 2001

Austin SL, Godleski LS: Therapeutic approaches for survivors of disaster. Psychiatr Clin North Am 22:897–910, 1999

Bisson JI, Shepherd JP, Joy D, et al: Early cognitive-behavioral therapy for post-traumatic stress symptoms after physical injury. Br J Psychiatry 184:63–69, 2004

Breslau N: The epidemiology for posttraumatic stress disorder: what is the extent of the problem? J Clin Psychiatry 62 (suppl 17):16–22, 2001

Coley KC, Saul MI, Seybert AL: Economic burden of not recognizing panic disorder in the emergency department. J Emerg Med 36:3–7, 2009

Deacon B, Lickel J, Abramowitz JS: Medical utilization across the anxiety disorders. J Anxiety Disord 22:344–350, 2008

Ehlers A, Clark DM, Hackmann A, et al: A randomized controlled trial of cognitive therapy, a self-help booklet, and repeated assessments as early interventions for posttraumatic stress disorder. Arch Gen Psychiatry 60:1024–1032, 2003

Fleet RP, Lavoie KL, Martel JP, et al: Two-year follow-up status of emergency department patients with chest pain: was it panic disorder? CJEM 5:247–254, 2003

Foa E, Hembree E, Rothbaum B: Prolonged Exposure for PTSD: Emotional Processing of Traumatic Experiences, Therapist Guide. New York, Oxford University Press, 2007

Huffman JC, Pollack MH: Predicting panic disorder among patients with chest pain: an analysis of the literature. Psychosomatics 44:222–236, 2003

Kleim B, Ehlers A, Glucksman E: Early predictors of chronic post-traumatic stress disorder in assault survivors. Psychol Med 37:1457–1467, 2007

Lieberman MD, Eisenberger NI, Crockett MJ, et al: Putting feelings into words: affect labeling disrupts amygdala activity in response to affective stimuli. Psychol Sci 18:421–428, 2007

Litz BT, Maguen S: Early intervention for trauma, in Handbook of PTSD: Science and Practice. Edited by Friedman MJ, Keane TM, Resick PA. New York, Guilford, 2007, pp 306–329

Matar MA, Cohen H, Kaplan Z, et al: The effect of early poststressor intervention with sertraline on behavioral responses in an animal model of post-traumatic stress disorder. Neuropsychopharmacology 31:2610–2618, 2006

Milner KK, Florence T, Glick RL: Mood and anxiety syndromes in emergency psychiatry. Psychiatr Clin North Am 22:755–777, 1999

Reiss S, Peterson RA, Gursky DM, et al: Anxiety sensitivity, anxiety frequency, and the prediction of fearfulness. Behav Res Ther 24:1–8, 1986. Cited by Schmidt NB, Zvolensky MJ, Maner JK: Anxiety sensitivity: prospective prediction of panic attacks and Axis I pathology. J Psychiatr Res 40:691–699, 2006

Sadock BJ, Sadock VA: Synopsis of Psychiatry, 9th Edition. Philadelphia, PA, Lippincott Williams & Wilkins, 2003, pp 591–642

Schmidt NB, Zvolensky MJ, Maner JK: Anxiety sensitivity: prospective prediction of panic attacks and Axis I pathology. J Psychiatr Res 40:691–699, 2006

Shalev AY, Freedman S, Adessky R, et al: Prevention of PTSD by early treatment: a randomized controlled study. Preliminary results from the Jerusalem Trauma Outreach and Prevention Study (J-TOP) (poster), in American College of Neuropsychopharmacology 46th Annual Meeting General Program, Boca Raton, FL, December 9–13, 2007. Nashville, TN, American College of Neuropsychopharmacology, 2007, p 63

Solomon Z, Shklar R, Mikulincer M: Frontline treatment of combat stress reaction: a 20-year longitudinal evaluation study. Am J Psychiatry 162:2309–2314, 2005

Wulsin L, Liu T, Storrow A, et al: A randomized, controlled trial of panic disorder treatment initiation in an emergency department chest pain center. Ann Emerg Med 39:139–143, 2002

Suggested Readings

Craske MG, Barlow DH: Master of Your Anxiety and Panic: Therapists Guide, 4th Edition. New York, Oxford University Press, 2006

Stein MB, Goin MK, Pollack MH, et al: Practice Guideline for the Treatment of Patients with Panic Disorder, 2nd Edition. January 2009. Available at: http://www.psychiatryonline.com. Accessed September 30, 2009.

Wells A: Cognitive Therapy of Anxiety Disorders. Chichester, UK, Wiley, 1997

8

The Cognitively Impaired Patient

James A. Bourgeois, O.D., M.D., F.A.P.M.

Tracy McCarthy, M.D.

Case Example

Mr. A, a 75-year-old male with multiple vascular risk factors, presented to the emergency department a few days after having an outpatient cardiac catheterization that revealed severe coronary artery disease. There were no immediate complications to the procedure; however, shortly after his return home, he experienced motor agitation, confusion, and disorientation. He did not appear to have any new neurological deficits. When seen in consultation, he had a variable level of consciousness, was grossly confused and disoriented, and was seeing "animals." Collateral history from family members revealed a gradual onset of mild problems, including memory and word-finding difficulties, even prior to the catheterization. He also was "depressed" and had mild sleep, energy, and appetite disturbances.

The patient with cognitive impairment, like Mr. A, presents unique challenges in emergency psychiatry. Many discrete psychiatric illnesses are associated with cognitive impairment. Thus, the differential diagnosis of cognitive impairment is broad, covering many, often overlapping diagnostic categories and forcing the physician to consider many possibilities. In addition, the "core deficit" of cognitive impairment may be less dramatic in its emergency presentation than the more "disruptive" clinical states (e.g., psychosis, mania, motor agitation, violence against self and/or others) that may be the initial focus of clinical attention. Therefore, the clinician encountering numerous disruptive clinical states in an emergency setting must keep in mind the possibility of an underlying cognitive disorder as explanatory for the bulk of the patient's clinical problems.

Prompt assessment requires an integrative approach, including the analysis of the clinical history (from both the patient and collateral sources), clinical examination (including validated "bedside" formal cognitive testing), neuroimaging, clinical laboratory, physical examination, electrocardiogram, and, on occasion, electroencephalogram (EEG).

Clinical disposition of the emergency presentation of cognitive impairment may be quite varied and sometimes challenging, and may include the emergent use of psychopharmacology, medical or surgical admission with psychiatric psychosomatic medicine consultation, medical-psychiatric unit admission, psychiatric unit admission, or placement in alternative models of supervised living. By necessity, the definitive psychiatric diagnosis and longtem management plan may not always be achievable in the emergency setting; initial assessment and intervention, however, remain crucial to the eventual definitive disposition of these cases.

As the population has aged, the prevalence of cognitive disorders has increased (Blennow et al. 2006). Simultaneously, increasing numbers of patients are not covered by appropriate health insurance. The convergence of these trends will inevitably lead to more patients with cognitive impairment being seen in emergency settings. Therefore, mastery of the emergency management of these patients is a clinical imperative.

Case Example *(continued)*

Mr. A had an admission score of 12 on the Mini-Mental State Exam, with clear impairments in attention span and orientation. He was diagnosed with delirium and was admitted to the medicine service for further evaluation. On physical examination at admission, his catheter wound site was found to be surrounded by an erythematous ring and was warm and tender to touch. There was no pus from the wound. Complete blood count revealed a leukocytosis. Head computed tomography (CT) did not demonstrate evidence of a recent infarct but did show some diffuse cortical atrophy and small vessel white matter disease.

Evaluation of the Patient

Safety and Restraint

Safety and restraint must be considered early in the case of cognitive impairment, often before a firm diagnosis is made. In addition to being a danger to themselves, patients who are agitated and cognitively impaired are very disruptive to the operation of an emergency service (not to mention potentially dangerous to other patients). As a result, emergency departments must have well-developed as-needed procedures to provide sitters for, seclude, restrain, and medicate disruptive patients with cognitive impairments. Once safety is assured, clinical management may proceed.

Workup

The emergency workup of the patient with cognitive impairment is a graphic illustration of the integrative biopsychosocial approach. The triad of examination, laboratory, and neuroimaging should be kept in mind in these evaluations.

Examination

As in other areas of clinical practice, examination begins with history taking. Because patients with cognitive impairments are invariably poor historians, collateral history from family, caregivers, other physicians, social service agencies, and others with an interest in the patient should be solicited (Robert et al. 2005), especially in an emergency setting. However, privacy regulations must be followed; the clinician must be circumspect about telling the collateral sources private information about the patient. Items to address in the history include but are not limited to those listed in Table 8–1.

The examination needs to include the physical and mental status items listed in Table 8–2. A number of brief cognitive screening tests are available to clinicians that can serve as useful tools in assessment and in following the

Table 8–1. History

History of present illness
Prior psychiatric history
Prior medical history
History of head trauma, seizures, stroke, other central nervous system events
Recent level of cognitive function
Substance abuse history
Highest level of educational and vocational attainment
Medications (prescription, over the counter, herbal supplements)
Family history of cognitive disorders and other psychiatric illness

course of cognitive disorders. The most popular instrument is the Mini-Mental State Examination (MMSE; Folstein et al. 1975). The MMSE is validated, has been translated into multiple languages, and is quick to administer. Disadvantages include its limited ability to assess frontal lobe executive function and inability to distinguish definitively between delirium and dementia. A modified shorter version, the Mini-Cog, consists of the three-item recall from the MMSE and the clock draw (Borson et al. 2000). It can be a useful quick screening tool for dementia. Another commonly used tool is the Confusion Assessment Method (CAM; Inouye et al. 1990). Used in assessing delirium, the CAM can also be administered in very little time and is geared toward use by general medical clinicians for the evaluation of acute delirium. Based on DSM-III-R (American Psychiatric Association [APA] 1987), the CAM also is validated, with high sensitivity and specificity. Executive functioning can be evaluated with the Frontal Assessment Battery, which includes tests of motor sequencing, verbal fluency, response inhibition, and other functions (Dubois et al. 2000). Of note, these tests are often less useful in evaluating subcortical disorders. An oral version of the Trail Making Test—Part B, called the Mental Alternation Test, is more useful for patients with subcortical disorders and has been validated in dementia associated with the human immunodeficiency virus (HIV). This simple test requires the patient to alternate saying numbers and letters (1, A, 2, B, 3, C, etc.). The number of correct alternations in 30 seconds is the score, with a maximum score of 52 and a cutoff score of approximately 14 (Billick et al. 2001).

Table 8–2. Examination

Physical examination

Vital signs

Pulse oximetry

Head, ears, eyes, nose, and throat (including thyroid)

Cardiovascular and abdominal examination (including fecal occult blood)

Genitourinary and/or gynecological examination (as appropriate)

Neurological examination

Mental status examination

General appearance

Psychomotor activity

Speech

Mood and affect

Thought process and content

Psychotic symptoms, suicidality, and homicidality

Judgment and insight

Formal cognitive examination (e.g., MMSE)

Frontal lobe testing

Note. MMSE = Mini-Mental State Exam (Folstein et al. 1975).

Laboratory Assessment

Laboratory assessment is crucial in the assessment of cognitive impairment. Because the acute presentation of cognitive impairment often represents over-lapping syndromes of delirium, dementia, and amnestic disorders, a wide laboratory net needs to be cast to be thorough. Table 8–3 lists laboratory tests commonly used in patients with cognitive impairment; individual items on this list may be omitted if clinical suspicion is low.

Table 8–3. Laboratory tests in cognitive impairment

Chemistry panel	Creatine phosphokinase	Urine drug screen
Complete blood count	Ammonia	Blood alcohol level
Urinalysis	Vitamin B_{12}	Quantitative drug levels
Arterial blood gases	Cultures	Acetaminophen level
Liver enzymes	HIV	Heavy metal screen
Thyroid panel	VDRL or RPR	Chest X ray
Rheumatological panel	Hepatitis panel	12-lead electrocardiogram

Note. RPR = rapid plasma reagin; VDRL = Venereal Disease Research Laboratory.

Neuroimaging

Because the workup for altered mental status is in many cases the same as a workup for dementia, neuroimaging is increasingly commonly included. The debate of CT versus magnetic resonance imaging (MRI) is a useful one; however, for most purposes, CT is easier to obtain, lower cost, easier for the patient to tolerate, and not subject to patient contraindications (e.g., claustrophobia, indwelling metallic devices). In addition, with CT there is usually no need for intravenous contrast dye to acutely evaluate cognitive disorders. Although the clinician needs to be mindful of repeated radiation exposure and thus not obtain CT scans excessively, the threshold for CT scanning in the emergency setting needs to be appropriately low so as not to miss reversible causes of cognitive impairment.

EEG and Lumbar Puncture

The EEG may be helpful in the delirium-versus-dementia workup, because it reliably reveals diffuse slowing in delirium cases and has a characteristic pattern in Creutzfeldt-Jakob disease (Engel and Romano 2004). However, because the EEG is not as useful in subtyping of delirium, it is not routinely obtained in typical delirium cases. Similarly, lumbar puncture is considered if there is high clinical suspicion of central nervous system (CNS) infection, but the yield is not adequately high for the procedure to be recommended routinely in all cases of altered mental status.

> ### Case Example *(continued)*
>
> Although Mr. A was initially diagnosed with delirium, the reports of gradual prehospitalization decline in cognitive functioning were concerning for a comorbid diagnosis of major depression or a dementia. Given the imaging findings, a diagnosis of vascular dementia was considered, but definitive diagnosis was deferred until Mr. A's delirium had a chance to clear.

Psychiatric Disorders Characterized by Cognitive Impairment

The issue of psychiatric diagnosis of cognitive impairments warrants a general discussion of semantics and classification. The formal diagnosis of cognitive disorder may not be adequately inclusive of all of the psychiatric disorders characterized by cognitive impairment seen in the emergency setting. The majority of patients who present with cognitive impairment in the emergency setting will have an illness classified in DSM-IV-TR (APA 2000), under "Delirium, Dementia, and Amnestic and Other Cognitive Disorders." In addition to delirium, dementia, and amnestic disorders, this group includes cognitive disorder not otherwise specified. This classification can be applied elastically to conditions such as postconcussive syndrome and the psychiatric sequelae of traumatic brain injury, which may be subsyndromal for more impairing disorders or may present in a mixed picture that bridges the constructs of dementia and delirium (Mooney and Speed 2001). A smaller percentage of patients with cognitive impairment, including adults, will have illnesses classified in DSM-IV-TR under "Disorders Usually First Diagnosed in Infancy, Childhood, or Adolescence." Even these two broad categories will not capture all cognitive impairments seen in an emergency setting, because some patients with psychotic disorders, dissociative disorders, and substance use disorders may also present with cognitive impairment.

Delirium

According to DSM-IV-TR, delirium is a subacute to acute-onset condition characterized by circadian disturbances, cognitive impairment, altered level of arousal and attention, and a variable course. It is the psychiatric consequence of systemic disturbance(s) and may follow a myriad of systemic disorders (see Table 8–4). The keys to a diagnosis of delirium are the acute or subacute onset and the fluctuating course. Although delirium is invariably the consequence of one or more systemic disturbance(s), the most important "static" risk factor for the development of delirium is preexisting dementia, a concept that can be understood as the "vulnerable brain" or "decreased cognitive reserve" (Engel and Romano 2004). Even though delirium presents with an acute or subacute onset, it can become chronic if the underlying systemic cause is not reversed. Examples of conditions associated with chronic delirium include disseminated cancer and end-stage liver disease.

Although the dementia patient is highly vulnerable to the development of delirium, delirium occurs in patients without dementia as well. Therefore, emergency presentation of delirium mandates an efficient but thorough clinical search for the implicated systemic disturbance(s). The associated systemic disturbance(s) in delirium may not be evident initially; however, delirium

Table 8–4. Causes of delirium

Brain tumor	Infection
Cardiopulmonary disease	Kidney disease
Electrolyte or fluid imbalance	Liver disease
Head trauma	Seizures
Hypercarbia	Substance intoxication
Hypoalbuminemia	Substance withdrawal
Hypoglycemia	Thiamine deficiency
Hypoxia	Other systemic illness

should be managed actively and syndromally while the search for systemic precipitants proceeds apace. Due to the myriad causes of delirium, the workup must be thorough and is ideally initiated in the emergency department. Because delirium is the psychiatric manifestation of systemic illness, the focus of clinical inquiry must cover many possible organ systems.

Treatment of delirium must be initiated promptly, even before the systemic disturbances associated with its onset are determined and reversed. Patients may remember the delirium episode, and delirium is often quite frightening to family members.

Delirium Superimposed on Dementia

A common presentation to the emergency room is the patient with premorbid dementia who subsequently develops acute delirium (Fick et al. 2002). Often, the premorbid dementia has not been clinically appreciated and treated. The delirium episodes may be recurrent, which may point to dementia as a risk factor.

Neuroleptic Malignant Syndrome

A particularly dangerous form of delirium is the iatrogenic syndrome of neuroleptic malignant syndrome (NMS). This constellation of delirium, rigidity, and increased creatine phosphokinase (CPK) should be suspected in any patient who presents with altered mental status and has had access to antipsychotic agents. In recent years, NMS has been increasingly commonly reported with the use of atypical antipsychotics. Prior episodes of validated NMS are an important part of the patient's history. Management requires an appropriately high index of suspicion, a prompt determination of CPK level, supportive care, and withholding of antipsychotics until the CPK has renormalized for at least 2 weeks, at which point antipsychotic therapy may be cautiously restarted with CPK monitoring. In some cases, dantrolene, bromocriptine, and electroconvulsive therapy may be considered. This condition is discussed in further detail in Chapter 4, "The Catatonic Patient."

Dementia

Dementia is a syndrome of global cognitive impairment that, according to the DSM-IV-TR definition, must include anterograde and/or retrograde amnesia and at least one other area of cognitive dysfunction, such as aphasia, apraxia, agnosia, or executive dysfunctions. Dementia presents with full alertness, which is crucial in distinguishing dementia from delirium, with which it is frequently comorbid. Most dementia syndromes have an insidious onset and a course characterized by slow progression, but the physician must bear in mind that this course, although prototypical for dementia and common in the majority of cases, is not uniform (Engel and Romano 2004). Acute presentation of a large decrement in cognitive function may result from a critically located CNS lesion (e.g., a dominant-hemisphere middle cerebral artery cerebrovascular accident [CVA] in a case of poststroke vascular dementia) (Román 2002). Dementia syndromes may be quite rapidly progressive (e.g., Creutzfeldt-Jakob disease) or may be somewhat reversible with clinical intervention (e.g., hypothyroidism, vitamin B_{12} deficiency) (Boeve 2006; Engel and Romano 2004). The distinction between dementia and delirium, while a crucial clinical concept, is in some ways a false dichotomy in clinical practice, because previously undiagnosed dementia patients will often present with delirium simultaneously. Dementia is the most tangible and important risk factor for the later development of delirium. Many patients will experience several episodes of delirium during the tragic course of a degenerative dementia.

In addition, dementia is associated with a range of other psychiatric comorbid conditions that episodically may dominate (and in a sense even define) the clinical picture. Mood disorders, most commonly depressive states, are very common in patients with dementia (Lyketsos et al. 2002; Robert et al. 2005). A patient who is acutely significantly depressed and chronically mildly demented may well present to the emergency room with depressed mood, neurovegetative signs, and even suicidal crisis, even though the underlying psychiatric illness is dementia. Many patients with comorbid dementia and depression will experience an episode of depression more in the cognitive realm (e.g., decreased memory or concentration) than in the emotional realm, and may interpret their clinical situation as one of increasing cognitive impairment, likely triggering even more seriously depressed mood, setting up a vicious cycle.

Even more disruptive, and leading to many emergency presentations of dementia patients, is the pernicious relationship between dementia and psychosis. Common comorbid psychotic symptoms in dementia include delusions, particularly paranoid delusions, and hallucinations (Leverenz and McKeith 2002). The delusions in dementia may be a defensive attempt to "cover up" cognitive impairment. For example, the patient who has lost a valued object because of cognitive impairment may instead believe that a family member has stolen the object. Indeed, the onset of psychotic symptoms in a patient with dementia is both disruptive and dangerous to the patient and the family, and is a common context of emergency presentation (Robert et al. 2005). Therefore, the differential diagnosis of acute psychosis must necessarily include a rule-out of dementia syndromes. Less frequently, a dementia patient may present to the emergency room with an episode of comorbid acute hypomania or mania (Román 2002).

Dementia patients may present with the phenomenon of sundowning, wherein the patient develops increased confusion and motor agitation in the evening and at night. These patients may or may not meet criteria for an episode of comorbid delirium for these episodes; nonetheless, these patients can become very dangerous and unsafe to manage at home or in noncontrolled living situations.

Finally, the emergency presentation of dementia patients may be due to social factors rather than clinical ones. Patients with mild to moderate dementia can usually live in the community, if they have adequate supervision and the provision of basic needs by helpful others. When a support person is ill or dies, however, the now-unsupervised dementia patient may be brought to the emergency department solely because of the inability to care for himself or herself. The clinician should routinely inquire into the stability of the social system, especially the loss of primary support figures, in the timing of emergency presentation of a patient with dementia.

Dementia of the Alzheimer's Type

Dementia of the Alzheimer's type (DAT) is the most common dementia syndrome in Western societies. It represents the majority of dementing illness in the United States (Blennow et al. 2006). Onset of DAT is generally after age 65, and the population incidence increases with age. DAT is characterized by insidious onset and slow but steady loss of multiple domains of cognitive function. Clinically, patients may present with amnesia and various other cognitive deficits, including disorientation, aphasia, anomia, apraxia, disturbed executive functioning, and loss of capacity for activities of daily living. Presentation to the emergency room is rarely for loss of cognitive function per se, but more commonly for the onset of decreased self-care behavior or for psychiatric comorbidity (e.g., depression, psychosis, agitation, violence).

Vascular Dementia

Vascular dementia is a dementia syndrome resulting from CNS infarction(s) encountered in patients with multiple vascular risk factors, usually a combination of hyperlipidemia, hypertension, smoking, and/or diabetes mellitus. The pattern of cognitive deficits may resemble those in DAT, although the course of illness tends to vary. Patients with vascular dementia may have relative stability of deficits over time, with occasional abrupt losses in cognitive function; this stepwise progression differs from the continuous progression in DAT (Román 2002). Less frequently (e.g., following a dominant-hemisphere CVA), a patient with vascular dementia may present who has not had prior cognitive impairment but who is suddenly experiencing an acute loss of a substantial number of cortical functions. Although following large CVAs patients may present with delirium acutely, once the delirium has cleared these patients are best understood as having vascular dementia.

Lewy Body Dementia/Lewy Body Variant of Dementia of the Alzheimer's Type

Lewy body dementia and Lewy body variant of DAT, although somewhat distinct conditions neuropathologically, are overlapping clinically. Neuropathically, Lewy body dementia and Lewy body variant of DAT feature distinctive Lewy bodies; Lewy body variant of DAT has characteristic neuropathology of Alzheimer's disease as well. Both are clinically distinct from (and best understood as being more severe than) DAT. Compared with DAT, Lewy body dementia and Lewy body variant of DAT are characterized by a younger age at onset, a more rapidly progressive course, fluctuations in mental status, and early-onset and clinically prominent hallucinations, typically visual hallucinations (Boeve 2006;

Leverenz and McKeith 2002). The emergency presentation of these patients is often driven by the disruption caused by the dramatic onset of the visual hallucinations, which is a prominent and often defining clinical feature.

Frontotemporal Dementia

Frontotemporal dementia is a dementia syndrome characterized by, relative to DAT, more prominent frontal lobe deficit–related decrements in appropriate social behavior with relatively preserved memory function. These patients present early in their illness with disruptive social behavior, such as sexual inappropriateness, aggressiveness, impulsivity, and emotional dysregulation (Boeve 2006; Kertesz and Munoz 2002). All of these behaviors tend to be quite disruptive to the caregivers; indeed, the caregiver distress is often much greater than that of the patient. When evaluated clinically, these patients have the above-noted frontal lobe deficit states but otherwise have a remarkably preserved cognitive examination, often including MMSE scores in the nonimpaired range.

Dementia Due to HIV Disease

Dementia due to HIV disease may result from direct effects of the HIV virus on CNS tissue and does not necessarily require clinical evidence of immunosuppression in general, although HIV patients with systemic immunocompromise will be at risk for other opportunistic CNS infections (e.g., toxoplasmosis) and CNS lymphoma, which further complicate the clinical picture. Because patients with HIV may occasionally present a somewhat ambiguous picture, with concurrent signs of delirium and dementia, HIV dementia needs to be on the differential diagnosis of any new dementia syndrome (and HIV testing should thus be strongly considered for new dementia cases). New-onset cognitive impairment in a known HIV patient should primarily be considered to be HIV dementia until other causes can be definitively established. HIV dementia is important to identify early, because aggressive treatment with highly active antiretroviral therapy agents can result in some reversibility of dementia symptoms. In addition, persistence of cognitive impairment can be a significant problem in established HIV patients, whose ability to self-manage their medications may be significantly affected.

Neurodegenerative Illness

Neurodegenerative illness due to several causes is characterized by cognitive impairment. Graphically illustrating the whole-brain concept that "neurological" and "psychiatric" illnesses commonly co-occur in patients with CNS degenerative disease, familiar neurological illnesses with a progressive course (e.g., Parkinson's disease, Huntington's disease, multiple sclerosis) are associated with a significant risk of dementia (on the order of 50% or more sometime during the course of illness; Boeve 2006). Subsequently, these patients are prone to delirium as well. The presentation of cognitive impairment in a patient with known neurological illness should lead the clinician to make these connections; indeed, in cases of multiple sclerosis, in particular, acute mental status changes may reflect a "flare" of the background neurological illness.

Amnestic Disorders

Amnestic disorders may occur in "isolation" in a few specific circumstances (e.g., transient global amnesia, Korsakoff syndrome, carbon monoxide poisoning). The hallmark of these interesting disorders is the focal deficit in declarative or semantic memory (i.e., memory for facts as opposed to learned motor acts). According to DSM-IV-TR, other cortical deficits (as in dementia) or any changes in circadian rhythm, level of consciousness, or attention (as in delirium) are absent. The memory deficit may be anterograde (an inability to learn new semantic material), retrograde (an inability to recall previously learned material), or a combination of both. Some of the amnestic disorders (described below) may have an acute onset; because they are very disruptive to the patient's functioning, they are likely to lead to the need for emergency assessment. In addition to the amnestic disorders specified among the cognitive disorders, dissociative amnesia (anterograde and/or retrograde amnesia following a psychosocial stressor) may phenomenologically resemble the other amnestic disorders; because of its likelihood of psychosocial disruption, it may also present emergently.

Transient Global Amnesia

Transient global amnesia is an acute-onset global amnesia that is reversible. It usually occurs in middle-aged patients with no prior psychiatric history. Other aspects of cognitive function are unimpaired. The cause is unclear but may be a temporary disturbance in temporal lobe function. Because of its precipitously acute onset and the preservation of other cognitive function, transient global amnesia is very disturbing to the patient and often leads to an emergency presentation. Full workup, including neuroimaging and assessment for vascular disease, is needed. Whether these patients have increased risk for cognitive impairment in the future is unclear.

Korsakoff Syndrome

Korsakoff syndrome is a usually acute-onset amnestic disorder in the context of alcohol dependence. It is attributed to thiamine deficiency. It may occur in isolation or as part of a larger picture of alcohol dementia. It is treated with intravenously administered thiamine and subsequent nutritional supplementation.

Carbon Monoxide Poisoning

Carbon monoxide poisoning may result in focal hippocampal injury and thus amnesia in the absence of more global cognitive impairment. It may be seen in patients who attempted suicide by rerouting of vehicular exhaust or in fire victims. If emergently available, hyperbaric oxygen treatment may be considered.

Childhood-Onset Syndromes Characterized by Cognitive Impairment

Although often relatively neglected in the adult psychosomatic medicine literature, several childhood-onset illnesses are discussed in this chapter because they are characterized by cognitive impairment. When patients with these illnesses are seen in the emergency room, their cognitive impairment will likely be an important clinical aspect of the case. In addition, because mental retardation is a risk factor for the later development of dementia, all of the considerations of dementia may also apply to these patients.

Mental Retardation

Mental retardation, although classified in DSM-IV-TR as an Axis II disorder, is by definition a disorder of cognitive impairment. In addition to the impairments due to the baseline cognitive deficits, these patients have increased risk of dementia (even from their impaired baseline) as they age. In addition, they may have other psychiatric comorbidity, such as autism spectrum disorders, which may cloud the clinical emergency presentation.

Down Syndrome

Down syndrome is due to trisomy 21. The majority of patients with Down syndrome will have mild mental retardation. However, as they age, there is a high likelihood of dementia superimposed on their mental retardation.

Fragile X Disorders

Fragile X syndrome is the most common cause of mental retardation due to a single genetic defect. In addition to having cognitive impairment, patients with fragile X syndrome often have autism spectrum disorders with associated impaired social function.

Fetal Alcohol Syndrome

Fetal alcohol syndrome is a mental retardation syndrome due to in utero exposure to alcohol in the children of alcohol-dependent women. These patients may have the characteristic facial features of fetal alcohol syndrome and various degrees of mental retardation.

Other Clinical Syndromes of Cognitive Impairment

Dissociative Amnesia

In dissociative amnesia, one of the dissociative disorders listed in DSM-IV-TR, the clinical emergency manifestations are cognitive. This will be a case of an acutely amnestic patient who has experienced a psychologically troubling or even traumatic event and defends against this reality by a dissociative defense, resulting in amnesia for the painful aspects of the experience. This history, however, may not be in the patient's awareness, so a collateral source is needed to establish the temporal connection.

Subdural Hematoma/Subarachnoid Hemorrhage

Subdural hematoma (often following head trauma) and subarachnoid hemorrhage (often associated with untreated hypertension) are vascular lesions that may lead to changes in mental status, resulting in an emergency presentation. These lesions may present in an emergency picture consistent with acute delirium, progressive dementia, or a combination of both.

Alcohol and/or Drug Disorders

Various substance-related conditions may present with cognitive impairment. Alcohol or drug intoxication may result in temporary cognitive impairment. Alcohol "blackouts" (brief periods of amnesia associated with alcohol dependence) may lead to emergency evaluation. Withdrawal from alcohol, sedatives, or hypnotics may present with frank delirium and autonomic instability (Engel and Romano 2004).

Traumatic Brain Injury

Traumatic brain injury (TBI) is a common injury in the emergency setting. Critical variables to address are the period of unconsciousness, degree of post-traumatic amnesia, and cognitive status at the time of evaluation. Acutely, TBI patients may present with a picture more consistent with delirium, whereas over time, some may maintain a clinical appearance of dementia. The dementia associated with TBI may take extended periods of time to improve (even months to years), and precise estimation of prognosis is difficult. Many TBI cases have elements of both delirium and dementia that can be understood as existing on the boundary of dementia and delirium. Still other TBI cases are clinically milder and subsyndromal for other cognitive disorders; these are sometimes called postconcussion syndrome.

Depressive Pseudodementia

The overlap of mood and cognitive function is dramatically illustrated by the condition of depressive pseudodementia. In this condition, which is usually seen in older patients, the manifestation of depression is primarily cognitive, not emotional. Patients are often quite distressed by the insidious onset of cognitive impairment and are concerned that they are developing dementia. Formal cognitive examination usually reveals mild deficits in orientation, recall, and concentration. In addition, other symptoms of depression may be elicited. Treatment with an antidepressant and reassessment of cognitive function and mood symptoms after the patient is at a therapeutic level for an adequately long clinical trial of antidepressant (which may take as long as 2 months) will often be associated with improved cognitive performance.

Clinical Management

Case Example *(continued)*

Mr. A was treated with a low-dose antipsychotic for agitation in his delirium. He received intravenous antibiotics for the wound infection. Opioids were minimized, and anticholinergic medications and benzodiazepines were held. Over the next several days, his delirium improved. His score was 22 when re-administered the MMSE, and family members assured the treatment team that he was at his recent cognitive baseline. He was discharged to the community for further outpatient workup for dementia and depression.

Treatment

The first step in treatment of cognitive impairment is the management of systemic factors, as guided by the results of physical examination, laboratory, and imaging results. To treat behavioral symptoms, a range of psychotropic medications are now in common use. Antipsychotics, both typical and atypical, are now standard in emergency care (Carson et al. 2006; Kile et al. 2005; Lacasse et al. 2006; Meagher 2001; Tune 2001; Weber et al. 2004). Most commonly used in emergency settings are the typical antipsychotic haloperidol (most other typical antipsychotics are rarely used in the emergency setting) and several atypical antipsychotics.

Due to their sedative/hypnotic properties, benzodiazepines alone should be used for delirium due to alcohol or sedative-hypnotic withdrawal, which are often associated with signs of autonomic hyperarousal. Benzodiazepines are often combined with typical antipsychotics or atypical antipsychotics for the management of delirium due to other causes (Meagher 2001). They should be used with caution, however, because they may exacerbate many cases of delirium and may increase cognitive impairment in dementia. The most important difference among benzodiazepines is in their pharmacokinetic properties—short-half-life agents will work more quickly but require more frequent dosing than long-half-life agents.

Although less frequently used in the emergency setting to treat patients with cognitive impairment, other agents are sometimes useful. Anticonvulsants may be used in a supplemental fashion to control agitation. One useful agent is Depacon, an intravenous form of valproate. It can be loaded at 15–20 mg/kg/day with monitoring of liver function, platelets, serum ammonia, and valproate serum levels (Kile et al. 2005). If anticholinergic toxicity is confirmed and/or if a history of premorbid dementia can be established, early use of cholinesterase inhibitors (donepezil, rivastigmine, or galantamine) may be initiated (Coulson et al. 2002). Finally, in cases of cognitive impairment with dangerous agitation, anesthetic agents such as propofol can be used emergently for a brief period, but the patient receiving this agent must be in an intensive care unit, receiving close clinical observation and airway management.

An important consideration is that medications used to control agitation in a patient with cognitive impairment also risk contributing to delirium, thereby worsening the patient's cognitive functioning. Therefore, medications should be used cautiously, and the minimum effective dose should be used, especially in elderly patients.

Disposition

Disposition of patients with cognitive impairment, once stabilized, from an emergency setting can be accomplished to a number of receiving institutions. These disposition decisions are often complicated, and no one type of institution will optimally manage all of the needs of these patients (Meagher 2001). Table 8–5 summarizes some possible disposition options, with associated advantages and disadvantages.

Legal Issues in Cognitive Impairment

Although not always a critical concern while patients are in the emergency setting, many legal issues may arise in the management of patients with cognitive impairment (see Table 8–6). The clinician needs a useful methodology to address these issues in the acute presentation of cognitive impairment.

Table 8–6.   Legal considerations in the management of patients with cognitive impairment

Decisional capacity for procedures, placement, do-not-resuscitate order, estate management, other decisions

Assignment of surrogate decision maker

Informed consent for off-label medications

Interface with social service agencies (e.g., adult protective services)

Participation in clinical trials

Confidentiality

Insurance issues

Financial issues

Table 8–5.   Considerations in disposition of patients with cognitive impairment

Disposition	Advantages	Disadvantages
Medical admission	Full medical workup Access to consultants	Limited psychiatric care
Psychiatric admission	Full psychiatric care 24-hour supervision	Limited medical care May refuse cognitive disorder patients
Medical-psychiatric admission	Comprehensive care 24-hour supervision	Rarely available May refuse cognitive disorder patients
Rehabilitation admission	Familiar with cognitive impairment	Limited medical care May not have comprehensive psychiatric care
Structured placement (skilled nursing facility)	Safe for impaired patients 24-hour supervision	Minimal medical care Minimal psychiatric care

Key Clinical Points

- Cognitive disorders are among the most common categories of psychiatric illness in the emergency department setting.

- Patients with cognitive impairment may present with various behavioral symptoms (e.g., psychosis, agitation, violence) in the emergency department.

- Cognitive disorders are an important part of the differential diagnosis of the presentation of agitated states.

- The "smoke" of delirium often leads to the discovery of the "fire" of dementia.

- Workup of the agitated patient with cognitive impairment requires neuroimaging, clinical laboratory, and physical assessment.

- Acute management of the patient with cognitive impairment may require typical antipsychotics, atypical antipsychotics, benzodiazepines, and other sedatives; chronic management requires the use of many classes of psychopharmacology.

- Thorough mental status examination and quantitative cognitive assessment are required for initial workup and serial assessments.

- Emergency department presentation of cognitive impairment is more often due to psychosis, agitation, and disruption in the care model than to progression of cognitive impairment per se.

References

American Psychiatric Association: Diagnostic and Statistical Manual of Mental Disorders, 3rd Edition, Revised. Washington, DC, American Psychiatric Association, 1987

American Psychiatric Association: Diagnostic and Statistical Manual of Mental Disorders, 4th Edition, Text Revision. Washington, DC, American Psychiatric Association, 2000

Billick SB, Siedenburg E, Burgert W, et al: Validation of the Mental Alternation Test with the Mini-Mental Status Examination in geriatric psychiatry patients and normal controls. Compr Psychiatry 42:202–205, 2001

Blennow K, de Leon MJ, Zetterberg H: Alzheimer's disease. Lancet 368:387–403, 2006

Boeve BF: A review of the non-Alzheimer dementias. J Clin Psychiatry 67:1985–2001, 2006

Borson S, Scanlan J, Brush M, et al: The Mini-Cog: a cognitive 'vital signs' measure for dementia: screening in multi-lingual elderly. Int J Geriatr Psychiatry 15:1021–1027, 2000

Carson S, McDonagh MS, Peterson K: A systematic review of the efficacy and safety of atypical antipsychotics in patients with psychological and behavioral symptoms of dementia. J Am Geriatr Soc 54:354–361, 2006

Coulson BS, Fenner SG, Almeida OP: Successful treatment of behavioral problems in dementia using a cholinesterase inhibitor: the ethical questions. Aust N Z J Psychiatry 36:259–262, 2002

Dubois B, Slachevsky A, Litvan I, et al: The FAB: a frontal assessment battery at bedside. Neurology 55:1621–1626, 2000

Engel GL, Romano J: Delirium, a syndrome of cerebral insufficiency. J Neuropsychiatry Clin Neurosci 16:526–538, 2004

Fick DM, Agostini JV, Inouye SK: Delirium superimposed on dementia: a systematic review. J Am Geriatr Soc 50:1723–1732, 2002

Folstein MF, Folstein SE, McHugh PR: "Mini-mental state": a practical method for grading the cognitive state of patients for the clinician. J Psychiatr Res 12:189–198, 1975

Inouye S, van Dyck C, Alessi C, et al: Clarifying confusion: the confusion assessment method. Ann Intern Med 113:941–948, 1990

Kertesz A, Munoz DG: Frontotemporal dementia. Med Clin North Am 86:501–518, 2002

Kile SJ, Bourgeois JA, Sugden S, et al: Neurobehavioral sequelae of traumatic brain injury. Applied Neurology 1:29–32, 2005

Lacasse H, Perreault MM, Williamson DR: Systematic review of antipsychotics for the treatment of hospital-associated delirium in medically or surgically ill patients. Ann Pharmacother 40:1966–1973, 2006

Leverenz JB, McKeith IG: Dementia with Lewy bodies. Med Clin North Am 86:519–535, 2002

Lyketsos CG, Lopez O, Jones B, et al: Prevalence of neuropsychiatric symptoms in dementia and mild cognitive impairment: results from the Cardiovascular Health Study. JAMA 288:1475–1483, 2002

Meagher DJ: Delirium: optimising management. BMJ 322:144–149, 2001

Mooney G, Speed J: The association between mild traumatic brain injury and psychiatric conditions. Brain Inj 15:865–877, 2001

Robert PH, Verhey FR, Byrne EJ, et al: Grouping for behavioral and psychological symptoms in dementia: clinical and biological aspects. Consensus paper of the European Alzheimer Disease Consortium. Eur Psychiatry 20:490–496, 2005

Román GC: Vascular dementia revisited: diagnosis, pathogenesis, treatment, and prevention. Med Clin North Am 86:477–499, 2002

Tune LE: Anticholinergic effects of medication in elderly patients. J Clin Psychiatry 62:11–14, 2001

Weber JB, Coverdale JH, Kunik ME: Delirium: current trends in prevention and treatment. Intern Med J 34:115–121, 2004

Suggested Readings

Blennow K, de Leon MJ, Zetterberg H: Alzheimer's disease. Lancet 368:387–403, 2006

Kile SJ, Bourgeois JA, Sugden S, et al: Neurobehavioral sequelae of traumatic brain injury. Applied Neurology 1:29–32, 2005

Lacasse H, Perreault MM, Williamson DR: Systematic review of antipsychotics for the treatment of hospital-associated delirium in medically or surgically ill patients. Ann Pharmacother 40:1966–1973, 2006

9

Substance-Related Psychiatric Emergencies

Iyad Alkhouri, M.D.

Patrick Gibbons, D.O., M.S.W.

Divy Ravindranath, M.D., M.S.

Kirk Brower, M.D.

Ms. P, a female in her 50s, had been brought into the emergency department with severe and persistent depression. She had been treated unsuccessfully for a few months. She presented with suicidal ideation, psychomotor retardation, and decline in functioning. Upon hospitalization, she had a drug screen, which showed positive for barbiturates. Ms. P admitted to purchasing barbiturates over the Internet for several years.

Ms. G, a 42-year-old married female with a history of alcohol dependence, was seen by her therapist for a routine follow-up appointment. She had been a patient of his for 2 years because of intermittent bouts of depression. At the visit, she was observed to be pressured and expansive, reportedly spending significant amounts of money on trivial purchases. She insisted on remaining naked at home and frequently complained that a neighbor was peeping at her, using a tree for cover. A drug screen was negative, and she was transferred to the emergency department for an evaluation of new-onset mania. In the emergency department, Ms. G admitted to consuming two 8-ounce bottles of cough syrup containing dextromethorphan daily for many years. She also reported a serious attempt to stop, and went through withdrawal featuring depression, low energy, nausea and vomiting, and repeated relapse.

Emergency departments around the country manage over 110 million visits annually (Centers for Disease Control 2005). In the emergency department, substance-related presentations constitute a substantial number of patient encounters (D'Onofrio et al. 1998a). Training in emergency psychiatry, therefore, must include a systematic review of substances, including potential toxicities and withdrawal syndromes. Knowledge about substances and their effects on psychiatric symptoms, as well as an understanding of the added risk of suicide for patients who are using substances, is also essential. For many patients with substance use disorder, the emergency department visit may be the first and/or only chance to find a path to treatment (Rockett et al. 2006).

In this chapter, we provide a review of substances of abuse in the emergency context to help the busy clinician work through a differential diagnosis of common "syndromes." For a more in-depth review of mechanistic issues and pharmacology and specific up-to-date treatment algorithms, the reader is referred to textbooks of emergency medicine, psychiatry, toxicology, and addictions (e.g., Glick et al. 2008).

Epidemiology, Prevalence, and Impact of Substance-Related Emergencies

Over 85,000 Americans lose their lives annually because of alcohol (Mokdad et al. 2004), and 25,000 die because of illicit drugs (Hoyert et al. 2006). A 2006 review of information obtained from emergency departments in 21 counties nationwide found that for patients visiting for substance use issues, 28% were for suicide-related reasons (with death in 0.2% of all patients) and 36% because of dependence on the drug in question. Of those taking one drug, 65% were seen for withdrawal symptoms and 35% for help with detoxification. When alcohol was involved, 30% of patients were intoxicated, 16% were in withdrawal, and 43% were injured (Substance Abuse and Mental Health Services Administration 2008).

Initial Evaluation of Patients

The key to diagnosis is a thorough history using available sources and performing a physical and psychiatric examination of the patient. All patients presenting to the psychiatric emergency department must be asked specifically about substances of abuse. Vigilant interviewers must inquire about the use and abuse of prescribed or over-the-counter drugs, as well as botanicals, nutritional supplements, and substances obtained over the Internet. Physical examination may reveal signs of drug use, such as track marks over veins.

The physical examination should be followed by the appropriate laboratory and imaging studies. Elevated liver enzymes, for example, may raise suspicion of substance abuse. It is important to rule out commonly encountered substance-related medical complications, such as subdural hematoma in alcohol intoxication, cerebral vascular accident or myocardial infarction in cocaine abuse, and severe lung injury and rhabdomyolysis in opioid intoxication.

Except in unusual circumstances, most intoxication and withdrawal symptoms are relatively easy to manage (Mayo-Smith 1997). The clinician should be aware of some variables that can predict a difficult course. In general, withdrawal and intoxication syndromes are more complex in medically compromised patients. Management is particularly problematic with specific substance–medical condition combinations, such as heart disease with cocaine abuse, alcohol dependence with seizure disorder, and opioid or sedative-hypnotic dependence with chronic obstructive pulmonary disease or sleep apnea.

Whenever possible, patients should be approached about drug screening in a matter-of-fact manner and in the spirit of helping. If a urine sample can be obtained with the patient's cooperation, then bladder catheterization can be avoided. In a true medical emergency situation, it is not necessary to obtain the patient's consent for a drug screen.

Urine drug detection tests commonly use enzyme-linked immunosorbent assay (ELISA) technology, in which an antibody contained in the test strip recognizes the structure of a specific molecule and binds to it to produce a color change. The practical constraints of this technology include a limited number of substances that can be tested, false positives due to cross-reactivity, and false negatives due to either nonspecificity for the substance present or substance concentration below the detection threshold.

Serum toxicology, often using gas chromatography–mass spectrometry, can be helpful in multidrug overdose and for some psychotropic medications (tricyclic antidepressants, lithium) but may require hours to days for the result, depending on the drugs tested and laboratory availability. This test should be reserved for situations in which certain results are essential, in which a positive finding is contested, or with a forensic interest. Drug screening results should be interpreted within the context of the overall presentation and not be considered a definitive diagnostic tool. The clinician should become familiar with the hospital laboratory cutoff values and with the drugs that are on the detection panel.

When collecting urine for a drug screen, one should take precautions to minimize manipulation of the sample, although manipulation tends to be infrequent in the emergency department because the required planning on the part of the patient is usually not possible in an emergency. Regardless, personal items should never be carried into the bathroom where a sample is being collected. The proximity of a same-sex staff member might be indicated for monitoring, particularly with adolescents. Adding blue food dye to the toilet bowl minimizes the chance that a patient will dilute the sample.

Syndromes of Substance-Related Emergencies

Substance-related emergency presentations can be divided in several ways. In the following subsections, we consider those that decrease, or depress, levels of consciousness, as in Ms. P, versus those that increase psychomotor activity and cause agitation, as in Ms. G (the cases described at the beginning of the chapter). One could also examine these syndromes by category of drug ingested, or by intoxication versus withdrawal syndrome. The key for the emergency clinician is maintaining a high level of suspicion and recognizing the patient's behavior as a syndrome of intoxication or withdrawal.

The Neurophysiologically Depressed Patient

Neurophysiologically depressed patients are those whose mental status and physiological states are mostly manifested by "slowness" or "depression" in the broad sense. This category refers not only to patients who are acutely sedated, lethargic, or even comatose, but also to those whose history suggests a recent downward trend in mental status. The common substance-related manifestations of depressed function are intoxication with central nervous system (CNS) depressants or withdrawal of CNS stimulants.

The most commonly abused CNS depressants are alcohol, barbiturates, benzodiazepines and analogs (BZDs), other sedatives-hypnotics, and opioids. Over-the-counter medications such as antihistamines, decongestants, dextromethorphan (cough suppressant), and inhalants are frequently abused by adolescents.

Alcohol Intoxication

Alcohol intoxication is the most common cause of substance-related emergency presentations. Some studies have shown that up to 40% of emergency department patients have alcohol detected in their blood. Alcohol acts by increasing the responsivity of gamma-aminobutyric acid (GABA) type A receptors to GABA and inhibiting the effects of glutamate at some of its receptors. The onset of intoxication may be experienced as disinhibition, which can result in agitation, combativeness, and, in rare cases, psychosis. Intoxication results in an overall depression of CNS function, with a dose-dependent decrease in motor control, diminished coordination, slurred speech, ataxia, and finally respiratory depression and coma. Very high blood alcohol levels (BALs) can cause a lethal respiratory arrest (e.g., BAL>400 mg/dL in nontolerant individuals). Alcohol will usually cause vascular dilation, hypothermia, and lowered blood pressure with reflexive tachycardia. Although alcohol intoxication is easy to diagnose, some coma presentations (i.e., hyperglycemic coma with ketosis) can mimic it.

Treatment of alcohol intoxication is supportive (Reoux and Miller 2000). Gastric lavage is not useful because alcohol is rapidly absorbed from the gastrointestinal tract. Toxic levels should be monitored serially for an expected gradual drop. Chronic alcoholics may metabolize ethanol at a rate of 15–20 mg/dL per hour, which in addition to intravenous fluids, thiamine, and correction of hypoglycemia, gradually results in decreasing signs of intoxication over a few hours. If this does not occur, the clinician should consider other explanations for alteration in consciousness, including other toxins, metabolic dysfunction, or subdural hematoma, which can present without any external evidence of trauma.

Alcohol is frequently consumed in overdoses with other substances. For example, tricyclic antidepressants not only enhance the CNS depression of alcohol but also delay its metabolism (Kerr et al. 2001). Concomitant use of cocaine can result in a metabolite (cocaethylene) with 3–5 times the half-life of cocaine, increasing the risk of sudden death up to 20 times compared with when cocaine is used alone (Farré et al. 1997).

When alcohol is consumed in the presence of disulfiram, the history is obvious unless the patient was unaware that what had been consumed contained alcohol (Fuller et al. 1986). For example, so-called nonalcoholic beers still contain sufficient alcohol to precipitate a disulfiram reaction. Symptoms are attributable to an accumulation of acetaldehyde, with intense flushing, chest pain/pressure, tachycardia, nausea/vomiting, and weakness. The combination can be life threatening in patients with serious underlying cardiac disease.

Benzodiazepine and Other Sedative-Hypnotic Toxicity

Benzodiazepine and other sedative-hypnotic toxicity develops not only in acute overdose but also in less obvious circumstances, such as when patients exceed their scheduled doses or when other CNS depressants (alcohol, opioids, or over-the-counter drugs) are used concomitantly. Accumulation can also result when BZDs are injected intramuscularly or when metabolism of mainly "oxidized" BZDs is affected by liver compromise, advanced age, or drug interactions, resulting in accumulation of active metabolites (D'Onofrio et al. 1999). Temazepam, oxazepam, triazolam, alprazolam, and lorazepam are metabolized primarily by conjugation (glucuronidation), making them less likely to accumulate in patients with liver impairment.

BZDs exhibit dose-dependent effects on coordination, memory, and cognitive functioning. BZDs affect level of consciousness, leading to somnolence and, in the extreme case or in combination with other toxins, to coma. In some instances, paradoxical agitation and excitement can occur, but this is a manifestation of drug-induced disinhibition plus external "stimulating" factors. Gastrointestinal symptoms, such vomiting, diarrhea, and urinary incontinence, can occur and tend to differentiate BZD toxicity from opioid toxicity, which is associated with urinary retention and not with diarrhea.

Flumazenil given intravenously in doses not to exceed 1 mg acts quickly to reverse the effects of BZDs. However, it should be administered with great caution to patients known to be physiologically dependent on BZDs because of the likelihood of precipitating seizures.

BZDs are rarely lethal by themselves but can be lethal due to synergism with other respiratory depressants, especially alcohol, barbiturates, or opioids. BZDs can also worsen ventilation in patients who have preexisting serious underlying cardiorespiratory problems such as sleep apnea, chronic obstructive pulmonary disease, or congestive heart failure.

The clinician should maintain a high index of suspicion for concomitant BZD use in patients with a history of alcohol misuse, because these patients are highly susceptible to cross-dependence. Patients dependent on methadone or other opioids also misuse BZDs, as do cocaine users, who value BZDs to medicate postcocaine jitteriness.

In a young individual (especially female) taken ill in proximity to attending a party or a club gathering, particular consideration should be given to possible unknowing exposure to gamma-hydroxybutyrate or flunitrazepam, so-called date rape drugs. These drugs can be lethal, particularly in combination with alcohol. Toxicity with these agents can be differentiated from other depressant toxicity by "sudden" awakening, myoclonus, hypothermia, fecal and urinary incontinence, and bradycardia. The coma induced by these substances is attended by episodic agitation upon stimulation. The main interventions are vigorous supportive care and monitoring for bradycardia, which is generally responsive to intravenously administered atropine (Robert et al. 2001).

Barbiturate use is consistently declining but remains among the most important causes of poisoning in the United States (Bronstein et al. 2007), and about 50% of these cases are due to intentional overdose. Barbiturate toxicity is more likely than BZD toxicity to cause coma and cardiac effects. Barbiturates are more lethal than BZDs when taken as single agents due to respiratory depression, particularly if the dose is more than 10 times the hypnotic dose. Pupil size, blood pressure, nystagmus, and reflexes are variable, but with serious poisoning, most patients develop hypothermia, apnea, and shock. A distinctive feature is the relative preservation of protective reflexes, such as sneezing and coughing, despite obvious respiratory depression. Treatment is supportive, including warming for hypothermia, volume expansion for cardiovascular shock, and mechanical ventilation for apnea. Removal of drug can be hastened with alkalinization of the urine and diuresis. CNS stimulants, flumazenil, and naloxone are not effective (Wilensky et al. 1982).

Opioid Toxicity

Opioid toxicity is readily recognizable by the feature of miosis in the presence of CNS and respiratory depression. This feature is persistent unless overdose results in significant hypoxia, in which case pupil dilation is possible. However, not all opioids cause significant miosis, and normal to even enlarged pupils have been reported with use of propoxyphene, meperidine, morphine, and pentazocine, in part due to the anticholinergic properties of some of these agents (Estfan et al. 2005). In intoxication, patients are minimally responsive or nonresponsive to physical stimulation and have slow, shallow respiration. Gastrointestinal sounds are absent, and urinary retention is common.

Opioids can be especially dangerous in combination with other medications, such as monoamine oxidase inhibitors. Also, prescription opioid formulations are frequently combined with acetaminophen or nonsteroidal anti-inflammatory drugs (NSAIDs). Therefore, toxicity in intoxication or overdose may come from these agents as well.

Naloxone is a specific antidote for opioid toxicity. It should be used with caution in patients known to be opioid dependent because it can precipitate full-blown withdrawal, resulting in acute agitation, confusion, or combativeness. Relatively high doses might be needed to treat long-acting oxycodone toxicity (Schneir et al. 2002), and repeated doses may be necessary due naloxone's short half-life.

Over-the-Counter Cough and Cold Medications

Over-the-counter cough and cold medicines are frequently abused by adolescents and may contain mixtures of various antihistamines, sympathomimetics with or without dextromethorphan, and acetaminophen. They are used alone or in combination specifically to produce a mood change ("high") and to self-manage detoxification. They are difficult to detect in urine, but the presence of amphetamine analogs such as pseudoephedrine may screen positive for amphetamine.

Inhalant Intoxication

Inhalants include a wide variety of aliphatic, aromatic, and halogenated hydrocarbons, including toxic solvents, causing an initial stage of disinhibition, excitement, or sense of drunkenness. (Anesthetic gases [e.g., nitrous oxide] and short-acting vasodilators [e.g., amyl nitrite] are classified separately from inhalants in DSM-IV-TR [American Psychiatric Association 2000].) With mounting inhaled concentrations, the picture changes to restlessness, then decreased consciousness and ataxia, after which coma, respiratory depression, and death may occur. Acute hazards include myocardial sensitization to epinephrine, with risk of arrhythmias, possible hepatic injury, and longer-term effects on cognition and concentration.

CNS Stimulant Withdrawal

CNS "depression" that seems to have evolved subacutely can also be a manifestation of CNS stimulant withdrawal (e.g., the cocaine "crash"). The hallmark of withdrawal from CNS stimulants is severe depression that may be accompanied by suicidal ideation, dysphoria, and sleep disturbance, along with severe drug craving. Increased appetite may also be observed as a rebound effect to the appetite-suppressant effects of stimulants.

The Agitated, Aggressive, and Psychotic Patient

The range of agitated behavior in the emergency department is rather wide, spanning from belligerence to physical aggression, at times complicated by full-blown psychosis. These problems can represent CNS stimulation or activation and can be caused by withdrawal from CNS depressants or intoxication with prescription or illicit stimulants or phencyclidine (McCarron et al. 1981). Paradoxical excitement can also be caused by intoxication with alcohol, sedative-hypnotics, and inhalants.

Alcohol Withdrawal

Alcohol withdrawal is the most common presentation in this category and may be complicated both by the possibility of high blood alcohol levels and by concomitant stimulant use or simultaneous withdrawal from another substance. Combativeness and aggression can be seen in both alcohol intoxication and withdrawal, yet the typical return of stability in a severely intoxicated alcohol-dependent patient as the BAL normalizes is a familiar picture to those working in the emergency department.

The BAL at which withdrawal appears varies from patient to patient and can begin in as little as 6 hours from the last drink in chronic alcoholics. The withdrawal syndrome is characterized by autonomic instability with elevated blood pressure, tachycardia, and profuse sweating; gastrointestinal symptoms with nausea, vomiting, and diarrhea; and CNS activation with anxiety and tremor. Hallucinations and seizures, typically single grand mal events, can herald more serious withdrawal complications. After 48–72 hours, about 5% of patients in alcohol withdrawal will develop a syndrome known as delirium tremens (DTs), which includes hallucinations (usually visual), delirium, and severe autonomic instability. Early, aggressive treatment of emerging alcohol withdrawal can prevent progression to DTs, which can be lethal in 5%–10% of patients despite treatment and in 20%–35% without treatment. Consumption of large quantities of alcohol, concomitant medical illness such as pneumonia, and a history of DTs increase the risk that a patient will enter into DTs during the course of withdrawal (Ferguson et al. 1996).

The optimal strategy for treating alcohol withdrawal is substituting a physiologically equivalent agent, such as BZD, that has a longer half-life, and then gradually tapering it off. This avoids an abrupt shift in equilibrium from the compensated intoxicated state to the uncompensated abstinent state. Even shorter-acting BZDs, such as lorazepam (1–2 mg iv or po every 1–2 hours), can be titrated to produce a mild state of sedation. Longer-acting BZDs, such as chlordiazepoxide, have the advantage of being self-tapering but may also accumulate in the presence of significant liver impairment (Greenblatt et al. 1978). BZD accumulation may, in turn, lead to a delirium that can be indistinguishable from the original presentation.

The use of antipsychotic medications, usually with low or no anticholinergic activity (e.g., haloperidol), can be used for severe hallucinations not responding to BZDs or for severe aggression and agitation. Central α_2 adrenergic agonists such as clonidine or a beta-blocker such as metoprolol can be used for hypertension or tachycardia if autonomic symptoms are prominent. All these medications are capable of causing toxicity (Battaglia et al. 1997). Given the potential lethality of alcohol withdrawal, caution should be exercised to avoid overmedication but not to the point of risking undertreatment.

The common practice of hydrating patients and providing them with thiamine and folic acid has helped to decrease long-term functional and neurological consequences of alcohol dependence, such as Wernicke's encephalopathy and Wernicke-Korsakoff syndrome. Hence, they continue to be essential in the treatment.

Sedative-Hypnotic Withdrawal

Sedative-hypnotic (e.g., BZD) withdrawal occurs within the first few hours to days after discontinuation of a GABAergic sedative-hypnotic agent following a period of regular use. Phenomenologically, withdrawal is very similar to that produced by alcohol withdrawal except that it can be extended over days to weeks (instead of hours to days), depending on the sedative-hypnotic's half-life. Patients may initially identify themselves as experiencing a withdrawal reaction with mostly or all subjective complaints, particularly if they are using BZDs chronically. Depending on the drug used, physiological symptoms may not be evident for several days. The syndrome may progress from this anxious prodrome to include tremor, tachycardia, hypertension, diaphoresis, gastrointestinal upset, mydriasis, sleep disturbance and nightmares, tinnitus, and increased sensitivity to sound, light, and sometimes tactile stimulation. Confusion or frank delirium can develop along with hyperthermia if the reaction is severe. CNS irritability may progress to generalized tonic-clonic seizures, which can appear up to 2 weeks following the last dose. With severe withdrawal, delirium and seizures tend to occur more frequently than with alcohol, and once the syndrome is actively evolving, it can be difficult to restore CNS equilibrium despite large doses of sedatives.

Significant anxiety, sleep disturbance, and mild to moderate autonomic symptoms can occur with abrupt discontinuation of long-term therapeutic doses. These symptoms may persist at some level for many months, and can be indistinguishable from disabling generalized anxiety or panic symptoms. Because of these features, it is rarely if ever a good strategy to abruptly stop these agents after a long period of use at therapeutic doses of sedative-hypnotics such as benzodiazepines.

Optimal management includes transition to an agent with a long half-life for stabilization, followed by very gradual taper as tolerated. Carbamazepine also has evidence to support its use in attenuation of protracted BZD withdrawal symptoms. Oxcarbazepine is less supported by evidence but has the advantage of being relatively nontoxic. Adjunctive treatment of protracted withdrawal symptoms with beta-blockers such as propranolol has also been modestly helpful in some patients.

Opioid Withdrawal

Opioid withdrawal is a distinctive entity with typical signs and symptoms that rarely cause changes in mental status (except for marked anxiety), including the presence of pupillary dilation, lacrimation, rhinorrhea, diaphoresis, piloerection, arthralgia/myalgias (hyperalgesia and aches), diarrhea, yawning, and serious drug craving/drug seeking.

Withdrawal is heralded by anxiety, craving/preoccupation, and vague discomfort (hyperalgesia). With short-acting agents, such as heroin, this begins within 6–18 hours after the last dose and is followed by a period of increasing withdrawal symptoms. The syndrome reaches a peak at 2–4 days, followed by rapid resolution. Symptoms are usually minimal to absent after 7–10 days. Significant withdrawal from long-acting agents, such as methadone or buprenorphine, may not emerge for 1–3 days. This withdrawal syndrome includes anxiety that can amplify the physical experience of withdrawal, so patient education and reassurance may be useful in moderating symptom intensity.

Although not life threatening in an otherwise healthy patient, opioid withdrawal can be lethal in the presence of significant medical compromise, such as recent myocardial infarction, diabetes, or congestive heart failure. Symptomatic treatment of withdrawal is appropriate because it is neither therapeutic nor humane to insist that an addict quit "cold turkey." Effective symptom relief promotes an alliance, thus opening a window for engagement in the treatment of a condition having wide-ranging morbidity and high mortality.

Buprenorphine, which is a partial agonist for μ-opioid receptors with high affinity, will effectively and quickly treat acute withdrawal from any opioid agent and can be continued as a maintenance drug, except in patients receiving methadone maintenance treatment of more than 30 mg/day. Because it acts as a partial agonist in comparison with other opioids, buprenorphine can precipitate acute withdrawal if given to an opioid addict who is not already in withdrawal. Given sublingually, buprenorphine can generate rapid and dramatic relief. However, the Drug Addiction Treatment Act of 2000 (P.L. 106-310) requires that patients receiving this drug for maintenance of sobriety receive the prescription from a provider with special training and also be enrolled in psychosocial treatment for opioid dependence. Lack of follow-up can limit its use after discharge from the emergency department (Brigham et al. 2007).

Other medications are useful for symptomatic relief to varying degrees, but none is as effective as an opioid. Clonidine, a central α_2 agonist, reduces sympathetic outflow at the locus coeruleus and spinal cord level and can attenuate some symptoms. NSAIDs can help with myalgias. Loperamide is useful for diarrhea. Sedating neuroleptics such as quetiapine are sometimes used for anxiety and restlessness, and trazodone at bedtime can aid sleep; however, some substance-dependent patients dislike the effects of either or both. BZDs or other controlled sedative hypnotics should be used with great caution or not at all because they are readily abusable, cause cross-dependence, interact with opioids, and tend to be difficult to discontinue once started in these patients.

CNS Stimulant Intoxication

CNS stimulants, such as amphetamines, sympathomimetics, cocaine, and so-called stimulant-hallucinogens such as 3,4-methylenedioxymethamphetamine (MDMA, commonly known as Ecstasy), cause a variety of symptoms, mostly varying in magnitude and duration as a function of potency, dose, and the user's susceptibility to the drug effect. Other symptoms of intoxication that are more specific to the particular agent may occur, such as mild psychedelic effects with MDMA and formication (i.e., the sensation of bugs crawling under the skin), particularly with cocaine and methamphetamine intoxication.

Physical signs of catecholamine excess include tachycardia, tachypnea, hypertension, mydriasis, myoclonus, hyperreflexia, tremor, movement disorders, nausea and vomiting, possible seizures, increased respiratory rate, and hyperthermia. The distinctive presence of these signs can help differentiate between drug-related toxicity and primary psychotic states.

When psychotic content occurs, it is frequently confined to paranoid delusions. Hallucinations, if they occur, are typically tactile (i.e., formication) or visual (e.g., simple geometric patterns or shapes). Evidence of a formal thought disorder or severe, bizarre delusions is rare. The history and time course of psychiatric symptomatology can be helpful in distinguishing substance-induced versus primary psychiatric presentations, because substance-induced symptoms can appear abruptly and resolve quickly (i.e., within days). Substance users may be less likely to have a family history of psychosis and frequently have no significant prodromal symptoms. With a patient presenting with psychotic-like symptoms, the clinician should explore the patient's insight around what is happening. Substance users are typically but not always aware of the effects of their drug use on their perception, and lack of insight is a typical feature of primary psychosis. The results of a drug screen can influence the clinician's suspicion that a psychosis is a result of a substance.

Stimulant toxicity can be fatal in severe cases, often from cardiovascular or cerebrovascular causes. When a patient has a neurological deficit, rapid imaging to rule out possible intracranial lesion or bleeding is essential. When a patient has chest pain, myocardial infarction needs to be ruled out.

Symptoms and signs of CNS stimulant toxicity can initially be masked by the concomitant use of CNS depressants, and may become clearer over time when one class of substance is eliminated from the body.

Sedation with a BZD is an appropriate initial intervention for CNS stimulant intoxication. Sedation with BZDs can help with seizures and confers some protection against the toxic effects of cocaine. To provide sedation in paranoid states, BZDs are preferable to neuroleptics, which are usually contraindicated due to the potential for lowering the seizure threshold, precipitating disturbances in cardiac rhythm, and increasing the risk of hyperthermia due to their anticholinergic effects.

For stimulant-induced tachycardia and hypertension, beta-blockers should never be used. They tend to produce unopposed α-adrenergic effects.

Physical restraints should be avoided if at all possible. Adequate sedation is usually sufficient to have a "peaceful" course in the emergency department.

Hallucinogen Intoxication

Physical symptoms resulting from the use of hallucinogens may include changes in body temperature, seizures (which may be resistant to treatment unless hyperthermia is treated), and psychosis that is typically accompanied with a relatively preserved insight. Anxiety symptoms may be prominent with "bad trips" and include panicky feelings and fear of losing one's mind. The management of these reactions is similar to those used for stimulant-induced psychiatric states, where minimization of stimulation and the presence of calm, reassuring personnel are helpful. Exploration of a previous similar experience with hallucinogens that resolved later can be helpful both to reassure the patient and promote reality testing.

Marijuana Intoxication

A common presentation in chronic high-dose marijuana users is the experience of hypervigilance and depersonalization/derealization. The presence of conjunctival injection, orthostatic hypotension, dry mouth, and increased heart rate can help differentiate marijuana-related presentations from other causes of psychiatric symptomatology. The frequent use of marijuana in a patient having known psychiatric illness can cause a dramatic exacerbation of symptoms and may be a factor in poor response to medication management.

The Drug-Seeking Patient

The types of substances patients seek during emergency department visits range from BZDs for "anxiety" and opioids for the treatment of pain (often out of proportion to objective findings) to medicines for which the patient says the prescription was "lost" (usually on the weekend or after pharmacy hours). To obtain painkillers, some patients have mimicked kidney stones by adding a drop of blood from a finger prick to their urine.

A clinician should suspect drug-seeking behavior when a patient is specific about what medication he or she needs, stating that the provider is not immediately available, or claims to be allergic to a list of alternate medications that might otherwise treat the symptoms. If available, a statewide audit register, such as the Michigan Automated Prescription System, can help identify a patient's prescription-filling habits by generating a record of all controlled substance prescriptions filled under that patient's identification within a 12-month period. This can be helpful in identifying drug-seeking behavior but may not be available in a timely manner.

Drug-seeking behavior may represent either 1) treatment seeking for a legitimate, medical disorder or 2) drug seeking to maintain an addiction. Although addiction is also a legitimate medical disorder, it requires a very different approach to treatment. Discerning the difference between treatment seeking for a nonaddiction disorder and drug seeking to maintain an addiction is not always easy. Even patients with legitimate pain, for example, may sometimes use pain medicine for emotional reasons. It is not unusual for those patients to ask for higher doses in a demanding or hostile manner. A patient who is anxious and depressed might be so fearful of receiving a reduced pain medication dosage that he or she will never report a pain score lower than 5–6.

Guiding Patients With Substance Use Disorders to Make a Change

Motivational interviewing is more a manner of approaching the patient than a specific technique. The essential feature is that the patient's own perceptions are used as a platform on which to build a treatment approach. Behavioral and attitudinal change in this model is approached as a goal that has meaning for the patient (Longabaugh et al. 2001).

The following are essential elements:

- Understanding the patient's views of his or her situation, especially by the use of reflective listening statements
- Affirming and accepting the patient as the overriding tone of the conversation
- Eliciting and selectively reinforcing the patient's own descriptive statements of problem recognition, concern, desire to change, benefit to self through change, and so on
- Having patience and allowing the patient to come to the awareness of a problem, rather than telling, diagnosing, or describing a problem to the patient, which is likely to elicit resistance
- Affirming the patient's freedom to choose not only the problem(s) identified, and the associated consequence(s), but also the treatment (requiring reflection on the outcome)

An excellent review of these techniques is provided by Miller and Rollnick (2002).

Disposition Issues

A working knowledge of recovery resources available for patients with substance use disorders and their families is essential for the clinician to take advantage of the window for intervention that the emergency encounter can produce. These resources might include social service agencies, child or adult protective services, charities within the community, shelters, and institutionalized treatment programs providing various levels of care. Local directories of Alcoholics Anonymous, Narcotics Anonymous, and Al-Anon meetings are helpful. Larger Alcoholics Anonymous communities coordinate service groups that can arrange for members to visit with the alcohol-dependent individual to share the experience of recovery (a "Twelfth-step call") (D'Onofrio et al. 1998b). Resource options are discussed further in Chapter 13.

One of the greatest challenges faced by emergency psychiatrists is the disposition of the patient who voices suicidal ideation while intoxicated (Rothschild 1997). While sober, these patients often deny any thoughts of self-harm, yet the fact that they abuse substances adds to the risk that they will indeed take their own life. Even if the evaluating psychiatrist is worried about the patient's safety, hospitalization may be difficult to arrange if the patient denies thoughts or plans for self-harm. The emergency evaluator must consider the patient's entire life situation in deciding whether it is safe to discharge the patient: Has the patient lost all social supports, employment, or housing? Does the patient have a concomitant psychiatric diagnosis? Is the patient at all hopeful? Is the patient able to articulate plans for the future, or does the patient seem helpless to figure out ways to help himself or herself? Has the patient attempted suicide before? If prior attempts have occurred, was the patient intoxicated at that time? Does the patient have a safety plan that includes staying sober? Is this plan realistic? Who can support the patient with this plan? For more information, the reader should see Chapter 2, "The Suicidal Patient."

Key Clinical Points

- Familiarity with acute presentations related to substance use disorders is an essential component of training in emergency psychiatry. Such training should include the general management of acute changes in behaviors, along with medical knowledge of complications of the habitual or occasional use of substances of abuse.

- In the initial evaluation, acute life support issues should be ensured, and a working diagnosis of major intoxication or withdrawal states can be made, with a decision regarding the appropriateness of treatment in a general emergency department, where medical equipment and expertise are immediately available, or in a psychiatric emergency department, where expertise can focus on behavioral management and use of psychotropic drugs and/or seclusion.

- The judicial use of antidotes or detoxification agents as indicated for intoxication and aspects of withdrawal should then be followed by an assessment of the patient and determination of further disposition.

- Psychiatric emergency personnel should be familiar with community resources for substance use disorders.

- Psychiatric emergency staff should help patients begin the path to recovery.

- Safety issues for patients, family, and staff are paramount throughout the course of diagnosis, evaluation, and management.

References

American Psychiatric Association: Diagnostic and Statistical Manual of Mental Disorders, 4th Edition, Text Revision. Washington, DC, American Psychiatric Association, 2000

Battaglia J, Moss S, Rush J, et al: Haloperidol, lorazepam, or both for psychotic agitation? A multicenter, prospective, double-blind, emergency department study. Am J Emerg Med 15:335–340, 1997

Brigham GS, Amass L, Winhusen T, et al: Using buprenorphine short-term taper to facilitate early treatment engagement. J Subst Abuse Treat 32:349–356, 2007

Bronstein AC, Spyker DA, Cantilena LR, et al: 2006 Annual Report of the American Association of Poison Control Centers' National Poison Data System (NPDS). Clin Toxicol (Phila) 45:815–917, 2007

Centers for Disease Control, Division of Health Care Statistics: National Hospital Ambulatory Medical Care Survey: 2003 emergency department summary. May 26, 2005. Available at: http://www.cdc.gov/nchs/data/ad/ad358.pdf. Accessed October 5, 2009.

D'Onofrio G, Bernstein E, Bernstein J, et al: Patients with alcohol problems in the emergency department, part 1: improving detection. SAEM Substance Abuse Task Force. Society for Academic Emergency Medicine. Acad Emerg Med 5:1200–1209, 1998a

D'Onofrio G, Bernstein E, Bernstein J, et al: Patients with alcohol problems in the emergency department, part 2: intervention and referral. SAEM Substance Abuse Task Force. Society for Academic Emergency Medicine. Acad Emerg Med 5:1210–1217, 1998b

D'Onofrio G, Rathlev NK, Ulrich AS, et al: Lorazepam for the prevention of recurrent seizures related to alcohol. N Engl J Med 340:915–919, 1999

Drug Addiction Treatment Act of 2000, Pub. L. No. 106-310, sec. 3501, 21 USC 801

Estfan B, Yavuzsen T, Davis M: Development of opioid-induced delirium while on olanzapine: a two-case report. J Pain Symptom Manage 29:330–332, 2005

Farré M, De La Torre R, González ML, et al: Cocaine and alcohol interactions in humans: neuroendocrine effects and cocaethylene metabolism. J Pharmacol Exp Ther 283:164–176, 1997

Ferguson JA, Suelzer CJ, Eckert GJ, et al: Risk factors for delirium tremens development. J Gen Intern Med 11:410–414, 1996

Fuller RK, Branchey L, Brightwell DR, et al: Disulfiram treatment of alcoholism: a Veterans Administration cooperative study. JAMA 256:1449–1455, 1986

Glick RL, Berlin JS, Fishkind AV, et al: Emergency Psychiatry: Principles and Practice. Philadelphia, PA, Lippincott Williams & Wilkins, 2008

Greenblatt DJ, Shader RI, MacLeon SM, et al: Clinical pharmacokinetics of chlordiazepoxide. Clin Pharmacokinet 3:381–394, 1978

Hoyert DL, Heron MP, Murphy SL, et al: Deaths: final data for 2003. Natl Vital Stat Rep 54(13):1–120, 2006

Kerr GW, McGuffie AC, Wilkie S: Tricyclic antidepressant overdose: a review. Emerg Med J 18:236–224, 2001

Longabaugh R, Woolard RF, Nirenberg TD, et al: Evaluating the effects of a brief motivational intervention for injured drinkers in the emergency department. J Stud Alcohol 62:806–819, 2001

Mayo-Smith MF: Pharmacological management of alcohol withdrawal: a meta-analysis and evidence-based practice guideline. American Society of Addiction Medicine Working Group on Pharmacological Management of Alcohol Withdrawal. JAMA 278:144–151, 1997

McCarron MM, Schulze BW, Thompson GA, et al: Acute phencyclidine intoxication: incidence of clinical findings in 1,000 cases. Ann Emerg Med 10:237–242, 1981

Miller WR, Rollnick S: Motivational Interviewing: Preparing People for Change. New York, Guilford, 2002

Mokdad AH, Marks JS, Stroup DF, et al: Actual causes of death in the United States, 2000. JAMA 291:1238–1245, 2004

Reoux JP, Miller K: Routine hospital alcohol detoxification practice compared to symptom triggered management with an objective withdrawal scale (CIWA–Ar). Am J Addict 9:135–144, 2000

Robert R, Eugène M, Frat JP, et al: Diagnosis of unsuspected gamma hydroxyl-butyrate poisoning by proton NMR. J Toxicol Clin Toxicol 39:653–654, 2001

Rockett IRH, Putnam SL, Jia H, et al: Declared and undeclared substance use among emergency department patients: a population-based study. Addiction 101:706–712, 2006

Rothschild AJ: Suicide risk assessment, in Acute Care Psychiatry: Diagnosis and Treatment. Edited by Sederer LI, Rothschild AJ. Baltimore, MD, Williams & Wilkins, 1997, pp 15–28

Schneir AB, Vadeboncoeur TF, Offerman SR, et al: Massive OxyContin ingestion refractory to naloxone therapy. Ann Emerg Med 40:425–428, 2002

Substance Abuse and Mental Health Services Administration, Office of Applied Studies: Drug Abuse Warning Network, 2006: National Estimates of Drug-Related Emergency Department Visits (DAWN Series D-30; DHHS Publ No [SMA] 08-4339). Rockville, MD, Substance Abuse and Mental Health Services Administration, 2008

Wilensky AJ, Friel PN, Levy RH, et al: Kinetics of phenobarbital in normal subjects and epileptic patients. Eur J Clin Pharmacol 23:87–92, 1982

Suggested Readings

Hawkins SC, Smeeks F, Hamel J: Emergency management of chronic pain and drug-seeking behavior: an alternate perspective. J Emerg Med 34:125–129, 2008

Moeller KE, Lee KC, Kissack JC: Urine drug screening: a practical guide for clinicians. Mayo Clin Proc 83:66–76, 2008; erratum in Mayo Clin Proc 83:851, 2008

Rockett IR, Putnam SL, Jia H, et al: Declared and undeclared substance use among emergency department patients: a population-based study. Addiction 101:706–712, 2006

Schanzer BM, First MB, Dominguez B, et al: Diagnosing psychotic disorders in the emergency department in the context of substance use. Psychiatr Serv 57:1468–1473, 2006

10

Child and Adolescent Emergency Psychiatry

B. Harrison Levine, M.D., M.P.H.

Julia E. Najara, M.D.

Ms. Q is a 16-year-old girl with a diagnosis of bipolar disorder NOS (not otherwise specified) and has been taking sertraline and aripiprazole. Her mother has brought her into the emergency department for suspected suicidal ideation. Ms. Q told her mother that she wanted to kill herself after a fight between the two of them. Per the patient's mother, the patient subsequently locked herself in her room, where her medications are kept. When she finally let her mother in, she appeared fatigued, as if she had taken a few tablets of aripiprazole. Given the reported desire to kill herself, the patient's mother is very concerned that this was a suicide attempt and requests that the patient be hospitalized. The patient endorses moderate improvement in her depression since starting her medications and affirms the fight, but denies all suicidal ideation or attempts.

In a summary of statistics for pediatric psychiatric visits to U.S. emergency departments between 1993 and 1999, Sills and Bland (2002) reported that a relatively stable number of patients ages 18 years and younger were seen for psychotic symptoms and suicide attempts or self-injury, but that an increase occurred in the number of nonurgent complaints. These complaints included substance-related disorders, anxiety disorders, and attention-deficit and disruptive behavior disorders, as described in DSM-IV-TR (American Psychiatric Association 2000). No significant change has occurred in the delivery of mental health care in the outpatient setting to offset this long-term rising trend in overutilization of the emergency department for disruptive behavioral issues. Consequently, the emergency department clinician is more likely to be asked to evaluate children and adolescents with seemingly less acute symptoms in addition to the steady number of more severe psychiatric complaints, such as suicidal ideation, as in the case of Ms. Q. This chapter focuses on the approach to and treatment of these patients.

Goldstein et al. (2005) note that children and adolescents present with psychiatric emergencies according to the academic calendar, suggesting that school stressors may be significant sources of stress or may exacerbate underlying premorbid psychiatric conditions in the child or adolescent. Fewer young children may present to psychiatric emergency services during summer months, whereas adolescents, who by nature of their age and the natural development of more serious psychiatric disorders, will present year-round.

Children and adolescents who present repeatedly to psychiatric emergency services were found to have diagnoses that include adjustment, conduct, or oppositional disorder, and to be under the care of a child welfare agency. Additionally, these patients were more likely to be noncompliant with treatment and outpatient follow-up, to be admitted to the hospital more frequently, to demonstrate need for additional social services, and to be unmanageable in residential treatment facilities where, for a variety of reasons, they were unable to remain (Cole et al. 1991).

Basics

In approaching the patient, the clinician needs to keep in mind that a child or adolescent is by definition a minor and should not be unaccompanied, so there will necessarily be collateral informants from whom to obtain history. Often, especially during standard working hours, collateral information must also be obtained from agencies or institutions that are stakeholders in the welfare of the child, such as the child's school, teachers, treating clinicians, foster agencies, or child protective services.

The mental status categories remain fairly consistent across the age span, although child psychiatrists may use somewhat different labels and, particularly with young children, rely more on observation of the child's spontaneously emitted behavior in interactions with people (parents and/or examiner) and play materials, as well as with materials specifically designed to facilitate the assessment of developmental level, such as the ability to make a block tower or perform pencil-and-paper tasks (M. Herzig, personal communication, 2003). Ideally, any child age 12 years or younger should be seen by or referred to a child and adolescent psychiatrist who would be better prepared than an adult psychiatrist to address developmental issues.

Essential Principles

The following are important principles of emergency psychiatry involving a child or adolescent:

1. The psychiatrist acts as the patient's advocate.
2. The assessment of safety is the chief goal of emergency evaluation.
3. Any intervention considered should be appropriate to establish and maintain the safety of the patient and of those in the immediate surroundings of the patient.
4. Assessment tests, procedures, and interventions should be efficient, practical, and useful in contributing to establishment of the etiology of the patient's presentation, and in helping to establish the primacy of medical versus psychiatric conditions (Allen et al. 2005).

Safety First

To achieve safety, the evaluator must obtain knowledge of the following:

1. The population to which this patient belongs
2. Specific risk factors associated with this population
3. The appropriate level of intervention required to maintain both temporary and long-term safety

4. Resources available to the specific population served
5. State, federal, and regulatory agency mandates
6. Standard level of care

General Evaluation Considerations

Specific to children and adolescent patients, the evaluator must access and consider three spheres of functioning (home, school, and social). Relevant questions regarding these spheres are listed in Table 10–1.

Initial Assessment

Establish and Maintain Temporary Safety

The first priority in evaluating a child or adolescent in the psychiatric emergency service is to rule out any nonpsychiatric, general medical conditions that might be responsible for the patient's altered mental status or psychiatric symptoms. The patient should be triaged to the most appropriate setting, and if that means to a medical emergency room rather than the psychiatric emergency room, this quick evaluation is potentially life saving, especially with certain conditions such as nonobvious head trauma, hypoglycemia, or other potentially reversible causes of mental status changes. Regardless of the diagnosis, it is good practice to assume that the child and the child's parents or caretakers are frightened, worried, and/or confused.

Clear and tactful communication is essential. The clinician not only must appear to be empathetic and caring, but also must actively listen to the patient and whomever brought the patient to the emergency room. The clinician must be very clear about communicating the process of the psychiatric evaluation and potential interventions before, during, and after they occur. A patient who feels mistreated or unheard could rapidly escalate symptomatically, and parents or caretakers who feel they have been marginalized or left out of the process are more likely to become adversarial rather than allied with the clinician.

Medical Evaluation and Examination

Any change in a patient's mental status should alert the clinician to the possibly reversible causes of psychiatric symptoms, including delirium, drug intoxication or overdose, physical illness, trauma, child abuse, or a primary

Table 10–1.   Three spheres of functioning for child and adolescent assessment

Spheres of functioning	Assessment considerations
Home	**Nature of the patient's relationship with family/caretakers**

1. Parents
   a. Are they married? Recently separated?
   b. Do they have socioeconomic issues or stressors?
   c. Do they have psychiatric issues? Drug or alcohol abuse/dependence?
   d. Is there a history of domestic violence? Has the patient witnessed this?
   e. Is the patient afraid something bad will happen to his or her parents?
   f. What is the family's source of income?
   g. What is the nature of the patient's relationship with parents?
2. Siblings
   a. Are the siblings biological? Half-siblings? Foster or adopted siblings?
   b. What are the age differences?
   c. Where does the patient fall in the sibling hierarchy?
   d. What is the nature of the patient's relationship with siblings?
3. Caretakers
   a. If the parents are not the primary caretakers, who are?
   b. Are the caretakers relatives? Foster family? Adoptive?
   c. Is the child being cared for in an institutional setting? Residential home? Group home?

Patient's enjoyment and place within the family
1. Is there any aspect of the family system that antagonizes the patient?
2. Is the family system supportive of the patient? How?
3. Is the patient happy at home? Scared to be home? How does the family spend time together?
4. Is the patient allowed to have friends outside the family circle?

Supervision
Is there adequate supervision of the minors, including the patient, in this home?

Table 10–1. Three spheres of functioning for child and adolescent assessment *(continued)*

Spheres of functioning	Assessment considerations
Home *(continued)*	**Social supports for the family**
	1. Is the family system strict? Unsupervised?
	2. If there is more than one caretaker/parent, are the caretakers/parents in agreement about issues of child rearing?
	Bedtime/curfew
	1. When is bedtime/curfew for the patient? Is it enforced?
	2. How often does the patient use the computer, especially the Internet?
	3. Does the patient stay up all night playing on the computer and then feel fatigued and nonproductive the following day at school?
School	**Academic performance**
	1. Has there been a decline in functioning?
	2. Have the patient's grades deteriorated?
	3. Has the patient had excessive school absences?
	4. Have there been phone calls home from teachers?
	Friends
	1. Does the patient have friends at school?
	2. Is he or she a bully or the victim of bullies?
	3. Does the patient isolate himself or herself? Does the patient belong to a group? A gang?
	Teachers
	1. Was a psychoeducational evaluation performed on the child?
	2. Does the child have any learning disabilities or speech-language difficulties?
	3. Is the child in an appropriate classroom setting?
	4. Does the child require more structure or supervision? Further testing?
	Caretakers
	1. Are caretakers supportive of the patient's academic work?
	2. Do caretakers help the patient with assignments? With remembering to do homework?

Table 10–1. Three spheres of functioning for child and adolescent assessment *(continued)*

Spheres of functioning	Assessment considerations
School *(continued)*	**Caretakers** *(continued)*
	3. Are the caretakers involved in the patient's school?
	4. What method(s) do the caretakers use to help the patient perform to his or her academic level or behave appropriately in school? Do they use positive reinforcement? Negative reinforcement?
	Enjoyment/sense of achievement
	1. Does the patient enjoy school?
	2. Does the patient feel adequately challenged?
	3. Is the patient struggling to keep up with schoolwork?
Social	**Friends**
	1. Does the patient have friends outside of school?
	2. Does the patient limit himself or herself to "virtual" friends (i.e., friends made through the Internet on video games, chat rooms, etc.)?
	Hobbies
	1. Is the patient involved in after-school or extracurricular activities? Sports? Clubs?
	2. Does the patient have particular interests? Computer or video games? Playing a musical instrument? Singing? Dancing?
	Enjoyment/frequency
	1. Does the patient enjoy social interaction with peers?
	2. How often does the patient see friends? Engage in social activities?
	3. Does the patient have a sense of mastery?
	4. What is this patient's self-image?
	5. What is this patient's future outlook?

neurological disorder. Accordingly, the physical evaluations listed in Table 10–2 should be conducted as clinically indicated.

Psychiatric Evaluation

The clinician must ensure that the patient is not a danger to self or others, and must provide a safe and nonthreatening environment to avoid escalation of potentially dangerous behaviors. This may be as simple as providing a quiet, softly lit room, or the patient may need to be treated with medications or physically restrained to calm anxiety, reduce psychotic symptoms, or help the patient to regain control of his or her potentially dangerous behavior. The interaction between the patient and his or her caretakers must be quickly evaluated to determine if their physical proximity is likely to hinder, worsen, or improve the ability of the patient to remain safe.

When obtaining history in the course of examining an adult patient, a clinician makes many observations regarding mental status. Only later does the clinician supplement or augment by asking specific questions (e.g., about orientation, memory, psychotic symptoms). The most skilled psychiatric interviewers try to embed specific clarifying questions in the flow of conversation with the patient. Thus, in the assessment of adults, the patient is the primary source of information, both about his or her history, illness, symptoms, and so on, and about his or her mental status.

The evaluation of children is different in that history is frequently obtained from others and the mental status examination is based on observations of the child and his or her interactions with the evaluator and, especially when the child is young, with the parent (M. Herzig, personal communication, 2003). The evaluation is the summation of subjective and objective findings provided by the patient, the parents, and other caretakers in the patient's life.

1. Chief complaint and history of present illness: Elicit the specific reasons why the patient is in the emergency room. Obtain details about acute and chronic stressors and their temporal relationship to the onset of acute or chronic symptoms. Explore patient's strengths and weaknesses.
2. Psychiatric history

3. Family history

   a. Current stressors

   b. Intrafamilial stressors

   c. Familial coping abilities and strategies

4. Developmental history (as relevant)

5. Medical history (as relevant)

6. Social history (as relevant)

7. Mental status examination

Common Presentations

Although children and adolescents present to the emergency department for various reasons, some of the most common are suicidality; psychosis, agitation, or aggressiveness; child abuse; and eating disorders. We discuss these more common psychiatric issues in this section.

Suicidality

Assessment

Once safety has been established, the patient should be evaluated for suicidal ideation. In contrast to suicidal adults, suicidal adolescents account for a higher proportion of all deaths, suicidal ideation is more common, suicidal attempts are more common, disruptive behavior disorders increase risk, and contagion effects are more powerful (Ash 2008). According to epidemiological and clinical studies, risk factors for suicidality in children and adolescents are often comorbid with other psychiatric disorders, such as depressive, disruptive, anxiety, or substance abuse disorders. Other risk factors include adverse family circumstances, such as the caretaker's low satisfaction with the family environment, low parental monitoring, and parental history of psychiatric disorder. Low social and instrumental competence, which are thought to undermine self-esteem and hinder the development of supportive social affiliations, was found to be associated with suicidal ideation or behavior (King et al. 2001). Evaluation of the child's home environment and the parents' or caretakers' capacity to support an at-risk child must be considered, especially as the evaluation moves toward a disposition.

Table 10–2. Key laboratory studies

Basic labs

To help rule out *potentially reversible causes of delirium or mental status changes*, or for baseline assessment before the initiation of medications:

Complete blood count with differential

Blood glucose

General chemistry screen

Liver function tests

Thyroid function tests

Urinalysis

Urine toxicology screen

Alcohol level (if indicated)

Pregnancy screen (if applicable)

Electrocardiogram

New-onset psychosis labs

If at risk, or for *new-onset psychosis and atypical psychosis*, all the above plus:

Infectious disease screens: Lyme titers (endemic areas), human immunodeficiency virus, rapid plasma reagin (if at risk, such as runaways, delinquents, children of substance abusers)

Rheumatoid factor

Anti-nuclear antibodies

Erythrocyte sedimentation rate

Vitamin B_{12}/folate (if at risk, such as patients who have anorexia, are strict vegetarian, or have malnutrition)

Computed tomography, magnetic resonance imaging (if evidence of neurological dysfunction or new-onset psychosis)

Electroencephalogram (if history is suggestive of seizures or seizure-like events)

Lumbar puncture (if history is suggestive of central nervous system involvement)

Special labs

If patient is taking *valproic acid*:

Amylase

Lipase

Valproic acid—to rule out toxicity; to establish therapeutic levels, obtain trough level in the morning before A.M. dose of valproic acid

Table 10–2. Key laboratory studies *(continued)*

Special labs *(continued)*

If patient is taking *lithium*:

Lithium—to rule out toxicity; to establish therapeutic levels, obtain trough level in the morning before A.M. dose of lithium

If patient is taking *antipsychotics*:

Hemoglobin A_{1c} (if weight has increased)

Fasting blood glucose (if weight has increased)

Lipid profile (if already taking or if starting antipsychotics)

The clinician should keep in mind the suicide rates among adolescents while evaluating risk. Although completed suicide is known to be a rare event in preteen children, the risk begins to increase at age 13 years, and by the end of adolescence, the rates are similar to those of young adults. Girls make more frequent attempts than boys, but boys are more likely to successfully complete suicide. The suicide rate for children and adolescents has remained fairly stable (despite significant trends within this range), 9.48 to 6.78 per 100,000 persons between 1990 and 2003, with a recent upward trend of 8% to 7.32 per 100,000 persons by 2004 (Centers for Disease Control and Prevention 2007).

Assessing the intention of a youth to commit suicide is important. The clinician should ask questions related to the components listed in Table 10–3.

Interventions

The clinician needs to spend time educating the family and the patient about suicide, suicide prevention, and mental illness. It is important to listen carefully, reflect back concerns, and be sure the patient and his or her parents or caretakers fully understand everything the clinician wishes to convey.

If the patient's suicidal gesture seemed to be a cry for help, he or she may not require further hospitalization but rather close follow-up with an outpatient clinician. This determination should be based on the individual case, the resources available, the willingness of the family to engage in treatment, and other considerations. For a youngster who has made an apparent nonlethal suicide attempt or who has passive suicidal ideation, further exploration of the home environment is essential to determining where the patient will be safest. Alternative placements may be necessary if the parents are unable to

Table 10–3. Elements of the suicide assessment

Suicide component considerations	Evaluation questions
Wish to die	What does the patient expect will happen if he or she dies?
	How lethal are the means by which the patient chose to end his or her life?
Preparations	Was the attempt planned beforehand or impulsive?
	Did the patient write a note or make attempts to say good-bye?
Concealment	Did the patient plan the attempt in a manner by which he or she would not be found? (Investigate the timing of the attempt or selection of the location in terms of discovery by others.)
Communication	Did the patient make attempts to tell others, either directly or indirectly?
Precipitants	What led to the event or the wish to die?
	What degree of stress or anxiety preceded the event?
	Was there any relief of symptoms after the event?
	Was any degree of reconciliation between the patient and significant others achieved by the event?
	In the context of similar stressors or exacerbation of stressors, does the patient now deny suicidality?

adequately monitor the youngster; are known to be dangerous or to abuse alcohol or substances; do not fully comprehend the discharge instructions; or are considered by the youngster to be significant enough stressors that his or her safety at home cannot be guaranteed. If the patient's safety at home is in any way in doubt, the first option is to find other family members who may be willing and able to take the child temporarily. If this is not possible, the child should be admitted until appropriate placement can be arranged in a residential crisis center, with a foster care agency, or with a similar social service agency.

In the psychiatric emergency service, because the patient is not likely to be seen again, antidepressants are not typically started.

Medicolegal Concerns

The clinician needs to keep in mind various medicolegal concerns. Psychiatrists are mandated reporters for child abuse, which does include medical neglect. If the patient's legal guardians refuse to cooperate and the child is in danger of harming self or others, the clinician may be required to report the case. If faced with such a dilemma, the clinician should consult a supervisor regarding the reporting of the case. Additionally, although children may be signed into a locked unit without the need for legal commitment, if the guardians are not cooperative and the clinician believes the child is at risk of or has suffered child abuse, the clinician needs to know if his or her state law allows for detention of the patient by way of commitment. If the patient was injured "accidentally," for instance, by ingesting drugs or alcohol or by using a firearm, this may substantiate child abuse by neglect (Dubin and Weiss 1991).

Disposition

From what is learned about the patient in the emergency department, the clinician determines the next level of care. Possibilities include inpatient hospitalization; hospital emergency room–based services (crisis intervention); stepdown programs such as a day treatment program, home-based crisis intervention, or intensive case management intervention; standard outpatient care; or no follow-up at all. Another option is to contact child protective services or another social service agency.

Psychosis, Agitation, or Aggressiveness

Assessment

For the child or adolescent who presents with psychosis, agitation, or aggressiveness, the clinician needs to consider several questions.

1. Does the patient have accompanying symptoms suggestive of a psychiatric disorder or of a medical or neurological disorder? The clinician should attempt to rule out any possibly reversible cause of the mental status change (e.g., pain, infection, confused state from the infection, partial complex seizures, toxic states, medication intoxication/withdrawal syndromes).
2. Is the behavior volitional or done for secondary gain?
3. Is the behavior secondary to fear or anxiety, or is it in anticipation of hospitalization?

4. What is the patient's cognitive level? Some children with developmental disabilities appear to be agitated when in fact their behavior is a reflection of a soothing strategy or a slight exacerbation of baseline stereotypes.

5. Does the patient have hallucinations? It is vital to consider the difference between developmentally appropriate (primary) hallucinations and hallucinations in the presence of psychiatric disorders. Aug and Ables (1971) listed five factors that may predispose a child to experience so-called primary hallucinations in the absence of any diagnosable disease or disorder:

   • Age and limited intelligence are important factors. For a child, wish-fulfilling fantasy is a common mode of thinking. However, a child of average intelligence at age 3 years can usually distinguish between fantasy and reality.

   • Emotional deprivation can lead to increased fantasy thinking, and perhaps hallucinations, as a way of providing the gratifications that reality cannot provide.

   • Emphasis on a particular mode of perception may be important. Life experience may make it difficult to distinguish between vivid auditory imagery and auditory hallucinations in a child who is partially deaf or between visual imagery and visual hallucinations in a child whose parent is preoccupied about the health of the eyes.

   • Family religious and/or cultural beliefs may predispose children to have deviant perceptual experiences.

   • Strong emotional states at times of stress may lead to regression, hallucinations, and/or dissociative states.

   Primary hallucinations include the following:

• Hypnagogic hallucinations (transient, occur between true sleep and waking)

• Eidetic imagery (child's ability to visualize or auditorize an object long after it has been seen or heard; an ability typically lost by the time of puberty in a child with no developmental delays or history of trauma)

• Imaginary playmate (typical for children 3–5 years of age, and the child is aware that this companion is fantasy or not real)

• Dreams, nightmares

- Isolated hallucinations (fleeting illusions based on misinterpretations of shadows, colors, and movements)
- Hallucinosis (a number of hallucinations extending over a period of time but not related to any known cause)

To determine whether the patient has a secondary hallucination suggestive of a psychiatric or medical etiology, the clinician should consider the full context of the patient's presentation (Weiner 1961). Primary mood or psychotic disorders should be considered if the patient also presents with severe mood symptoms, either depressed or manic; if the patient's affect is incongruent, flattened, blunted, or grandiose; or if the patient has impaired memory, agitation, restlessness, a disturbed sleep-wake cycle, or disturbances of memory, attention, or concentration.. If the patient's hallucinations are accompanied by perceptual distortions, automatic and repetitive movements, partial loss of consciousness, or periods of confusion, or if they are preceded by a visual aura, then a primary neurological condition such as epilepsy or migraines should be considered.

Intervention

Because safety is of primary importance, the clinician should first deescalate the environment. If possible, familiar persons should remain nearby, and the child should be provided with food, fluids, and diversionary activities such as toys, games, or drawing materials.

When working with a cognitively limited patient who is verbally and physically aggressive, the clinician should try to ignore the patient (e.g., by avoiding eye contact, verbal responses, and touching). If the patient approaches a staff member while engaging in aggressive or disruptive behaviors, the staff member should move far away from the patient to limit interaction. However, the staff member must take immediate action if the situation is potentially dangerous to the patient or anybody else.

If the patient remains agitated, the clinician should consider one of the medications listed in Table 10–4. The following considerations should be taken into account in choosing medications:

- Other psychoactive medications or substances that the patient currently is receiving or has ever received

- The possible effect of psychotropic medication on the patient's medical illness
- Comorbid symptoms
- Route of administration
- Potential side effects and the patient's risk factors
- Desired rapidity of effect
- Dosing

The following important guidelines should also be followed:

- Do *not* order prn medications without physician reevaluation.
- Do *not* mix different types or classes of antipsychotic medications.
- Do *not* mix different types of benzodiazepines.

At times, restraints may be considered for patients who are psychotic, agitated, or aggressive. The use of restraints should be limited, however, to cases in which all interventions have failed and should be considered only temporary until an adequate level of behavioral control is gained by the patient.

Medicolegal Concerns

All interventions that require sedation or restraints should follow regulatory guidelines specific to the hospital and state. Additionally, parents must be included in all decisions.

Disposition

Any patient who presents with symptoms suggestive of a prodromal psychotic state, first-break psychosis, or exacerbation of psychotic symptoms that were previously well controlled should be hospitalized for safety, further evaluation, and management of symptoms. On occasion, some patients may present with mild psychotic symptoms that could be safely managed at home. If the family is able to provide appropriate supervision and outpatient follow-up, the home environment may be preferable. Patients with new presentations of mood, anxiety, or disruptive behavior disorders should be assessed for safety as previously described and the most appropriate level of care determined for disposition. Patients with developmental disabilities, however, do not respond well to changes in their environment and/or caretakers. The presence of a familiar caretaker at the point of arrival at the emergency room very often deescalates the patient's agitation by quickly reestablishing known routines. If the agitation is quickly controlled, the patient can be discharged home and hospitalization is avoided. The emergency services psychiatrist should be familiar with resources available for patients with developmental disabilities, and applications for external supports at school and home should be initiated at this point. Inpatient hospitalization should be used only as a last resort unless a unit with specialized interventions for children with disabilities is available. Specific therapeutic interventions catering to this population are limited or lacking in regular psychiatric units, and these patients, due to their behavioral difficulties, are too often isolated and overmedicated in this setting.

Child Abuse

Any behavior that harms the physical or psychological well-being or the normal growth and development of a child by an adult is considered child abuse. From October 2005 to September 2006, approximately 905,000 U.S. children were victims of maltreatment that was substantiated by state and local child protective service agencies (Centers for Disease Control and Prevention 2008). There are no specific ethnic or socioeconomic groups in which child abuse is more prevalent. Because child abuse typically occurs in the context of a family crisis, the clinician should be suspicious of the nature of the child's emergency but work hard to establish rapport with both the child and the parents, without demonstrating outwardly any preconceived thoughts or attitudes. A strong alliance will help the child to reveal sensitive information. Additionally, maintaining a professional stance will help if the intervention requires removal of the child from the family to the protective environment of an inpatient unit or other social service until details are evaluated.

According to the U.S. Department of Health and Human Services, Administration for Children and Families, risk factors for child abuse fall into the categories listed in Table 10–5 (Child Welfare Information Gateway 2006). In addition to recognizing the risk factors for child abuse, the clinician needs to know the types of child abuse and be aware of child abuse law. The clinician should also be aware of available hospital and community resources that deal specifically with this issue.

Table 10–4.   Commonly used psychotropic medications for pediatric population

Name	Dose	Onset of action	Elimination half-life (hours)
Lorazepam	0.25–2 mg po or im q 6–8 hours prn (maximum 2–3 doses in 24 hours)	im: 20–30 minutes po: 30–60 minutes	Children: 11 Adults: 13
Chlorpromazine	10–50 po or 12.5–25 im q 2–4 hours prn (maximum 2–3 doses in 24 hours)	im: 15 minutes po: 30–60 minutes	30
Haloperidol	0.25–5 mg po or im q 2–4 hours prn (maximum 2–3 doses in 24 hours)	im: 20–30 minutes po: 2–3 hours	18–40
Risperidone	0.125–2 mg po q 4–6 hours prn (maximum 2–3 doses in 24 hours)	po: 1–3 hours	20
Benztropine	0.25–2 mg po or im q 6–8 hours prn (maximum 2–3 doses in 24 hours)	im: ≤15 minutes po: ≤1 hour	6–48
Diphenhydramine	12.5–50 mg po or im q 4–6 hours prn (maximum 2–3 doses in 24 hours)	im: <2 hours po: 2–4 hours	2–8

Haloperidol and lorazepam

For extreme agitation, to achieve a higher level of sedation

Haloperidol, lorazepam and benztropine or diphenhydramine

For extreme agitation, to achieve a higher level of sedation and to prevent extrapyramidal symptoms

Haloperidol and diphenhydramine

To achieve a higher level of sedation and to prevent extrapyramidal symptoms (EPS)

To prevent or if patient develops EPS, provide oral dosage of diphenhydramine q 6–8 hours to cover up to 48 hours postexposure to one single dose of haloperidol.

Table 10–4. Commonly used psychotropic medications for pediatric population *(continued)*

Name	Dose	Onset of action	Elimination half-life (hours)

Haloperidol and benztropine

To prevent EPS

To prevent or if patient develops EPS, provide oral dosage of benztropine q 8–12 hours to cover up to 48 hours postexposure to one single dose of haloperidol.

Chlorpromazine is associated with orthostatic hypotension and cardiovascular collapse; use carefully and do not use in combination with diphenhydramine or benztropine.

Lorazepam is associated with respiratory depression; use carefully if pulmonary functions are compromised. Also, lorazepam is associated with paradoxical reactions (increased agitation) in small children and developmentally disabled children.

Other anxiolytic or antipsychotic medications

If patient is already receiving them with good results, you might consider giving an extra dose.

Source. Findling 2008; Schatzberg and Nemeroff 2004.

Types of Child Abuse

Child neglect. Child neglect is generally characterized by omissions in care that result in significant harm or risk of significant harm. Neglect is frequently defined in terms of a failure to provide for the child's basic needs, such as adequate food, clothing, shelter, supervision, or medical care. Typically, child neglect is divided into three types: physical, educational, and emotional neglect.

Sexual abuse. Sexual abuse includes both touching offenses (fondling or sexual intercourse) and nontouching offenses (exposing a child to pornographic materials) and can involve varying degrees of violence and emotional trauma. The most commonly reported cases involve incest, or sexual abuse occurring among family members, including those in biological families, adoptive families, and stepfamilies. Incest most often occurs within a father-daughter relationship; however, mother-son, father-son, and sibling-sibling incest also occurs. Other relatives or caretakers also sometimes commit sexual abuse.

Table 10–5.   Risk factors for child abuse

Parent or caregiver factors	Personality characteristics/mental health
	History of abuse
	Substance abuse
	Child-rearing approaches
	Teen parents
Family factors	Family structure
	Domestic violence
	Stressful life events
Child factors	Birth to age 3 years
	Disabilities
	Low birth weight
Environmental factors	Poverty and unemployment
	Social isolation and social support
	Violence in communities

Physical abuse.   Although an injury resulting from physical abuse is not accidental, the parent or caregiver may not have intended to hurt the child. The injury may have resulted from severe discipline, including injurious spanking, or physical punishment that is inappropriate to the child's age or condition. The injury may be the result of a single episode or repeated episodes and can range in severity from minor marks and bruising to death.

Psychological maltreatment.   On the "Emotional Abuse" page at the Child Welfare Information Gateway (2009) Web site, psychological maltreatment, or emotional abuse, is defined as "a repeated pattern of caregiver behavior or extreme incident(s) that convey to children that they are worthless, flawed, unloved, unwanted, endangered, or only of value in meeting another's needs." That Web site lists six categories of psychological maltreatment:

- Spurning (e.g., belittling, hostile rejecting, ridiculing)
- Terrorizing (e.g., threatening violence against a child, placing a child in a recognizably dangerous situation)
- Isolating (e.g., confining the child, placing unreasonable limitations on the child's freedom of movement, restricting the child from social interactions)

- Exploiting or corrupting (e.g., modeling antisocial behavior such as criminal activities, encouraging prostitution, permitting substance abuse)
- Denying emotional responsiveness (e.g., ignoring the child's attempts to interact, failing to express affection)
- Mental health, medical, and educational neglect (e.g., refusing to allow or failing to provide treatment for serious mental health or medical problems, ignoring the need for services for serious educational needs)

Evaluation

The patient's mental status examination may reveal a frightened youngster who may have unrealistic expectations about reunions with an abusive family or family member, or who may describe magical thinking about undoing the abuse. The child or adolescent may present in a variety of ways, such as being overly responsible, being impulsive, displaying extreme mood swings, misunderstanding personal boundaries, or being shy or withdrawn. The younger patient may experience nightmares or night terrors, and may be extra clingy with one person but refuse to be near another. Older children, especially adolescents, may become more withdrawn, change their clothing style to one that is more sexually provocative, or make efforts to hide their sexual development and attractiveness. The older child may also develop promiscuous behaviors or deviant sexual behaviors, run away, develop alcohol or substance abuse problems, or attempt suicide.

A child who is a suspected victim of abuse should be examined carefully by a pediatrician in the medical emergency department for signs of abuse. Labs, cultures, swabs, and imaging studies may be warranted to substantiate clinical findings.

Intervention

As always, in working with potential abuse victims, the clinician should maintain a professional stance, which requires being sensitive, thoughtful, empathetic, objective, and goal and action oriented. Child abuse cases may bring up strong countertransferential feelings in the clinician, who may feel anger toward the alleged offender and sympathy for the victim; however, the clinician must refrain from being confrontational or accusatory, and maintain a sense of calm and safety within the emergency department. The clinician should learn from both the patient and the patient's parents or caretakers the details of the alleged abuse and then consult with other members of the psychosocial team, hospital child abuse assessment team, or other supervisors to determine appropriate disposition.

Medicolegal Concerns

Whether there is suspected or confirmed child abuse, two reports must be filed: 1) a written legal form documenting the examination findings and 2) a telephone report to the child abuse agency to begin the disposition process and treatment plan for the child and family. The child abuse agency will subsequently manage further disposition issues once the patient is discharged from the hospital. Usually, when an at-risk child's family must be investigated by the child abuse agency, a full evaluation is conducted within 24 hours. On occasion, the clinician may need to provide courtroom testimony, or hospital administrators may need to step in and use legal authorities to protect or hospitalize a child or to remove family members who are threatening and violent.

In any event, the family members must be informed of their rights and responsibilities, including a full court hearing with legal representation and a continued duty to protect the child from further abuse (Ludwig 1983). In cases where suspected abuse is substantiated by physical findings (sexual or physical), the child should be admitted and the appropriate investigative authorities immediately involved. These include a hospital-based child abuse assessment team, the local social services office, or, at the very least, law enforcement. If there are no physical findings and the abuse is alleged by the child, the aforementioned investigative authorities must be contacted and the allegations reported. Typically, these officials will direct the clinicians regarding how to proceed.

Disposition

If the child's safety is of primary concern, he or she should be hospitalized to control the child's environment, provide safety and consistency, and facilitate further evaluation of the child and the allegations. Once the diagnosis of abuse is made, the parents or caretakers should be informed immediately and the disposition plans described.

Eating Disorders

Some of the more common presentations of anorexia nervosa to the emergency room include recent dizziness or fainting spells in school or at home or seizures; when the parent or caregiver is highly suspicious of an eating disorder after the patient is observed vomiting (and may also complain of a gastrointestinal illness); or when the parent or caregiver notes that the patient is dangerously restricting intake. A 2008 study found that about 16.9% of those with anorexia nervosa attempted suicide (Bulik et al. 2008). For the emergency psychiatrist, the question of whether to admit a patient with an eating disorder to either a medical unit or a psychiatric unit will be based on the available resources in the clinician's hospital. Following completion of a full physical and psychiatric evaluation, including a necessary evaluation of the family, inpatient medical hospitalization is warranted if any one of the following criteria is met:

- ≤75% of ideal body weight (patient in gown after voiding)
- Heart rate < 45 bpm, resting by lying down for at least 5 minutes
- Hypokalemia (on evaluation of plasma electrolytes)
- Hyponatremia (on evaluation of plasma electrolytes)

Given the significantly high suicide rate for patients with anorexia nervosa, some of their presentations will be similar to those of other psychiatric patients who require immediate hospitalization for stabilization and safety (American Psychiatric Association 2006):

- Severe suicidality with high lethality or intention (which under any circumstances warrants hospitalization).
- Worsening ability to control self-induced vomiting, increased binge eating, use of diuretics, and use of cathartics that may be considered life threatening.
- Weight changes related to altered or changed mental status due to worsening symptoms of mood disorder, suicidality, or psychotic decompensation.
- Preoccupation with weight and/or body image, accompanied by food refusal, or obsessive thoughts about body image or weight that cause the patient to be uncooperative with treatment and require a highly structured setting for rehabilitation.

Other presentations may not warrant inpatient hospitalization depending on the entire clinical picture and full psychiatric evaluation (American Psychiatric Association 2006):

- Recent precipitous or steady drop in weight and/or a total body weight that is <85% of normal healthy body weight. Body mass index (BMI; calculated as [weight in kilograms/height in meters]^2), is less useful in children than

adults and should not be used to estimate, except at extremes, a patient's nutritional status. Age-adjusted BMIs are available (Centers for Disease Control and Prevention 2006). Children below the 5th percentile are considered
underweight. However, other factors, such as abnormal muscularity, body
frame status, constipation, and fluid loading, will influence these results and
may be misleading. Additionally, specific individual BMIs may be better understood according to ethnic groups (Lear et al. 2003).

- Metabolic disturbances, including hypophosphatemia, hyponatremia,
  hypokalemia, or hypomagnesemia; elevated blood urea nitrogen in context of normal renal function.

- Hemodynamic disturbances in children and adolescents: heart rate in the
  40s; orthostatic changes (>20 bpm increase in heart rate or >10–20 mm
  Hg drop); blood pressure below 80/50 mm Hg.

Key Clinical Points

- Temporary safety is the chief goal of emergency evaluation.

- Any intervention considered should be appropriate to establish and
  maintain the safety of the patient.

- Assessment tests, procedures, and interventions should be efficient,
  practical, and useful for establishing the primacy of medical versus psychiatric conditions.

- Acute agitation should be managed first with environmental deescalation, before medications or physical restraints are used.

- Acute crisis intervention requires the clinician to maintain a professional stance, while demonstrating empathy, actively listening, and appropriately delivering education and instructions.

- Provisional psychopharmacological management should be attempted
  for patients with acute behavioral dyscontrol, agitation, aggressiveness,
  or psychosis.

- With children, especially those who are naïve to psychotropic medications, medications should be used only if necessary, starting with low
  doses.

- If a patient does not respond as expected after one or two doses, the clinician should discontinue the medication and review the case in detail.

- Provisional diagnoses should be established to guide treatment and preliminary disposition of a patient.

- The clinician should generate a sense of trust and alliance with the patient and his or her family. *The clinician should avoid promising something he or she is unsure of or cannot deliver.*

References

Allen MH, Currier GW, Carpenter D, et al; Expert Consensus Panel for Behavioral Emergencies 2005: The expert consensus guideline series: treatment of behavioral emergencies 2005. J Psychiatr Pract 11 (suppl 1):5–108, 2005

American Psychiatric Association: Diagnostic and Statistical Manual of Mental Disorders, 4th Edition, Text Revision. Washington, DC, American Psychiatric Association, 2000

American Psychiatric Association: Practice guideline for the assessment and treatment of patients with eating disorders, third edition. 2006. Available at: http://www.psychiatryonline.com/content.aspx?aID=138722. Accessed October 7, 2009.

Ash P: Suicidal behavior in children and adolescents. J Psychosoc Nurs Ment Health Serv 46:26–30, 2008

Aug RG, Ables BS: Hallucinations in nonpsychotic children. Child Psychiatry Hum Dev 1:152–167, 1971

Bulik CM, Thornton L, Pinheiro AP, et al: Suicide attempts in anorexia nervosa. Psychosom Med 70:378–383, 2008

Centers for Disease Control and Prevention: Tools for calculating body mass index (BMI). March 22, 2006. Available at: http://www.cdc.gov/nccdphp/dnpa/growthcharts/bmi_tools.htm. Accessed October 10, 2009.

Centers for Disease Control and Prevention: Web-based Injury Statistics Query and Reporting System (WISQUARS™). Atlanta, GA, U.S. Department of Health and Human Services, Centers for Disease Control and Prevention, 2007. Available at: http://www.cdc.gov/injury/wisqars/index.html. Accessed January 25, 2010.

Centers for Disease Control and Prevention: Nonfatal maltreatment of infants—United States, October 2005–September 2006. MMWR Morb Mortal Wkly Rep 57:336–339, 2008

Child Welfare Information Gateway: What is child abuse and neglect? 2006. Available at: http://www.childwelfare.gov/can/types. Accessed October 7, 2009.

Child Welfare Information Gateway: Emotional abuse. April 3, 2009. Available at: http://www.childwelfare.gov/can/types/emotionalabuse. Accessed October 7, 2009.

Cole W, Turgay A, Mouldey G: Repeated use of psychiatric emergency services by children. Can J Psychiatry 36:739–741, 1991

Dubin WR, Weiss KJ: Handbook of Psychiatric Emergencies. Springhouse, PA, Springhouse, 1991

Findling RL: Clinical Manual of Child and Adolescent Psychopharmacology. Washington, DC, American Psychiatric Publishing, 2008

Goldstein AB, Silverman MA, Phillips S, et al: Mental health visits in a pediatric emergency department and their relationship to the school calendar. Pediatr Emerg Care 21:653–657, 2005

King RA, Schwab-Stone M, Flisher AJ, et al: Psychosocial and risk behavior correlates of youth suicide attempts and suicidal ideation. J Am Acad Child Adolesc Psychiatry 40:837–846, 2001

Lear SA, Toma M, Birmingham CL, et al: Modification of the relationship between simple anthropometric indices and risk factors by ethnic background. Metabolism 52:1295–1301, 2003

Ludwig S: Child abuse, in Textbook of Pediatric Emergency Medicine. Edited by Fleisher GR, Ludwig S. Baltimore, MD, Williams & Wilkins, 1983

Schatzberg AF, Nemeroff CB: Textbook of Psychopharmacology, 3rd Edition. Washington, DC, American Psychiatric Publishing, 2004

Sills MR, Bland SD: Summary statistics for pediatric psychiatric visits to U.S. emergency departments, 1993–1999. Pediatrics 110:e40, 2002

Weiner M: Hallucinations in children. Arch Gen Psychiatry 5:544–553, 1961

Suggested Readings

Allen MH, Currier GW, Carpenter D, et al; Expert Consensus Panel for Behavioral Emergencies 2005: The expert consensus guideline series: treatment of behavioral emergencies 2005. J Psychiatr Pract 11 (suppl 1):5–108, 2005

Findling RL: Clinical Manual of Child and Adolescent Psychopharmacology. Washington, DC, American Psychiatric Publishing, 2008

Tardiff K: Medical Management of the Violent Patient: Clinical Assessment and Therapy. New York, Marcel Dekker, 1999

11

Seclusion and Restraint in Emergency Settings

Wanda K. Mohr, Ph.D., A.P.R.N., F.A.A.N.

Gem Lucas, D.O.

Mr. E, a 33-year-old male with a medical history of hepatitis C, hepatitis B, bipolar disorder with nonadherence with psychiatric medication, and a history of violence, was admitted to the emergency department. He was found walking in the middle of the street at 2:00 A.M. by the police, who brought him to the emergency department. On arrival, he was combative, disoriented, and visually hallucinating. Multiple intravenous (IV) puncture sites were noted. His history included three prior hospitalizations for cocaine intoxication and rhabdomyolysis. His urine drug screen was positive for cocaine. In the emergency department, the patient was calmed with a so-called cocktail of haloperidol 5 mg and lorazepam 2 mg. He was evaluated and admitted to the medical ward. On awakening, Mr. E pulled out his IV line, and spat at and threatened to bite staff. Physical restraints were ordered as the patient became increasingly more threatening and was throwing urine in his room. Involuntary chemical restraints were also ordered, and Mr. E was given chlorpromazine intravenously because he refused oral medication. The patient was then able to receive IV fluids and supportive care. He was discharged within 7 days in a medically stable condition. Prior to discharge, Mr. E was restarted on quetiapine for his bipolar disorder and given a follow-up appointment at the psychiatric clinic for that day.

Restraints and seclusion can be used appropriately as safety measures, or they can be misused. Mr. E's situation represents the appropriate use of chemical and physical restraints. Both measures were clearly necessary because this patient was a danger to himself, as well as to staff, by throwing around bodily fluids and threatening to bite them.

Until very recently, in-depth discussion of seclusion and restraint was not presented in psychiatric textbooks. The frequent absence of this topic is curious because perhaps no other procedures employed in psychiatry have been as controversial in the past decade as seclusion and restraint. This controversy is rooted in the facts that 1) seclusion and restraint, despite their long history of use in psychiatry, have no sound theoretical or research foundation as an intervention and 2) they pose significant risk to patients and staff. However, behavioral emergencies in all clinical settings can be dangerous situations. Specifically, violent patients in emergency departments can cause urgent situations that require medical intervention. In this chapter, we discuss the use of seclusion and restraint in behavioral emergencies occurring in clinical settings. We do not cover the use of devices used in medical settings for immobilization or for the primary purpose of restraint or isolation/seclusion that has a direct medical rationale. Because space limitations prevent us from including more than an overview, at the end of the chapter, we list Web sites that provide further information.

Definitions

In the United States, two national organizations regulate and set standards for the uses of seclusion and restraint: the Centers for Medicare & Medicaid Services (CMS) and The Joint Commission (JCAHO; formerly the Joint Commission on Accreditation of Healthcare Organizations). Various definitions of seclusion and restraint are used by different state and federal regulatory agencies and professional organizations. The Child Welfare League of America (2002a, 2002b) has compiled these definitions, and their Web site also contains a state-by-state comparison of regulations (http://www.cwla.org).

In short, physical restraints are procedures or devices that are employed to limit a person's mobility. These can range from the precautionary raising of a bed rail to prevent an incapacitated person from falling out of bed, to holding a person, to the more dramatic mechanical modalities of arm and leg cuffs (four point) and addition of a fifth point by tying a sheet across the person's midsection. Mechanical devices are rarely indicated or used; however, if they are employed, they should be devices manufactured expressly for the purpose of restraining patients and approved by the U.S. Food and Drug Administration. A number of devices have been made from a variety of different materials, such as leather or polyurethane with buckles or Velcro closures.

Most commonly in psychiatric settings, a restraint consists of trained people taking patients to the floor and holding them until they are calm. In the case of children, restraint may include something euphemistically called a "therapeutic hold." This refers to a brief physical holding technique used to restrict a child's freedom of movement for reasons of safety (Berrios and Jacobowitz 1998).

Seclusion refers to the temporary, involuntary confinement of a patient in a room or area from which the person is physically prevented from leaving. It can include locked and unlocked seclusion. Seclusion does not refer to a "time-out" intervention that may be consistent with a patient's treatment plan (JCAHO); a time-out should not exceed 1 hour.

Chemical restraint refers to the administration of a medication that is used to control behavior or freedom of movement but that is not a part of a patient's daily medication regimen.

Various deescalation and restraint procedures are taught by a number of vendors who sell their so-called aggression management programs to facilities; some facilities develop their own programs. There are approximately 47 multistate training programs, and the number of home-grown programs is not known. No national accreditation is available for such programs. Seclusion and restraint training and procedures are not taught in professional education programs as part of any curriculum (Gately and Stabb 2005; Schwartz and Parks 1999; Stillwell 1991).

Indications

The CMS's (2006) indications for the use of seclusion or restraint states that it is to be used only in emergency situations needed to ensure patients' physical safety and after less restrictive interventions have been determined to be ineffective to protect patient or others from harm. The JCAHO's (2000) indications are similar but include the phrase "where there is imminent danger." Both bodies indicate exclusions for the purposes of coercion, punishment, discipline, convenience, and retaliation by staff.

At this writing, the position statements of both the American Academy of Child and Adolescent Psychiatry (AACAP; Masters et al. 2002) and the American Psychiatric Association (1984) state that the indications for the use of seclusion and restraint are for reasons of safety. The patient must present as a clear danger to self or others, and less intrusive measures to control such behavior must have failed. Both organizations also include a statement indicating that restraint or seclusion may be used to prevent serious disruption of the treatment milieu or damage to property.

Bioethicist George Annas (1999) opined that restraint use can only be justified in emergency situations to prevent patients from hurting themselves or others, and then for the shortest time and with the least restriction possible.

The decision to place a patient in restraints ideally should be made by the attending physician. In emergencies, however, other qualified staff may initiate a restraint if a physician is not immediately available. The JCAHO and CMS regulations regarding ordering seclusion and restraint are summarized in Table 11–1.

Patient Assessment

A proper initial assessment of psychiatric patients should include identifying causes of violence (including a thorough differential diagnosis), history of violent behavior, early warning signs and triggers, relevant trauma history, and preexisting medical conditions that place individuals at risk of injury or death should safety measures such as seclusion, chemical restraint, and/or physical restraint be needed. Agitation that is seen in the emergency department is generally caused by one or more of the following categories: a general medical condition, substance intoxication or withdrawal, a primary psychiatric disturbance, and staff provocation.

Table 11–1.   Regulations regarding seclusion and restraint orders

MD/LIP to order [CMS]

Qualified trained staff may initiate before order obtained [JCAHO]

MD/LIP to see patient
    w/in 1 hr [CMS]
    w/in 4 hr (or less for children) [JCAHO]

Revaluation & renewed order by primary treating MD/LIP [CMS and JCAHO]
    q 4 hr for adults
    q 2 hr for 9–17 yo
    q 1 hr for under 9 yo

MD/LIP in-person reevaluation every 24 hr thereafter [CMS]

MD/LIP in-person reevaluation thereafter [JCAHO]
    q 8 hr for adults
    q 4 hr for under 18 yo

No prn medications or standing orders [CMS and JCAHO]

Can "reuse" existing order if has not expired [JCAHO]

Note: CMS = Centers for Medicare & Medicaid Services; hr = hours; JCAHO = Joint Commission on Accreditation of Healthcare Organizations; MD/LIP = physician or licensed independent practitioner; q = every; yo = years old.

Choosing Seclusion or Chemical or Physical Restraint

The treatment of acutely agitated individuals is a major issue in emergency psychiatry. The initial treatment of patients who are agitated or exhibit aggressive behavior should focus on calming them through a quiet and empathic but also firm approach. Such patients may elicit fear in staff members, making treatment and communication difficult; however, empathy is the most useful tool in clinicians' armamentaria.

There is little of an empirical nature in published standard practices to guide clinical decisions regarding seclusion and restraint; no overall benchmarks for their use; and no data about the appropriate mix of seclusion, restraint, and medication for various kinds of patients. Controversy exists across different settings concerning the proper use of emergency measures with patients who pose a threat to themselves or others. In emergency departments, physicians most often use physical or chemical restraints in the course of treating violent patients. In examining evidence for the treatment of patients in the emergency department, Zun (2005) concluded that some studies had examined the use of chemical restraints, but studies of the use of physical, chemical, or seclusion measures, alone or in combination, were sorely lacking.

It is important to note that each state, although covered by federal law, has its own set of laws governing the rights of patients. Also, each hospital has its own "restraint policy," which should be reviewed by all physicians and staff, because it may be very specific about how to restrain patients and may state who needs to be informed that the patient has been restrained.

Figure 11–1 is an algorithm based on our review of various descriptive literatures in this area that reflects clinical consensus of how decisions to restrain or seclude normally take place.

Training Requirements

According to both JCAHO and CMS, all staff with direct patient contact must have ongoing education and training in the proper and safe use of restraints. JCAHO requires that viewpoints of patients be incorporated into such training, and patients should be contributors or participants in such training whenever possible. Training elements must include assessment and debriefing skills, risk factors, recognizing and responding to causes of escalating behavior, conflict resolution, effective communication and deescalation techniques, and individual treatment planning with recognition of risk factors and early intervention. A number of technical assistance and training programs are based on best practices, with input from stakeholders, and teach prevention and avoidance of seclusion and restraint. Some of these are included in the section "Suggested Readings and Web Sites" at the end of this chapter.

Contraindications to Seclusion and Restraint

Nonphysical safety measures are always preferable to seclusion and restraint. Above all, no form of restraint should be used in the absence of rigorous staff training in some formal type of crisis prevention or management program, as well as cardiopulmonary resuscitation. The presence of an automatic external

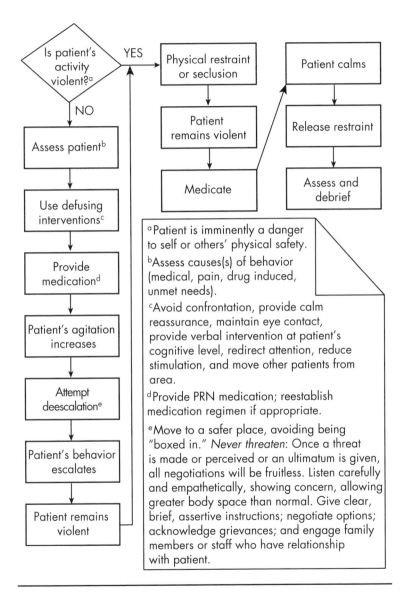

Figure 11–1.   Algorithm for decision making regarding use of seclusion and restraint.

defibrillator in psychiatric settings is advisable, and staff should know when and how to operate the device. According to the American Psychiatric Association (1985), the psychiatric use of seclusion and restraint are contraindicated in patients with any unstable medical conditions, those with delirium or dementia, or those who are overtly suicidal. The AACAP parameters warn that the use of restraints in children who have been sexually abused should be avoided (Masters et al. 2002). Mohr et al. (2003) suggested that prone restraint in particular should be avoided in patients who have increased abdominal girth, a condition common in patients who have been treated with atypical antipsychotics. According to JCAHO (2000), smokers are at higher risk of death when put in restraints; restraints should not be used with patients who have physical deformities that preclude the proper application of a restraint device; and prone restraints may predispose patients to asphyxia, and supine restraints may predispose them to aspiration.

Procedure

There are no overall professional standards that are empirically validated on how to deal with situations in which patients are violent. The psychiatric specialty organizations, nursing organizations, and emergency department physician organizations have issued consensus statements and parameters on the issue of seclusion and restraint; however, there are no guidelines as to how to handle such situations, and despite regulations, not all hospitals provide training in violence and aggression prediction (Peek-Asa et al. 2007). In general, the following scenario occurs in clinical situations: When a patient's behavior begins to escalate wherein he or she is in imminent danger—for example, if a patient becomes verbally threatening or moves to hurt himself or herself in any way—many institutions call some sort of code. Such codes are similar to those called for cardiac emergencies. This code triggers a response from trained designated staff, usually four or five people, who come to see if they can assist and deescalate the patient. One person is designated as the leader of this team. If physical restraint is necessary, the leader directs the restraint and talks with the agitated person. Each staff member is assigned an extremity, and they either hold the person, carry the person to a seclusion room, or apply mechanical restraints.

Some institutions call security guards as a "show of force." Several experts caution against this tactic because it is associated with increased escalation in patients who feel trapped and threatened. In a recent study, Peek-Asa et al. (2007) expressed concern that few hospitals had trained their security staffs in the management of violent disturbances. The authors speculated that hospital administrators may presume that security personnel previously received such training. Moreover, professional staff reported that security guards did not routinely try to deescalate or defuse situations, but were prone to use force as a means of controlling situations.

Forced Chemical Restraints: Indications and Controversy

The clinical use of forced medication is controversial and viewed as a departure from the usual ideal of a collaborative relationship between clinician and patient. The terms most often used to describe such actions—*chemical restraint* and *rapid tranquilization*—are not synonymous. As most commonly used, *chemical restraint* means a medication that is used to control behavior or restrict the patient's freedom of movement and that is not a standard treatment for a patient's medical or psychiatric condition. *Rapid tranquilization* refers to giving medication every half hour to every hour to target symptoms of agitation, hostility, and motor excitement (Schatzberg et al. 2007).

Indications

The indication for chemical restraint is to protect patients from harm to self or others when there is impending danger and measures to deescalate have failed. Medications can be given orally, intramuscularly, or intravenously. The selection of route depends, to some extent, on the cause of the agitation and the emergent situation. Chemical restraint can be used at a patient's request and ideally should be taken voluntarily rather than forced (Dorfman and Kastner 2004; Schatzberg et al. 2007). The JCAHO does not address the use of chemical restraints in their standards except to say that their use is inappropriate and needs to be addressed as part of a facility's performance improvement plan. The AACAP practice parameter states that the pro re nata (as-needed) use of chemical restraint is prohibited. Schatzberg et al. (2007) opined that administering a medication to patients involuntarily is more invasive than physically restraining them.

The least restrictive level of care must be used with aggressive patients and balanced against violating basic human rights. This is a medicolegal issue, and documentation must show that forced medication was used for the safety of the patient, the safety of others, or protection of the milieu from destruction. Ideally, prior to administration of a chemical restraint, patients should be assessed for the primary cause of their aggression, which may include change of mental status or another medical condition. Care must be taken to obtain a good medical history and to obtain a patient's most recent list of medications. Physicians need to be aware of a patient's possible overdose on unknown medications (prescribed or over-the-counter drugs) or intoxication with illicit drugs or alcohol. The incidence of potential drug-drug interactions is high in an unselected emergency department population; therefore, physicians should be vigilant for potential drug-drug interactions, especially among the most high-risk patients taking multiple medications. Clinicians also should be aware of what medications may be contraindicated with patients' comorbid medical conditions. As with all restraints, constant monitoring is necessary and should include vital signs and neurological checks until the patient is fully awake and ambulatory (Sorrentino 2004). Table 11–2 summarizes the most common medications used to manage agitation and aggression (as of 2008).

The ideal drug for restraint would 1) have efficacy in adults and children, 2) have multiple routes of administration, 3) be nonaddictive, 4) have minimal side effects with a good safety record, and 5) be cost-effective. This ideal has not been realized. In addition, high-quality, empirical data on the most effective and appropriate management of behavioral emergencies are limited (Allen 2000; Allen and Currier 2004; Allen et al. 2005). Generally, antipsychotic agents are not recommended for aggressive patients who do not have a diagnosis of a psychotic disorder or bipolar mania; for these patients, nonspecific sedating agents, such as lorazepam, are preferred. The two most common classes of medications employed for chemical restraint in agitated patients are benzodiazepines and antipsychotics. As of 2004, lorazepam was the most frequently used benzodiazepine for "rapid sedation" of the agitated patient, because it offers a quick onset (5–10 minutes with intravenous or intramuscular administration or 20–30 minutes with oral administration). Lorazepam is help-

ful in alcohol withdrawal; it has a short half-life, multiple routes of administration, and no active metabolites; and its metabolism is not cytochrome
P450 dependent. Lorazepam, like all benzodiazepines, can cause respiratory
depression; has a synergistic effect with other sedatives; and can cause sedation, dizziness, weakness, and unsteadiness (Sorrentino 2004). Studies suggest that benzodiazepines used at doses typical in emergency settings may be
more effective than haloperidol (Allen et al. 2005; Currier et al. 2004).

The antipsychotic effects of neuroleptics do not occur for 7–10 days;
however, these drugs are nonaddictive and have sedating properties that are
useful in calming agitated patients. At present, the high-potency group that
carries the greatest risk of extrapyramidal symptoms is the most frequently
used. It should be underscored that antipsychotic-induced akathisia can result
in further agitation. Haloperidol is most often used to calm patients, and it is
available in intramuscular and oral forms. The onset of action is 10–30 minutes for intramuscular haloperidol and 45–60 minutes for oral haloperidol.
Haloperidol is not approved for intravenous use by the FDA, but it is administered "off-label" through this route. The IV use of haloperidol has been associated with sudden death and has been the subject of an FDA alert (Yan
2007). The incidence of extrapyramidal symptoms has been reported to be
approximately 1%, with the most common dystonic reactions including oc-
ulogyric crisis, torticollis, and opisthotonos. There are possible benefits to
coadministering diphenhydramine or benztropine with haloperidol in the
clinical practice of using so-called cocktails to control aggression. Physicians
must always be alert for neuroleptic malignant syndrome when antipsychotic
medications are used (Sorrentino 2004).

Second-generation antipsychotics (SGAs) are playing an increasingly important role in the control of symptoms of patients with acute psychosis. Ziprasidone, olanzapine, and aripiprazole are available in intramuscular forms, and
risperidone is available in dissolvable oral tablets, although the dissolvable form
has not been reported to offer superiority over the tablet. The time to peak
concentration is significantly shorter for risperidone than for olanzapine. This
should be taken into account when rapid control of agitation is desired. The
standard initial dose of ziprasidone is 10–20 mg, taking effect in 15–20 minutes and having low incidence of extrapyramidal symptoms. The recommended interval between first and second injections is 4 hours (Ewing et al.
2004).

Table 11–2.   Medications used to manage agitation and aggression

Medication	Route	Dose	Onset of efficacy	Contraindications[a]	Adverse reactions[b,c]
Aripiprazole	IM Single-dose vials: 9.75 mg/1.3 mL Oral solution: 1 mg/mL	IM: efficacy demonstrated for 5.25–15 mg (no additional benefit with 15 mg dose vs. 9.75 mg dose) Repeat injections should not be given in less than 2 hours Maximum daily dose: 30 mg	30–60 minutes	Use caution in patients with a history of seizures	Dizziness, insomnia, possible activation
Haloperidol	PO/IM	IM: 2–5 mg every 30–60 minutes until sedation achieved IV: No recommendations (Haloperidol is not approved for intravenous use by the FDA, but it is administered "off-label" through this route. IV use of haloperidol has been associated with sudden death and has been the subject of an FDA alert; see Yan 2007.)	IM: 10 minutes IV: 5–30 minutes PO: 45–60 minutes	Parkinson's disease, caution in severe cardiovascular disease	Extrapyramidal symptoms, hypotension, anginal pain in cardiac patients Sudden cardiac death

Table 11–2. Medications used to manage agitation and aggression (*continued*)

Medication	Route	Dose	Onset of efficacy	Contraindications[a]	Adverse reactions[b,c]
Lorazepam	PO/IM	PO: 2–6 mg in divided doses, increasing as needed IM: initial 4 mg; after 10–15 minutes, may administer again; maximum generally 10 mg/day	5–30 minutes	Acute narrow-angle glaucoma, respiratory insufficiency, sleep apnea syndrome	Sedation, dizziness, weakness, unsteadiness
Olanzapine	PO/IM	PO: 5–10 mg initially, increasing up to 20 mg/day IM: initial dose of 10 mg, second dose of 5–10 mg 2 hours after first; no more than three injections per 24 hours	IM 15–30 minutes	Any unstable medical condition (e.g., acute myocardial infarction, sick sinus syndrome, recent cardiac surgery), prostatic hypertrophy, narrow-angle glaucoma, paralytic ileus	Somnolence, dry mouth, dysphagia, dizziness, asthenia, joint pain, postural hypotension

Table 11–2.   Medications used to manage agitation and aggression (*continued*)

Medication	Route	Dose	Onset of efficacy	Contraindications[a]	Adverse reactions[b,c]
Risperidone	PO Oral solution: 1 mg/mL Orally disintegrating tablets: 0.5 mg, 1 mg, and 2 mg	1 mg initially, increasing as tolerated up to dose of 3 mg bid; manufacturer recommends dose increases in no less than 24-hour period	Peak concentration achieved in 1 hour	Oral solution incompatible with cola or tea	Extrapyramidal symptoms, somnolence, nausea, hyperkinesias, orthostatic hypotension
Ziprasidone	IM	IM: 10–20 mg Maximum dose of 40 mg/day Doses of 10 mg may be administered every 2 hours; doses of 20 mg may be administered every 4 hours	15–20 minutes	Known history of QT prolongation, recent myocardial infarction, uncompensated congestive heart failure	Somnolence, nausea, headache, asthenia, orthostatic hypotension, seizures (rare), sudden death

Note.   IM = intramuscular; IV = intravenous; PO = oral.

[a]Hypersensitivity to the drug is always a contraindication.

[b]Increased risk of death from cerebrovascular accident reported with second-generation antipsychotic use in elderly patients.

[c]Neuroleptic malignant syndrome (rare) is always a consideration with antipsychotic medications; hyperglycemia, in some cases extreme and associated with ketoacidosis or hyperosmolar coma and death, has been reported in patients taking antipsychotic medication.

Source.   Stahl 2006.

Intramuscular olanzapine has been found to be more effective than either haloperidol or placebo for managing acute agitation in schizophrenia, and it is well tolerated (Breier et al. 2002; Wright et al. 2003). A potential drawback with the use of intramuscular olanzapine in emergency situations is the possibility of postural hypotension. In reducing agitation, olanzapine is effective in a dose-dependent relationship, with higher doses (10 mg) being more effective than lower (2.5 mg), although 5 mg doses may be sufficient in some adults (Breier et al. 2002). A second injection of 10 mg may be given as soon as 2 hours after the first, and additional injections may be administered every 4 hours if needed. The patient should not receive more than 30 mg in a 24-hour period.

Aripiprazole is the latest SGA to be available in injectable form and has been found to be comparable in effectiveness to intramuscular haloperidol, with significantly greater tolerability (Currier et al. 2007; Tran-Johnson et al. 2007).

Benzodiazepines and antipsychotics have been administered together as a chemical restraint with or without diphenhydramine or benztropine in cocktails. When benzodiazepines and antipsychotics are given together, lower doses of both medications can be used, resulting in decreased side effects from the individual agents. Symptoms of akathisia from the antipsychotic may be diminished by the benzodiazepine (Schatzberg et al. 2007). The use of olanzapine in conjunction with benzodiazepines has been shown to cause a hypoventilatory syndrome and is not recommended (Breier et al. 2002).

Special Populations

Pregnant Women

The U.S. Food and Drug Administration has established use-in-pregnancy risk categories (see, e.g., http://depts.washington.edu/druginfo/Formulary/Pregnancy.pdf); however, these categories have limitations and are considered inadequate. At this writing, benzodiazepines are category D, with possible complications of "floppy baby," withdrawal, and increased risk of cleft lip or palate especially with first-trimester exposure. Hypnotic benzodiazepines are category X, which means contraindicated in pregnancy. All antipsychotic medications, whether typical or atypical, are category C (meaning that risk cannot be ruled out) except clozapine. First-generation antipsychotics have been associated with rare anomalies, fetal jaundice, and fetal anticholinergic effects at birth. The SGAs have unknown possible effects in pregnancy and are category C. In the absence of data, it may be better practice during pregnancy to use high-potency typical antipsychotic agents, such as haloperidol, which has been available for many years and has a relatively good track record in pregnancy (Schatzberg et al. 2007).

Geriatric Patients

Antipsychotic use is controversial in geriatric patients, who may be more likely to develop adverse side effects. The use of SGAs in patients with dementia has been reported to be associated with increased mortality from cerebrovascular accidents and other causes; speculation is that SGAs are associated with the same risks in the elderly (Alexopoulos et al. 2005). Authorities recommend that nonpharmacological interventions be employed first in dementia patients exhibiting behavior dyscontrol. All typical antipsychotics may cause pseudoparkinsonism and akathisia in the elderly. In addition, there is an increased risk of tardive dyskinesia in the elderly. Atypical antipsychotics are preferred over benzodiazepines in patients with dementia (Schatzberg et al. 2007).

In geriatric patients, as in all patients, it is critical to treat the underlying cause of agitation (Piechniczek-Buczek 2006). Because geriatric patients are likely to have increased comorbid medical conditions, the clinician must be on the alert for drug-drug interactions. When combined with calcium channel blockers, thiazide diuretics, and prazosin, antipsychotic medications may increase hypotension. When antipsychotics are given with beta-blockers, the combination may cause increased antipsychotic levels. When given with class 1A or 1C antiarrhythmics, antipsychotics may prolong cardiac conduction. Antipsychotics may increase digitalis levels (Schatzberg et al. 2007).

Children and Adolescents

Low-dose antipsychotic medication is used to control agitated behavior in inpatient children and adolescents. However, the use of even low-dose antipsychotic medication, as well as of benzodiazepines and antihistamines, to decrease agitation in children can cause side effects or adverse reactions. Typical and atypical agents may cause tardive dyskinesia, and SGAs as a class are associated with weight gain and metabolic syndrome, although some atypical antipsychotics (e.g., risperidone) appear more weight neutral when given in lower doses. A higher rate of dystonic reactions with antipsychotics has been seen in adolescent males early in treatment. Antipsychotic medication may cause cognitive blunting and interfere with learning. Benzodiazepines have been found to aggravate behavioral disorders or increase activity, especially in children with attention-deficit/hyperactivity disorder. Continued use of sedative antihistamines may have anticholinergic side effects and may cause cognitive blunting (Schatzberg et al. 2007).

Observation (Including the 1-Hour Rule)

When patients are restrained by staff members using any technique, the JCAHO and CMS require that a staff member be designated to observe the patient continually for any signs of physical distress. Staff members must be directed never to disregard a patient's statement that he or she cannot breathe or to explain away such statements as manipulation. Too often, such pleas have been disregarded with tragic consequences (Nunno et al. 2006).

When a patient is in restraint or seclusion, the CMS requires the patient to be continually monitored face to face. The JCAHO states that patients who are in seclusion should be continually monitored face to face, but that after the first hour in seclusion, patients may be monitored continually using video and audio equipment. The JCAHO directs that a patient should be monitored every 15 minutes while in either restraint or seclusion for readiness to discontinue the procedure and to assure his or her comfort. Comfort refers to, among other things, vital signs, range of motion, proper body alignment, circulation, and need for toileting and/or hydration, as well as psychological comfort. Such monitoring should be conducted by a qualified staff member who is able to recognize when to contact a medically trained licensed independent practitioner or emergency medical service. Restraint use should also be documented. Clinicians are cautioned that it is imperative that patients be continually monitored and that the "15-minute checklist" should not be used as a pro forma exercise in paperwork.

The clinician, either a physician or other licensed independent practitioner, works with the staff and patient to identify ways to help the patient gain behavioral control. A new order is provided for seclusion and restraint if necessary. These orders must adhere to the regulations as explicated in Table 11–1.

Within 1 hour of the application of a restraint or placing a patient in seclusion, a physician or a licensed independent professional must conduct a face-to-face evaluation of an individual. This "1-hour rule" was promulgated by CMS at the urging of professionals and advocates who were concerned about the misuse and overuse of seclusion and restraint, and about the number of deaths and injury that were accompanying them (see section "Death and Other Adverse Effects").

Release From Restraint and Debriefing

Patients should be released from restraints when they are calm and no longer pose a threat to themselves or others. Early in the restraint process, patients should have been apprised of the rationale for the restraint and the criteria for release. This information should be reiterated when patients are less agitated. Before release, patients should be oriented to the environment and should have ceased verbally threatening the staff. Facilities may have specific behavioral criteria articulated in operational terms to provide guidance to staff; some facilities may also require that a patient contract verbally for safety. Most facility policy and procedure manuals and training programs have specific procedures for releasing patients from mechanical restraints.

Following a patient's release from restraint, facilities are required to conduct a debriefing that includes staff and patient within 24 hours of the incident. The purpose of such debriefing is to determine how to avoid a similar event in the future. Discussion should focus on the circumstances resulting in the seclusion and restraint (e.g., precipitant), methods for more safely responding, helping staff to understand the precipitant, and developing alternative methods for helping patients and staff to cope and avoid future seclusion and restraint. The most important outcomes of such a debriefing should be reexamination of the treatment plan, an assessment of whether the procedure was done safely and was consistent with training, and a determination of whether the procedure was necessary.

Death and Other Adverse Effects

As mentioned, most often a physical restraint is employed in which staff members hold the patient until he or she becomes calm. There is no preferred position in which to hold a person. All restraints have significant morbidity and mortality risks. Prone restraints seem to bear the greatest risk. The JCAHO reviewed 20 cases of death in restraints; in 40% of the cases, the cause of death was asphyxia, most often resulting from factors such as placing excessive weight on the patient's back (JCAHO 1998).

If one surveys the psychiatric literature, death seems to be a relatively rare event. However, in the absence of any sustained data collection across diverse settings, deaths associated with restraint use may not be as rare as a first impression might suggest.

Mohr et al. (2003) identified asphyxiation as the most common reported cause of restraint-related death, but other causes included death by aspiration, blunt trauma to the chest (commotio cordis), malignant cardiac rhythm disturbances secondary to massive catecholamine rush, thrombosis, rhabdomyolysis, excited delirium with overwhelming metabolic acidosis, and pulmonary embolism. Evans et al.'s (2003) retrospective investigation of death certificates and records identified a large number of restraint-related deaths, further underscoring that restraint is not a benign procedure.

Nunno et al. (2006) found 45 child and adolescent fatalities related to restraints in institutions between 1993 and 2003. In over half of the deaths, asphyxia was the cause. In each case for which information was available, there was no evidence that the child's behavior met the standard of danger to self or others.

O'Halloran and Frank (2000) discussed 21 asphyxial deaths that occurred during prone restraints in health care facilities, detention centers, or jails; restrainers included police officers, security personnel, laypersons, custodial officers, and firefighters. From one to seven persons were engaged in the restraint, and the time of restraints from initiation to death was estimated to be 2–12 minutes.

The negative psychological impact of restraint and seclusion has been well documented. Studies conducted of patients' subjective experiences of restraints found that the experiences were generally viewed as punitive and coercive, had a negative impact on the therapeutic alliance, and were counterproductive in that they promoted unwanted behaviors (Kahng et al. 2001; Magee and Ellis 2001; Zun 2005). When in seclusion, patients described feeling neglected, fearful, isolated, vulnerable, and punished (Martinez et al. 1999).

Staff members are also injured during restraint. However, in states and institutions that have reduced their restraint use, not only have staff injuries decreased, but the institutions have realized significant financial savings because each restraint episode represents a good deal of expense (LeBel et al. 2004).

Reporting Patient Death

On July 2, 1999, the Patients' Rights Interim Final Rule was published (CMS 1999), requiring that a hospital must report to a CMS regional office any patient death that occurs while the patient is restrained or in seclusion for behavioral management. The CMS also stipulates that such reporting must include each death that occurs within 24 hours after a patient has been removed from seclusion and restraint and every death that occurs within 1 week of seclusion and restraint, if it is reasonable to assume that restraint use or placement in seclusion contributed directly or indirectly to a patient's death. The number of deaths reported from 1999 to 2002 was 75 (U.S. Department of Health and Human Services 2002). This number undoubtedly does not reflect the complete picture, because only institutions receiving CMS monies are required to report these deaths.

Paradigm Case of Child Restraint Leading to Death

A 9-year-old child weighing 56 pounds fell asleep in her chair at a therapeutic school. She was awakened by staff and told to sit up and sit straight, without feet crossed. She had been restrained for "oppositional behavior" twice that week for an hour each time; in her frustration, she kicked her foot, sending her shoe across the room. Staff members deemed her to be "out of control" and took her to the floor, restraining her in a prone position. A 250-pound staff member put the weight of his body over her torso. The child struggled against the restraint for 1 hour, during which time she cried that she could not breathe. She lost control of her bladder and bowels. When staff members deemed her to be quiescent, they turned her over. She was blue. Efforts at resuscitation were not successful. The cause of death was compressional asphyxia, and the manner of death was ruled homicide.

Unlike the case presented at the beginning of this chapter, in which restraint was successfully used, this case, which happened in Wisconsin in 2004, represents the use of unnecessary restraint that resulted in an unnecessary death. It is a typical scenario of the kind that was studied by Nunno et al. (2006) and reflects poor staff training and judgment.

Documentation and Legal Considerations

Documentation serves as an important source of information for other professionals. It is imperative that clinicians document as clearly and accurately as possible the rationale for restraint or seclusion and chronicle precisely what has transpired. The documentation should include the nature of the emergency or the reason that restraint was considered necessary, the measures enacted to deescalate the patient to prevent the need for restraint, antecedents to the violent behavior if assessed by staff, the type of restraint employed, the staff members who were involved, the length of time of the restraint, and the patient's condition both during the restraint and after termination of the restraint. Although some of this documentation may be delegated to staff members, physicians should be mindful that many clinical staff, even those with college educations, have little formal education in clinical psychiatry, and the only training they may have in restraint and seclusion is what they have been taught "on the job." Many staff members may not understand the proper way to document incidents appropriately in the medical record. Even with checklist documentation, which is becoming increasingly popular, they may not have a good understanding of the terms that are presented in the checklist. This can pose potential difficulties should legal problems arise (Mohr 2006).

Clinicians should be aware of legal considerations pertaining to restraint of psychiatric patients and document carefully and thoroughly. Physicians are especially vulnerable from a legal standpoint because they have ultimate responsibility for patients' treatment, they must write the order for restraint or seclusion, and they must narrate the course of a patient's history and treatment, as well as the rationale for and outcomes of treatment (Northcutt and Shea 2006).

In the past, claims of constitutional violations were a common response to systemic overuse of seclusion and restraint. Constitutional claims include violations of the fourteenth-amendment right to freedom from restraint and violation of the fourth-amendment right to be free from unreasonable search and seizure. The use of restraints is supported by the 1982 Supreme Court decision in *Youngberg v. Romeo*, which affirmed that a patient could be restrained to protect others or self. Challenges to this decision may reemerge, because professional judgment in the field strongly supports significant reduction in the use of restraint.

In recent years, forensic pathologists have developed a conventional standard wherein if an asphyxial death happens during a restraint episode, the manner of death is always listed as homicide, regardless of the intent of the procedure (National Association of Medical Examiners 2002). This has prompted criminal investigations that might not have happened in the past. Tort claims have also been more common. They can involve a number of different causes of action: excessive force, medical malpractice, failure to protect, assault and battery, and failure to maintain a safe environment. Attorneys are also examining the application of the Americans With Disabilities Act of 1990 to the use of seclusion and restraint under the *Olmstead v. L.C.* (1999) decision, in which the U.S. Supreme Court ruled that unjustified isolation of individuals with disabilities is properly regarded as discrimination based on disability.

Because of legal and liability considerations, unusual terminology and jargon should be avoided. Also, to the extent possible, operational definitions and descriptions should be employed.

Key Clinical Points

- Behavioral emergencies are dynamic, complex events requiring assessment and rapid intervention.

- Seclusion and physical and chemical restraints are tools in the arsenal for managing behavioral emergencies.

- Use of seclusion and physical restraints is regulated by the Centers for Medicare & Medicaid Services and The Joint Commission (formerly the Joint Commission on Accreditation of Health Care Organizations), and regulations vary from state to state.

- The use of physical restraints is fraught with risks for staff and patients.

- High-quality empirical data on effectively managing behavioral emergencies are lacking.

References

Alexopoulos GS, Jeste DV, Chung H, et al: The expert consensus guideline series: treatment of dementia and its behavioral disturbances. Postgrad Med (Special Report), January 2005, pp 6–22

Allen MH: Managing the agitated psychotic patient: a reappraisal of the evidence. J Clin Psychiatry 61 (suppl 4):11–20, 2000

Allen MH, Currier GW: Use of restraints and pharmacotherapy in academic psychiatric emergency services. Gen Hosp Psychiatry 26:42–49, 2004

Allen MH, Currier GW, Carpenter D, et al; Expert Consensus Panel for Behavioral Emergencies 2005: The expert consensus guideline series: treatment of behavioral emergencies. J Psychiatric Pract 11 (suppl 1):5–108, 2005

American Psychiatric Association: The American Psychiatric Association Task Force Report 22: The Psychiatric Uses of Seclusion and Restraint. Washington, DC, American Psychiatric Association, 1984

Americans With Disabilities Act of 1990, 42 U.S.C. § 12101 et seq.

Annas G: The last resort: the use of physical restraints in medical emergencies. N Engl J Med 341:1408–1412, 1999

Berrios CD, Jacobowitz WH: Therapeutic holding: outcomes of a pilot study. J Psychosoc Nurs Ment Health Serv 36:14–18, 1998

Breier A, Meehan K, Birkett M, et al: A double-blind, placebo-controlled dose-response comparison of intramuscular olanzapine and haloperidol in the treatment of acute agitation in schizophrenia. Arch Gen Psychiatry 59:441–448, 2002

Centers for Medicare and Medicaid Services: Final Rule: Medicaire and Medicaid Programs: Hospital Conditions of Participation: Patients' Rights. 42 CFR Part 482, December 8, 2006

Child Welfare League of America: Advocacy: seclusion and restraints, 2002a. Fact sheet. Available at: http://www.cwla.org/advocacy/secresfactsheet.htm. Accessed January 25, 2010.

Child Welfare League of America: CWLA Best Practice Guidelines: Behavior Management. Washington, DC, Child Welfare League of America, 2002b

Currier GW, Allen MH, Bunney EB, et al: Safety of medications used to treat acute agitation. J Emerg Med 27(suppl):S19–S24, 2004

Currier GW, Citrome LL, Zimbroff DL, et al: Intramuscular aripiprazole in the control of agitation. J Psychiatr Pract 13:159–169, 2007

Dorfman DH, Kastner B: The use of restraint for pediatric patients in emergency departments. Pediatr Emerg Care 20:151–156, 2004

Evans D, Wood J, Lambert L: Patient injury and physical restraint devices: a systematic review. J Adv Nurs 412:274–282, 2003

Ewing J, Rund D, Votaloto N: Evaluating the reconstitution of intramuscular ziprasidone into solution. Ann Emerg Med 43:419–420, 2004

Gately LA, Stabb SD: Psychology students' training in the management of potentially violent clients. Prof Psychol Res Pr 36:681–687, 2005

Joint Commission on Accreditation of Healthcare Organizations: Preventing restraint deaths. Joint Commission Sentinel Event Alert. November 18, 1998. Available at: http://www. jointcommission.org/SentinelEvents/SentinelEventAlert/sea_8. htm. Accessed October 11, 2009.

Joint Commission on Accreditation of Healthcare Organizations: Comprehensive Accreditation Manual for Hospitals: The Official Handbook. Oakbrook Terrace, IL, Joint Commission on Accreditation of Healthcare Organizations, 2000

Kahng S, Abt KA, Wilder DA: Treatment of collateral self-injury correlated with mechanical restraints. Behavioral Interventions 16:105–110, 2001

LeBel J, Stronmberg N, Duckworth K, et al: Child and adolescent inpatient restraint reduction: a state initiative to promote strength-based care. J Am Acad Child Adolesc Psychiatry 43:37–45, 2004

Magee SK, Ellis J: The detrimental effects of physical restraint as a consequence for inappropriate classroom behavior. J Appl Behav Anal 34:501–504, 2001

Martinez RJ, Grimm M, Adamson M: From the other side of the door: patient views of seclusion. J Psychosocial Nurs Ment Health Serv 37:13–22, 1999

Masters K, Bellonci C, Bernet W, et al: Practice parameter for the prevention and management of aggressive behavior in child and adolescent psychiatric institutions with special reference to seclusion and restraint. J Am Acad Child Adolesc Psychiatry 41(suppl):4S–25S, 2002

Mohr WK: Psychiatric records, in Medical Legal Aspects of Medical Records. Edited by Iyer P, Levin BJ, Shea MA. Tucson, AZ, Lawyers and Judges Publishing, 2006, pp 691–705

Mohr WK, Petti TA, Mohr BD: Adverse effects associated with physical restraint. Can J Psychiatry 48:330–337, 2003

National Association of Medical Examiners: A Guide for Manner of Death Clarification. Atlanta, GA, National Association of Medical Examiners, 2002

Northcutt CL, Shea MA: Generating and preserving the medical record, in Medical Legal Aspects of Medical Records. Edited by Iyer P, Levin BJ, Shea MA. Tucson, AZ, Lawyers and Judges Publishing, 2006, pp 3–10

Nunno M, Holden M, Tollar A: Learning from tragedy: a survey of child and adolescent restraint fatalities. Child Abuse Negl 30:1333–1342, 2006

O'Halloran RL, Frank JG: Asphyxial death during prone restraint revisited: a report of 21 cases. Am J Forensic Med Pathol 21:39–52, 2000

Olmstead v L.C. 527 U.S. 581 (1999)

Peek-Asa C, Casteel C, Allareddy V, et al: Workplace violence prevention programs in hospital emergency departments. J Occup Environ Med 49:756–763, 2007

Piechniczek-Buczek J: Psychiatric emergencies in the elderly population. Emerg Med Clin North Am 24:467–490, 2006

Schatzberg AF, Cole JO, DeBattista BM: Manual of Clinical Psychopharmacology, 6th Edition. Washington, DC, American Psychiatric Publishing, 2007

Schwartz TL, Park TL: Assaults by patients on psychiatric residents: a survey and training recommendations. Psychiatr Serv 50:381–383, 1999

Sorrentino A: Chemical restraints for the agitated, violent, or psychotic pediatric patient in the emergency department: controversies and recommendations. Curr Opin Pediatr 16:201–205, 2004

Stahl SM: Essential Psychopharmacology: The Prescriber's Guide. New York, Oxford University Press, 2006

Stillwell EM: Nurses' education related to the use of restraints. J Gerontol Nurs 17:23–26, 1991

Tran-Johnson TK, Sack DA, Marcus RN, et al: Efficacy and safety of intramuscular aripiprazole in patients with acute agitation: a randomized, double-blind, placebo-controlled trial. J Clin Psychiatry 68:111–119, 2007

U.S. Department of Health and Human Services,, Centers for Medicare & Medicaid Services: Patients' Rights Interim Final Rule. July 2, 1999. 42 CFR 482.13 (1999)

U.S. Department of Health and Human Services, Centers for Medicare & Medicaid Services: Medicare and Medicaid programs; hospital conditions of participation: clarification of the regulatory flexibility analysis for patients' rights. Fed Regist 67(191):61805–61808, October, 2, 2002

Wright P, Lindborg SR, Birkett M, et al: Intramuscular olanzapine and intramuscular haloperidol in acute schizophrenia: antipsychotic efficacy and extrapyramidal safety during the first 24 hours of treatment. Can J Psychiatry 48:716–721, 2003

Yan J: FDA warns of serious side effects from IV haloperidol. Psychiatric News 42(21):14, 2007. Available at: http://pn.psychiatryonline.org/content/42/21/14.2.full?sid=f7a37a04-25e6-4033-ae73-466c082c955f. Accessed January 25, 2010.

Youngberg v Romeo, 457 U.S. 307 (1982)

Zun LS: Evidence-based treatment of psychiatric patients. J Emerg Med 28:277–283, 2005

Suggested Readings and Web Sites

American Academy of Child and Adolescent Psychiatry (AACAP)

http://www.aacap.org

Presents issue briefs on the use of seclusion and restraint with children and adolescents, and summaries of proposed legislation.

American Academy of Physician Assistants (AAPA)

http://www.aapa.org/advocacy-and-practice-resources

Includes position statement on reducing seclusion and restraint usage.

American Nurses Association (ANA)

http://www.nursingworld.org

Contains position statement on reducing seclusion and restraint usage from the nursing perspective.

Centers for Medicare & Medicaid Services

http://www.hcfa.gov/publications/newsletters/restraint

Offers information on restraint reduction including archived copies of the HCFA National Restraint Reduction Newsletter.

Judge David L. Bazelon Center for Mental Health Law

http://www.bazelon.org

Provides current information on legislation and court decisions affecting the use of seclusion and restraint in psychiatric facilities. Also contains information on the Americans With Disabilities Act (ADA), and Olmstead v. L.C.

National Alliance on Mental Illness (NAMI)

http://www.nami.org

Features position statement on seclusion and restraint and chart summarizing abuse of restraint usage across the country from October 1998 through March 2000.

National Association of Consumer/Survivor Mental Health Administrators (NAC/SMHA)

http://www.nasmhpd.org/nac_smha.cfm

Provides history of abuse in mental health settings and contact information for national consumer affairs officials.

National Association of Protection and Advocacy Systems (NAPAS)

    http://www.napas.org

    Offers information on federally mandated protection and advocacy programs that protect the rights of persons with disabilities, including psychiatric disabilities. Also contains a special report on seclusion and restraint.

National Association of Psychiatric Health Systems (NAPHS)

    http://www.naphs.org

    Provides guidelines on the use of seclusion.

National Association of State Mental Health Program Directors (NASMHPD)

    http://www.nasmhpd.org

    Features a position statement, legislative updates, and free online publications.

National Mental Health Consumers' Self-Help Clearinghouse

    http://www.mhselfhelp.org

    Includes information on restraint reduction and other issues from a consumer advocate perspective.

U.S. General Accounting Office

    http://www.gao.gov/archive/1999/he99176.pdf

    Provides 1999 report, "Improper Restraint or Seclusion Use Places People at Risk," which was provided to Congressional requesters.

12

Legal and Ethical Issues in Emergency Psychiatry

Nancy Byatt, D.O., M.B.A.
Debra A. Pinals, M.D.

Emergency psychiatry can be an exciting, fast-paced environment in which medical decisions are often made without the luxury of long periods of time for deliberation. From the moment a patient presents to the psychiatric emergency services (PES) setting, important issues surface that are critical for mental health staff to understand so that they operate within the constraints of law, ethics, and regulations. For example, a duty of care exists for patients who present themselves to the emergency room. Refusing care could incur allegations and liability related to patient abandonment. A patient who walks into a lobby but decides not to register may not fall under this duty of care. Once a patient is known to have presented, the mental health staff may have certain obligations related to treatment. From that point forward, legal, regulatory, and system issues related to confidentiality, informed consent, emergency restraint, and utilization management are commonplace. Having an understanding of common legal and ethical underpinnings of emergency psychiatric practice is important in the PES setting. In this chapter, we review some of the common legal themes encountered in emergency psychiatry and provide information on their management.

Confidentiality

> While working as a mental health professional in the psychiatric emergency department, you answer an outside call. A woman on the line states, "I think my sister, Ms. X, is in the psychiatric emergency room. How is she doing?" How do you respond?

Trust is the foundation of a therapeutic relationship. A physician's maintenance of confidentiality assures patients that their autonomy is respected and valued. In adolescent populations, the lack of willingness to seek medical care and to disclose pertinent history has been linked directly to perception and fear of disclosure (Mermelstein and Wallack 2008). Patients have also reported choosing to change or withhold pertinent clinical information due to fear of a breach in confidentiality (Mermelstein and Wallack 2008). It is incumbent on psychiatrists to respect patients' confidentiality by making every effort to assure the highest degree of privacy possible.

One might argue that in no other field of medicine is the need for confidentiality as paramount as in psychiatry. Psychiatrists ask patients not only to reveal their innermost feelings, but also to discuss problems that many people may find shameful or stigmatizing. Patients are placed in the precarious position of being vulnerable and dependent on psychiatrists to protect the same information that needs to be shared for treatment to take place.

The importance of confidentiality in psychiatric communication has been recognized in case law and codified in statute (Mermelstein and Wallack 2008). The U.S. Supreme Court, in the landmark case *Jaffe v. Redmond* (1996), recognized the importance of a psychotherapist-patient privilege. Other changes in medical privacy have taken place. For example, the Health Insurance Portability and Accountability Act of 1996 (HIPAA; U.S. Department of Health and Human Services 2009) is a set of rules enacted by the federal government to systematically respond to threats to medical privacy. HIPAA mandates that patients authorize release of information and be informed as to how their medical information will be used.

Exceptions

Although important, the right to privacy is not absolute; exceptions arise that require confidentiality to be broken. Even though it may be clinically necessary and legally sound to break a patient's confidentiality in certain circumstances, one must carefully consider and document the necessity to do so for patient care, the effect of the communication, and the benefit-risk ratio of and alternatives to any such approach. A common example in the emergency department involves the need to contact family or other treatment providers to gather information about a patient who has presented. If a patient consents to such communication, the issue of breach of confidentiality is moot. However, emergency psychiatrists and clinicians often need to contact family members, friends, or other persons, without patient consent, to ascertain clinical background information that could ultimately help mitigate risk of harm to the patient or others. In an emergency, the PES clinician should proceed with obtaining the needed information and be sure to explain to the family member or other collateral contact the rationale for requesting the information without patient consent (Mermelstein and Wallack 2008).

A risk of harm to a third party raises another important potential exception to the obligation to maintain confidentiality of patient information (Herbert 2002). Most states have adopted legal rules, either through case law or legislation, that impose provisions stemming from California's Supreme Court decision in *Tarasoff v. Regents of the University of California* (1976). Some states impose an actual and explicit duty to protect a potential third party who may be at risk of being harmed by a person under the care of a psychiatrist or other mental health clinician, whereas other states have less specific requirements. Thus, local laws may or may not impose a liability protection against claims of breach of confidentiality in such circumstances. At times, actions a clinician may ethically or legally take, depending on the clinical scenario and jurisdiction, include warning third parties of the potential for harm, but at other times, and important to the final California Supreme Court analysis of the original *Tarasoff* case (*Tarasoff v. Regents of the University of California* 1974), actions to protect a potential victim may extend beyond warning the potential victim toward taking actions to protect the person(s) at risk of harm. For example, protection of a third party may be better executed by taking other actions, such as hospitalization of the patient (Herbert 2002).

Sharing Information With Providers and Emergency Department Staff

PES staff often struggle to maintain confidentiality while obtaining information from or giving information to other providers and emergency department staff in the interest of patient care. Additional challenges result when certain components of mental health record information are to be shared with other general health care providers, whose limitations related to confidentiality may not be held in the same regard. A bidirectional flow of necessary information between providers is essential, because it allows PES staff to work in a patient's best interests and to maintain a collaborative relationship with other providers. Free sharing of information cannot, however, be done merely for staff convenience. An emergency exception to confidentiality allows for the communication to occur.

PES staff generally follow a crisis model that focuses on acute issues, such as safety and symptom relief, with the goal of transferring the patient to an inpatient hospital setting for stabilization or return to outpatient care. PES staff, therefore, should concentrate on obtaining and sharing information needed for acute patient care. In PES settings, where mental health clinicians work side by side with other clinicians, it is important to consider the physical setting and risk of incidental disclosure when discussing cases with referring clinicians (Mermelstein and Wallack 2008).

Asking for Releases, Time Permitting

HIPAA addresses authorization for release and permits disclosure of medical information in the interest of providing appropriate care for patients, unless requested otherwise. If time permits, PES staff ideally should educate the patient about the relevant issues and request consent before releasing information. In the case of Ms. X, one should obtain patient consent before acknowledging to others that the patient is in the emergency department. Given that this is often not feasible in the PES setting, staff should use discretion and limit what they discuss to what is necessary for acute patient care

(Mermelstein and Wallack 2008). For example, although it may be important to share that a patient is in the emergency room with certain family members to be able to gather information from them, it may not be reasonable to share with them all patient information (e.g., the circumstances of a patient's recent breakup of a relationship).

Hospitalization

Ms. X has been evaluated in PES, and it is abundantly clear that she would benefit from a psychiatric hospitalization given the lack of outpatient psychiatric and psychosocial support available for her, as well as her severe depression, passive suicidal ideation, and psychotic symptoms that are significantly impacting her ability to function. You are, however, reassured because she is denying any intent or plan to act on her suicidal thoughts and states many reasons why she would not want to die. Also, although her family members are concerned about her functioning and prefer a psychiatric hospitalization, they feel that she would be safe if discharged home. Based on your assessment, you feel that a psychiatric hospitalization is indicated but do not feel that Ms. X meets criteria for involuntary commitment because she does not appear to be at imminent risk of harm to self or others. How do you proceed?

Psychiatric hospitalization is generally intended to stabilize and provide a therapeutic environment for patients, yet it can be perceived as a violation of one's civil liberty when done involuntarily. Psychiatry is distinct from other specialties in that it routinely uses involuntary civil commitment as a means to provide intensive, hospital-level care in certain circumstances when persons are in need of such intervention but are refusing voluntary hospitalization. PES staff must ensure that proper restrictions on hospitalization are used to preclude the abuse of power related to civil commitment (Lidz et al. 1989).

Voluntary Admissions

Voluntary admission is preferred over involuntary because it can foster the development of a therapeutic alliance and recognizes an individual's autonomy. For a voluntary psychiatric admission, some states have as part of statutory language the requirement that the facility is capable of providing care and that the patient is in need of psychiatric care. As in the case of Ms. X, PES clinicians must assess whether a voluntary admission is clinically indicated or whether a less restrictive alternative for psychiatric treatment (e.g., a crisis stabilization placement) would be appropriate and more therapeutic (Simon and Goetz 1999).

There are different types of voluntary status, and the procedure for discharge varies with each type (Appelbaum and Gutheil 2007).

Pure Voluntary Admission

Under a pure voluntary status, the patient is free to leave the hospital at any time, much like in medical settings. Many states limit pure voluntary status in psychiatric settings, given the higher likelihood that patients who exercise their right to leave might raise enough clinical concern to warrant petitioning for their civil commitment (Appelbaum and Gutheil 2007).

Conditional Voluntary Admission

The conditional voluntary status allows the admitting facility to detain patients in the hospital for a period of time, often up to several days, after the patient has announced his or her desire to leave. This period of detainment may be used to allow the patient to change his or her mind, for evaluation of the patient and a determination about whether it is clinically indicated to initiate proceedings for involuntary commitment, or for discharge planning. If the facility decides to seek commitment, the patient can be held in the hospital until the hearing takes place. If a patient decides to leave and criteria for involuntary commitment are not met, then the patient is free to go, even if further inpatient treatment is clinically indicated (Appelbaum and Gutheil 2007). The discharge in this case is often granted against medical advice (AMA) and documented as such, after a discussion that involves an attempt to address the patient's reasons for leaving and reviews risks for leaving versus benefits of further hospitalization. Regardless of whether the patient leaves AMA, follow-up treatment and referrals should be provided (Brook et al. 2006).

"Coerced Voluntary" Admission

Although patient advocates have articulated concern that vulnerable persons with mental illness may be coerced into a conditional voluntary admission, research indicates that the legal status on admission is not a reliable indicator of whether patients experience coercion during the hospital admission process

(MacArthur Research Network on Mental Health and the Law 2001). PES clinicians, however, should be cautious not to coerce patients into agreeing to a voluntary hospitalization when there is no intention or rationale that would justify hospitalizing the patient involuntarily. In *Zinermon v. Burch* (1979), a person was committed to a state hospital voluntarily although he lacked the capacity to give informed consent to the hospitalization. The U.S. Supreme Court held that the failure to identify patients who lack the capacity to give informed consent is a violation of patients' rights. What this means in clinical practice is complex, because capacity to consent to inpatient psychiatric hospitalization may require a low threshold. In assessing a patient's competence to consent to psychiatric hospitalization, PES clinicians balance the desire to make voluntary hospitalization and its benefits widely available (even to those who may have limited capacity for making a choice toward voluntary hospitalization) with the need to ensure that patients without decisional capacity are not hospitalized involuntarily without appropriate legal grounds to do so (Lidz et al. 1989; Simon and Goetz 1999).

Emergency Holds/Detention

Psychiatric patients presenting to the emergency department are often escorted against their will by police officers. In many states, police officers have the power to transport patients involuntarily based on information obtained from a treating professional or family member that indicates that the patient is at imminent risk of harming self or others. Jurisdictions often have statutes allowing police officers to "emergency petition" patients to be transported to the nearest emergency department for further evaluation. Some emergency holds can last hours, some longer. While evaluating patients, PES clinicians need to consider how the petition was obtained and the circumstances that led to the petition. As noted, the PES evaluation may or may not lead to an involuntary psychiatric hospitalization (Simon and Goetz 1999).

Persons who have ingested substances may present to the emergency department in an apparent state of acute psychiatric decompensation. Individuals who are intoxicated or abusing substances, for example, are often brought to the emergency department secondary to dangerousness to self or others. Patients with alcohol dependence and a high tolerance for alcohol may not present with slurred speech or ataxia and may disclose suicidal intent while appearing sober. A toxicology screen and cognitive screening examination should be completed to ensure that such a patient, and patients who have less tolerance, are not evaluated for involuntary psychiatric hospitalization while still intoxicated. Once sober, these patients may not fit the criteria for an involuntary psychiatric hospital admission (Simon and Goetz 1999).

Involuntary Hospitalization

The power to commit a patient to the hospital involuntarily represents a significant limitation on the individual's liberty and should be only be used with extreme care (Byatt et al. 2006). Involuntary hospitalization should be sought only when less restrictive means are not available (Simon and Goetz 1999).

The standards that the patient, as a result of having a mental illness, must meet to be committable generally include some combination of several of the following criteria: 1) danger to others, 2) danger to self, 3) inability to care for self, 4) danger to property, 5) need of psychiatric treatment, and 6) risk of deterioration. The emphasis on the dangerousness criteria (i.e., the first three criteria listed here) since the mid-1970s has created a tension related to trying to hospitalize patients who are in need of treatment but who are not putting themselves or others at risk. Some states have expanded commitment parameters, therefore, to allow the latter two possible criteria, although this is less common.

The state's general power to use civil commitment for psychiatric hospitalization is described as limited to individuals who have a mental disorder, often itself defined by state regulations, statutes, or case law. The debate about the scope of civil commitment is at times posed as a problem of defining the kind of mental disorder that is required to justify commitment (Byatt et al. 2006). Patients who are determined to be potentially violent toward others but who do not have mental illnesses do not generally meet criteria for involuntary commitment to a psychiatric hospital (Simon and Goetz 1999).

The ability to institute involuntary short-term psychiatric hospitalization for patients with mental illness in emergency situations is an important intervention used until a court hearing can be held. The period that a person can be held involuntarily varies across jurisdictions. The criteria that must be met to continue to hold a psychiatric patient are often those required for court-ordered commitment. At the end of the emergency commitment period, facilities must decide whether to release the patient or to petition for court-ordered hospitalization. The strict time limits on emergency commitment are sometimes subverted secondary to delays in scheduling hearings at the court level. As a result, patients may be involuntarily held for psychiatric reasons for weeks or longer before a hearing (Byatt et al. 2006).

Capacity to Make Medical Decisions

A brief mental status examination completed on Ms. X reveals attention and memory deficits consistent with delirium. Discharge home no longer seems a possibility given her delirium and the fact that her mental status appears significantly different from her baseline. Ms. X is now demanding to leave. How do you proceed?

Assessment

Determining whether a patient has the capacity to make medical decisions involves respecting the autonomy of patients who are capable of making decisions and protecting those who do not (Appelbaum 2007). Competence is usually presumed, and patients are afforded autonomy in their decisions to accept or reject recommended medical treatment unless their competence is questioned. The terms *capacity* and *competency* are often interchanged; however capacity is based on a clinical judgment, whereas competence is a legal determination made by a judge (Appelbaum 2007; Byatt et al. 2006).

Capacity Versus Commitment

Patients are frequently hospitalized involuntarily in the emergency department or medical inpatient unit who have acute medical problems and desire to leave or attempt to leave but lack the capacity to decide to leave AMA. To have decision-making capacity related to medical decisions, one must be able to appreciate the reasonably foreseeable consequences of a decision or lack of decision. Capacity is specific to particular decisions and can change over time. Patients who lack the capacity to make medical decisions may reject recommended treatment. In such cases, clinicians need to determine the appropriate course of action. Approaches to assessment and treatment planning should take into consideration what is the expectation of recovery and whether some type of advanced directive for health care decisions may come into play (Byatt et al. 2006). It is important to consider that a patient who lacks capacity to make medical decisions is not necessarily committable to a psychiatric inpatient setting. Similarly, patients who appear to meet criteria for civil commitment due to risk of harm to themselves or others may not lack the capacity to make medical decisions.

Patients must be allowed to leave AMA if they have decisional capacity and choose to forgo recommended treatment. A patient who has such decisional capacity cannot be forced to accept unwanted treatment even if the treatment being refused could save the patient's life. The medical team, however, must take the necessary steps to keep a patient in the emergency department if the patient lacks decisional capacity and wants to leave AMA. At times, the steps to take to ensure that such patients stay in the hospital are not clear. Documents to initiate psychiatric civil commitment may not be appropriate to keep in the emergency department those patients who do not fit criteria for commitment to a psychiatric facility (Byatt et al. 2006).

As with Ms. X, when a patient requests to leave the emergency department AMA, the emergency department team should contact appropriate consultants as needed to help ascertain a patient's decision-making capacity and appropriateness for civil commitment. Documentation should ideally include a general psychiatric evaluation and a capacity evaluation, indicating whether the patient has a primary psychiatric issue or a psychiatric issue secondary to a general medical condition. The involvement of next of kin is helpful to obtain guidance in making medical decisions. Unless a health care proxy or equivalent type of authorization is in place, next of kin cannot legally override a patient's refusal to stay in the hospital but can provide guidance with treatment decisions. Where there is no legal authority for family to make decisions for the patient, it is important to balance confidentiality and attempts at obtaining guidance in the particular emergency by providing family with only the information needed to manage the medical situation (Byatt et al. 2006).

The medical team may need to hold patients who lack decisional capacity involuntarily in an emergency department or medical floor but may not be able to treat patients against their will except in acute emergency situations where lack of treatment may result in a hastening of death or result in serious deterioration of health.

The medical or psychiatric team should try to use the least restrictive methods to keep the patient in the emergency department. The medical or psychiatric team may call the police or security to restrain the patient so as to mitigate safety risks if attempts to manage the patient without physical or mechanical restraints fail. Initiation of legal or administrative review can help attend to the legal rights of patients when the need for mechanical restraints arise and can also serve to address ethical concerns related to possible inappropriate coercive treatment of patients. Input from hospital legal, administrative, or ethics personnel can be critical when sorting through issues related to coercion in treatment. The medical treatment team may consider pursuit of guardianship if lack of capacity is suspected to persist; while guardianship is pending, the medical or emergency team may engage in emergency-based treatment (Byatt et al. 2006).

Informed Consent

> Ms. X's delirium cleared after a brief admission. She returned to the emergency department a week later. She continues to be depressed and is reporting auditory hallucinations and delusions that parts of her body are rotting. The physicians indicate that she is in need of antipsychotic medications.

Elements of informed consent include disclosure, competence, and voluntariness (Appelbaum and Gutheil 2007; Pinals 2009). The doctrine of informed consent requires that a physician disclose certain information to a patient so that the patient can make a decision about his or her own care. Determining how much information is disclosed can be complicated; in general, topics should include information related to risks and benefits of the recommended treatment and alternatives to that recommended treatment, as well as risks of no treatment (American Medical Association 2008). In addition, for a valid informed consent process to unfold between a doctor and a patient, the patient must be in a situation in which he or she is making a voluntary choice among alternatives, and in which coerced treatment, except under certain legally and ethically permissible circumstances, would not be reasonable.

The doctrine of informed consent also is premised on the idea that a valid informed consent requires the patient to be competent to make treatment decisions. Persons are presumed to be competent unless certain circumstances exist whereby they are thought to lack capacity to make decisions for themselves (see above for specific situations relevant to the emergency department). Laws related to health care proxies, for example, generally allow a previously designated health care proxy or durable power of attorney to make medical decisions for a patient who is assenting to treatment once a physician determines that a patient no longer has the capacity to make decisions for himself or herself. Guardianship may be sought for patients who lack capacity to make treatment decisions, which allows the court to make a formal adjudication around the patient's capacity and also allows a formal surrogate decision maker to make medical decisions on behalf of the patient whether or not the patient is assenting to the proposed treatment. Guardianship determinations often take time to obtain, but they can also be obtained in emergency medical situations. In an emergency room setting, it is important to identify whether a patient has a previously designated health care proxy or guardian who is legally authorized to make medical decisions on behalf of the patient. The involvement of family, if available, can also be helpful in the informed consent process, especially when the emergency department patient lacks the capacity to make decisions autonomously. As noted above, there may be ethical and legal limitations to the role of family that require balancing.

An exception to the requirements of informed consent is the emergency exception. A physician is permitted to medicate a patient involuntarily and without engaging in a full informed consent dialogue in a situation that involves a psychiatric emergency in which risk of harm to self or others could not be averted in the absence of this intervention, and in which less restrictive alternatives to emergency medication would not be sufficient (Appelbaum and Gutheil 2007; Pinals 2009).

Another exception to the requirement for an informed consent dialogue with the patient is after a guardian has been appointed for the patient. Nevertheless, even in situations where a patient is under guardianship, a discussion about treatment recommendations with an incompetent patient can still be an important component of psychiatric care in the emergency department setting, and can help alleviate a patient's concerns and work toward building a foundation of a therapeutic alliance for a patient who may need long-term treatment and may return to the emergency room for treatment in the future. To the extent that such dialogue may need to be carried out in terms understandable to the incompetent patient, the information provided may be offered in a more limited manner to the ward, though full disclosure to the guardian would be part of the informed consent process (Pinals 2009).

A complicated exception to providing informed consent involves a therapeutic waiver whereby a competent patient states that he or she is agreeing to treatment but does not wish to hear the information about the treatment that the physician would be providing. Such an exception to informed consent would generally require documentation that the patient waived the informed consent process and was capable of doing so.

Another complicated exception is that of therapeutic privilege, which is when a physician elects not to provide a full informed consent disclosure because the physician believes that the information would be harmful in and of itself or create a situation for the patient wherein the opportunity for rational dialogue would be foreclosed if a disclosure related to the medical condition and recommended treatment is given in full. This exception is considered to be very narrow and should not be exercised simply because one believes that a patient would refuse a particular treatment if he or she heard about all the risks involved. In fact, the belief that psychiatric patients will refuse treatment if its risks are disclosed can be a problematic assumption. One study, for example, showed that information related to tardive dyskinesia did not specifically harm patients or even lead to refusal of treatment (Munetz and Roth 1985). Although this exception is not commonly used, if the therapeutic privilege exception is being considered, the rationale for not providing informed consent for the particular patient situation should be contemporaneously documented. In the case of Ms. X, the clinician should recommend the needed medication, using language that the patient will understand about the condition that is being treated. The emergency department physician should also review with the patient the recommended treatment's risks and benefits, the risk of no treatment, and any alternative treatments available. If Ms. X is unable to engage in the discussion, the clinician should consider and document if any of the above exceptions to informed consent apply, prior to administering the recommended medication.

Transfer of Care

A few hours later, the emergency department physician states that Ms. X has been medically cleared for transfer to a nearby freestanding psychiatric hospital. Ms. X has not had labs drawn and now appears confused. Is it appropriate to transfer Ms. X at this time?

In the past decade, much attention has been paid to creating legislation and policies to protect patients and health care providers from the financial, institutional, and political demands that may interfere with the ability to evaluate and treat patients in a PES setting (Quinn et al. 2002; Saks 2004).

Abandonment

In the 1980s, reports emerged of inappropriate transfers of medically unstable patients, with a resultant increase in morbidity and mortality. Such inappropriate transfers were believed to be in response to increasing financial pressures, triggering private hospitals to discharge patients to the streets or to public hospitals before adequate evaluation or stabilization. In response, Congress initiated the Emergency Medical Treatment and Active Labor Act of 1986 (EMTALA; see http://www.cms.hhs.gov/EMTALA/ for overview) as part of the Consolidated Omnibus Budget Reconciliation Act of 1985 (COBRA). EMTALA mandated that all hospitals receiving Medicare funds must adequately screen, examine, stabilize, and transfer patients, regardless of the patients' ability to pay. Prior to transfer, patients must be evaluated and stabilized, and the receiving hospital must agree to the transfer and have the facilities to provide needed treatment. It would not be appropriate to transfer Ms. X given that she has not been adequately evaluated and she is not stable for transfer. EMTALA applies to both medical and psychiatric conditions; therefore, PES staff would benefit from education to ensure that legal and ethical standards of care are upheld (Quinn et al. 2002; Saks 2004).

Communication

Appropriate transfer of patients requires proper documentation of medical and/or psychiatric evaluation and communication with the receiving facility. The transferring facility must ensure that the receiving facility has the appropriate space and personnel, that it is agreeing to accept the patient, and that all relevant records are sent. In addition, a transfer certificate clearly documenting the risks and benefits on which the transfer is based must accompany the patient and must be signed by the physician authorizing the transfer (Quinn et al. 2002; Saks 2004).

Transfer Problems

EMTALA requires hospitals with specialized capabilities, such as acute psychiatric units, to accept patients regardless of a patient's ability to pay, if the receiving facility has the capacity (Quinn et al. 2002; Saks 2004). Heslop et al. (2000) noted that psychiatric staff and patients are often frustrated with unacceptable standards of care due to the difficulties and delays encountered in securing access to suitable care.

Care may be hampered by stigmatization of certain psychiatric populations, such as those with personality disorders, agitated psychosis, or substance abuse, as well as by financial and practical problems, including lack of insurance and comorbid medical issues (Bazemore et al. 2005). Heslop et al. (2000) commented on the lack of communication and coordination of care between emergency services and psychiatric inpatient units. Further exacerbating the problem, delays in transfer often result in longer waits for other waiting patients (Heslop et al. 2000). If an identified hospital refuses to accept a patient when it has the capability and capacity, then EMTALA has been violated. If the statute is violated by physicians or an institution, civil liability can be imposed, possibly resulting in termination of the institution's Medicare provider agreement. This is noteworthy given the negative impact that refusal of transfer has on standard of care in PES settings (Quinn et al. 2002; Saks 2004).

Liability Management

> Ms. X's medical workup is complete, and she appears medically stable for a psychiatric admission. She acknowledges suicidal ideation, obsessive thoughts about death, and feeling hopeless, helpless, and overwhelmed. Ms. X's family requests urgent psychiatric treatment, yet they do not feel that she is at acute risk of harm to self. Ms. X is requesting to leave PES, denies any intent or plan for self-harm, and reports that she can maintain her safety outside the department. Although Ms. X is requesting discharge and denying any intent or plan for self-harm, you remain concerned about her welfare and feel strongly that an inpatient admission is indicated. How do you approach the patient and document your decision making?

Uncertainty is inherent in the practice of psychiatry, particularly in PES settings. As a result, psychiatrists are understandably concerned about facing malpractice lawsuits. Although negative outcomes often result in tragic suffering and harm, such outcomes are not synonymous with malpractice. Malpractice is a negligent civil (noncriminal) wrong committed by a physician that leads to damage. Even when outstanding care is provided, malpractice lawsuits remain a risk, and it behooves the PES clinician to anticipate and prepare for such lawsuits by practicing professionally, seeking consultation in difficult cases, documenting clearly, using adequate risk assessment, and arranging clear follow-up (Appelbaum and Gutheil 2007).

Documentation

Almost as important as the dictum to "do no harm" is the requirement to "write it down," because countless acts of litigation provide evidence that documentation is the primary determinant of legal outcome. Writing more does not necessarily decrease liability. Efficient documentation that entails risk-benefit analysis, reasoning for clinical decisions, and assessment of the patient's capacity to participate in treatment planning is most effective (Gutheil 1980). When a thoughtful risk-benefit analysis is documented, a claim of negligence is more likely to be refuted even if a negative outcome proves that the decision was wrong. PES clinicians should also record the thinking that goes into decision making and not only the final decision. At times, PES clinicians may feel they are expected to read minds or predict future events in order to reduce harm. Documentation of the risks and benefits and the patient's capacity to participate in treatment with brief quotes from the patient regarding his or her views of the treatment decisions may be helpful in demonstrating that an informed consent discussion took place (Appelbaum and Gutheil 2007).

Trend Toward Standard Risk Assessment Tools

A trend is growing toward a multidimensional approach to suicide and violence risk assessments commonly conducted in PES settings. The traditional approach has involved a clinical interview and clinical judgment, without as much attention to a standardized mechanism to consider risk factors that are shown to be statistically associated with increased suicide and violence risk. This approach has limitations given the complexity of risk assessment and the individual nature of each patient. Evidence suggests that formal risk assessment tools may reduce suicide risk by providing an assessment template that can assist with the vital aspects of the assessment (Cutliffe and Barker 2004). Similar tools have also been developed for violence risk assessment (Lamberg 2007). Before using such instruments, the clinician needs to know whether they are appropriate for the emergency department context.

Planning for Aftercare

Adequate arrangement and documentation of follow-up are powerful as a liability and risk prevention tool. Documentation of therapeutic approaches, interventions, and arrangement for follow-up after discharge can be important for demonstrating the attempt to maximize the possibility of ongoing quality of patient care. PES clinicians should be careful to identify appropriate aftercare when this is thought to be indicated after a careful evaluation, and to carefully document the rationale if no aftercare is recommended (Appelbaum and Gutheil 2007).

Managed Care

> After a meeting with Ms. X and her family, Ms. X agrees to a voluntary psychiatric admission. The PES clinician obtaining insurance approval informs you that Ms. X's insurance company will not approve an inpatient psychiatry admission without a doctor-to-doctor discussion. What will you tell the reviewer so that Ms. X gets the treatment you feel is warranted?

Financial Considerations

Managed care has had a dramatic impact on psychiatry and has led to unique ethical problems. A large proportion of insurance companies have mental health benefits managed under carve-out behavioral health care companies that contract to provide all mental health services and often substance abuse services. Many behavioral health care companies also provide services based on risk or capitations. In the risk model, payment or authorization of clinical services is approved only if there is evidence of enough acuity and risk to necessitate such treatment. Capitated services predetermine the hospital or clinical provider regardless of clinical situation, further exacerbating the issue (Lazarus and Sharfstein 2002).

Ethical and Legal Considerations

The financial arrangements associated with managed care prospective utilization review create unparalleled ethical dilemmas for health professionals. Clinicians often find themselves struggling with conflict of interest posed by utilization review, payors' focus on cost containment, and the demands of external regulatory bodies. Psychiatrists may encounter new challenges when providing patient care because of the recent emphasis on patient autonomy and informed consent as opposed to the previous more authoritarian physician role (Lazarus and Sharfstein 2002). Legal liability toward clinicians working within the constraints of managed care is important to understand, especially in the face of limited liability for managed care organizations (Appelbaum 1993).

Utilization Review

Utilization review creates many ethical dilemmas that raise issues related to confidentiality, conflict of interest, and informed consent. The process itself can also interfere with the doctor-patient relationship. Third-party reviewers ask psychiatrists to reveal patient information that can compromise confidentiality. It may be unclear as to whether the information requested is overly inclusive or unnecessary given that cost containment is the primary reason for review. Psychiatrists should develop parameters and practices that allow them to inform patients if needed care is unavailable or if qualified specialty providers are unavailable within the limits of their insurance plan. Referrals outside the system may be indicated if needed to ensure appropriate care. Clinicians also need to inform patients of options for treatment that extend beyond their benefits, because most insurance companies have mental health limitations. Furthermore, it is important to appeal adverse managed care decisions, and in some circumstances, it may be necessary to provide medically necessary treatment in the emergency department setting even if reimbursement from the managed care organization does not appear forthcoming (Appelbaum 1993). Although a PES clinician may be tempted to alter reports to obtain prior approval, honesty is fundamental to the doctor-patient relationship and should not be compromised (Lazarus and Sharfstein 2002). It is incumbent on psychiatrists and PES clinicians to adapt to the constraints of managed care while maintaining their clinical professional ethics (Lazarus and Sharfstein 2002).

Conclusion

Emergency mental health care is an exciting part of psychiatry. Clinical situations present a variety of complexities, including those related to ethics, policy, regulation, and law. Emergency mental health professionals need to have an awareness of these parameters to help achieve patient care that conforms to clinical practice and legal requirements.

Key Clinical Points

- PES clinicians need to operate within the constraints of law, ethics, and regulations and to be knowledgeable about these constraints as they apply to clinical practice.

- Psychiatrists can respect patients' confidentiality by making every effort to assure the highest degree of privacy possible.

- PES staff should ensure proper assessment and formulation of the issues relevant to the requirements for involuntary hospitalization in order to preclude the abuse of power related to civil commitment.

- Determining whether a patient has the capacity to make medical decisions involves respecting the autonomy of patients who are capable of making decisions and protecting those who do not.

- Elements of informed consent include disclosure, competence, and voluntariness. Informed consent requires that a physician disclose certain information to a patient and allow the patient to make a decision about his or her own care.

- Legislation and policies have been created to protect patients and health care providers from the financial, institutional, and political demands that may interfere with the ability to evaluate and treat patients in a PES setting.

- PES clinicians and psychiatrists can anticipate and prepare for malpractice lawsuits by practicing professionally, seeking consultation in difficult cases, documenting clearly, using adequate risk assessment, and arranging clear follow-up.

- Psychiatrists and PES clinicians often need to adapt to the constraints of managed care while maintaining their ethics.

References

American Medical Association: Informed consent. Available at: http://www.ama-assn.org/ama/pub/physician-resources/legal-topics/patient-physician-relation-ship-topics/informed-consent.shtml. Accessed March 3, 2008.

Appelbaum PS: Legal liability and managed care. Am Psychol 48:251–257, 1993

Appelbaum PS: Assessment of patients' competence to consent to treatment. N Engl J Med 357:1834–1840, 2007

Appelbaum PS, Gutheil TG: Clinical Handbook of Psychiatry and the Law, 4th Edition. Philadelphia, PA, Wolters Kluwer/Lippincott Williams & Wilkins, 2007

Bazemore PH, Gitlin DF, Soreff S: Treatment of psychiatric hospital patients transferred to emergency departments. Psychosomatics 46:65–70, 2005

Brook M, Hilty DM, Liu W, et al: Discharge against medical advice from inpatient psychiatric treatment: a literature review. Psychiatr Serv 57:1192–1198, 2006

Byatt N, Pinals D, Arikan R: Involuntary hospitalization of medical patients who lack decisional capacity: an unresolved issue. Psychosomatics 47:443–448, 2006

Cutliffe JR, Barker P: The Nurses' Global Assessment of Suicide Risk (NGASR): developing a tool for clinical practice. J Psychiatr Ment Health Nurs 11:393–400, 2004

Gutheil TG: Paranoia and progress notes: a guide to forensically informed psychiatric recordkeeping. Hosp Community Psychiatry 31:479–482, 1980

Herbert PB: The duty to warn: a reconsideration and critique. J Am Acad Psychiatry Law 30:417–424, 2002

Heslop L, Elsom S, Parker N: Improving continuity of care across psychiatric and emergency services: combining patient data within a participatory action research framework. J Adv Nurs 31:135–143, 2000

Jaffe v Redmond, 518 U.S. 1 (1996)

Lamberg L: New tools aid violence risk assessment. JAMA 298:499–501, 2007

Lazarus JA, Sharfstein SS: Ethics in managed care. Psychiatr Clin North Am 25:561–574, 2002

Lidz CW, Mulvey, EP, Appelbaum PS, et al: Commitment: the consistency of clinicians and the use of legal standards. Am J Psychiatry 146:176–181, 1989

MacArthur Research Network on Mental Health and the Law: MacArthur Coercion Study executive summary. February 2001. Available at: http://macarthur.virginia.edu/coercion.html. Accessed October 13, 2009.

Mermelstein HT, Wallack JJ: Confidentiality in the age of HIPAA: a challenge for psychosomatic medicine. Psychosomatics 49:97–103, 2008

Munetz MR, Roth LH: Informing patients about tardive dyskinesia. Arch Gen Psychiatry 42:866–871, 1985

Pinals DA: Informed consent: is your patient competent to consent to treatment? Curr Psychiatry 8:33–43, 2009

Quinn DK, Geppert CM, Maggiore WA: The Emergency Medical Treatment and Active Labor Act of 1985 and the practice of psychiatry. Psychiatr Serv 53:1301–1307, 2002

Saks SJ: Call 911: psychiatry and the new Emergency Medical Treatment and Active Labor Act (EMTALA) regulations. J Psychiatry Law 32:483–512, 2004

Simon RI, Goetz S. Forensic issues in the psychiatry emergency department. Psychiatr Clin North Am 22:851–864, 1999

Tarasoff v Regents of the University of California, 118 Cal Rptr 129, 529 P2d 553 (1974)

Tarasoff v Regents of the University of California, 17 Cal.3d 425 (1976)

U.S. Department of Health and Human Services: The Health Insurance Portability and Accountability Act of 1996 (HIPAA) privacy rule. Available at: http://www.hhs.gov/ocr/privacy. Accessed October 10, 2009.

Zinermon v Burch, 494 U.S. 418 (1979)

Suggested Readings

American Medical Association: Informed consent. Available at: http://www.ama-assn.org/ama/pub/physician-resources/legal-topics/patient-physician-relationship-topics/informed-consent.shtml. Accessed March 3, 2008.

Appelbaum PS: Assessment of patients' competence to consent to treatment. N Engl J Med 357:1834–1840, 2007

Appelbaum PS, Gutheil TG: Clinical Handbook of Psychiatry and the Law, 4th Edition. Philadelphia, PA, Wolters Kluwer/Lippincott Williams & Wilkins, 2007

U.S. Department of Health and Human Services The Health Insurance Portability and Accountability Act of 1996 (HIPAA) privacy rule. Available at: http://www.hhs.gov/ocr/privacy. Accessed October 10, 2009.

13

Disposition and Resource Options

Zoya Simakhodskaya, Ph.D.

Fadi Haddad, M.D.

Melanie Quintero, Ph.D.

Divy Ravindranath, M.D., M.S.

Rachel L. Glick, M.D.

Previous chapters of this book have dealt with issues of assessment and immediate management of psychiatric emergencies. The critical last step of any emergency department visit is disposition. Any gains made with emergency department interventions may unravel if the patient is not discharged to the correct environment with the right supports. Based on the assessment, the patient may require inpatient psychiatric treatment for further management of the ongoing psychiatric emergency or may be safely discharged back into the community, with or without additional social and psychiatric supports. More-over, subsets of patients may be particularly difficult to discharge from the emergency department. These are the topics addressed in this chapter.

Discharge to Inpatient Treatment

> Mr. F, a 26-year-old African American man, presented to the emergency de-partment accompanied by his mother. He stated that his "jaw was dislocated and it was affecting the whole body." The patient reported that he could no longer look at himself in the mirror and shave, did not leave the house, and had lost weight over the last several months. Although the patient had a his-tory of prior drug use, he denied any at present. The family psychiatric his-tory revealed depression, substance abuse, and schizophrenia. The patient's mother was distressed about the situation and requested hospitalization. The clinician felt that hospitalization was appropriate but not mandatory, and of-fered inpatient hospitalization to the patient.

As addressed in prior chapters, there are many indications for inpatient psychiatric treatment. Each of these indications shares psychiatric illness too severe to allow safe management in the outpatient setting. These indications include thoughts of harm to others and suicidal ideation that are resistant to interventions made in the emergency department; mood symptoms, persis-tent psychosis, or cognitive dysfunctions that impair self-care; or a lack of ca-pacity to understand the need for treatment.

After determining that the patient requires inpatient treatment, the emer-gency department provider's goals focus on maintaining the patient's psy-chiatric status while investigating options for further inpatient treatment. Actions may include obtaining serial reassessment; giving updates to the pa-tient; providing for basic needs, such as food, bathing, and grooming; and ad-ministering medications, with an emphasis on achieving stability within the emergency department. The focus should be on timely interventions to pre-vent worsening of the patient's symptoms.

In many communities, finding acute inpatient psychiatric treatment for patients can be very challenging. Even as outpatient psychiatric treatment has become more available, the number of acute psychiatric hospitals has decreased. Despite this decrease, bridging outpatient services, such as those described later in this chapter (see subsection "Comprehensive Psychiatric Emergency

Program"), have not increased in number to meet the demand for emergency psychiatric treatment (Salinsky and Loftis 2007).

Not all psychiatric hospitals are created equal. Some hospitals are associated with general hospitals, whereas others stand alone, without an associated medical hospital. Some hospitals specialize in treatment of psychotic disorders, whereas others specialize in the treatment of mood disorders. Electroconvulsive therapy may be available at one hospital but not at another. That being the case, it is vitally important for clinicians to match the anticipated needs of each patient with services available at psychiatric treatment units in the community.

One other consideration in selecting a hospital for a patient is whether that hospital will accept the patient's health insurance. If not, then at the end of the hospitalization, the patient may be unwittingly left with a large hospital bill that could have been avoided with a more appropriate disposition. Some insurance companies require prior authorization for hospital-based treatments. Therefore, a good practice is for the emergency department to attempt to contact the patient's insurance company before pursuing transfer to a psychiatric hospital. Many localities have hospitals (e.g., county hospitals) that will take patients who have no health insurance or who are unable to produce proof of insurance due to their mental state.

The patient should be presented over the phone to appropriate hospitals, and the request for transfer should be made. Although a physician will always accept the patient for transfer, the phone call requesting the transfer may be fielded by a nonphysician provider (e.g., social worker, nurse). After the relevant information is conveyed to the nonphysician provider at the inpatient facility, this person will either accept the patient for direct admission to the hospital on the physician's behalf or request that the referring emergency department physician speak directly to the inpatient facility's physician to clarify the details of the case. On occasion, the psychiatric hospital will ask for a transfer from the original emergency department to the psychiatric hospital's emergency department so that further face-to-face assessment can be made. This request should be made clear before the termination of the telephone call because it is critical information for the ambulance facilitating the transfer and may be relevant information for the patient.

Most hospitals will only provisionally accept a patient until they receive documentation of the details of the case and until they know that the patient is medically stable for transfer and for inpatient psychiatric treatment—that is, "medically cleared." A clear definition of this term is somewhat evasive and dependent on the specific situation. For example, a patient who has made a suicide attempt will require more medical attention than a patient who presents with suicidal ideation but without a recent suicide attempt. Moreover, newly psychotic patients may be psychotic because of a medical condition that should not or could not be treated in a psychiatric hospital. The same can be true of a patient in an extreme mood state, a patient who is cognitively impaired or delirious, or a patient who is severely anxious. Many psychiatric patients have medical comorbidities (e.g., diabetes mellitus) that may be exacerbated due to poor self-care, which is in turn driven by the patient's psychiatric condition. These comorbid conditions need to be assessed and stabilized prior to the patient's transfer to a psychiatric hospital. In general, medical clearance requires complete assessment of the patient such that the likelihood of the presence or development of a medical emergency is low. This process may require inpatient medical treatment with comanagement by a consulting psychiatric service. Medically cleared patients can still have medical conditions, but these conditions should be sufficiently stable that the patient can be safely treated as a medical outpatient.

Despite the assurances of an emergency department psychiatrist regarding medical clearance, some hospitals require additional steps, such as documentation of medical clearance from a medical provider or common serum and urine laboratory values, such as complete blood count, comprehensive metabolic panel, thyroid-stimulating hormone, urinalysis, urine pregnancy test, and urine drug screen, even if no indication for these studies was found in the general history and physical examination. Some hospitals also ask for other studies, such as a chest X ray or electrocardiogram. Interpretation of these studies may require the assistance of emergency physicians or other providers in the emergency department. Moreover, as discussed previously, further investigation and stabilization of patients with abnormalities found in studies may require inpatient medical treatment. This is all the more reason to maintain a good relationship with the general providers in the emergency department.

Because of prior abuses of patients with psychiatric illness, most states have laws governing the manner by which patients may be admitted to a psychiatric hospital. Even for patients who are requesting psychiatric hospitalization, most states require that the patients be told their rights with regard to inpatient treatment, and documentation of that discussion is necessary. Usually, a state-generated form is available for this reporting. Moreover, except in the case of threat of immediate dangerousness to self or others, consent for hospitalization does not imply consent for specific treatments. Each treatment option needs to be discussed separately with a patient.

Each state has a mechanism for involuntary treatment of a psychiatric patient in immediate risk of dangerousness to self or others or with psychiatric symptoms severe enough to impair self-care or the patient's understanding of the need for treatment. These mechanisms were developed to protect the patient's right to free movement and to prevent assault against members of a potentially vulnerable population. These mechanisms vary from state to state and may apply for a variety of psychiatric interventions, including 24-hour psychiatric holds, 72-hour psychiatric holds, psychiatric hospitalizations of varying duration, and court-ordered outpatient psychiatric evaluation and treatment. Given that the specific mechanisms vary from state to state, further discussion of this issue is deferred to community-specific sources.

Once the patient has been medically cleared, legal issues have been addressed, and insurance preauthorization has been obtained (if needed), the patient is ready for transfer. The emergency department provider remains liable until the patient arrives at the accepting hospital. The vast majority of patients require transfer to the accepting hospital by ambulance. Even a cooperative but suicidal patient is prone to changing his or her willingness for hospitalization en route to the hospital. That being the case, many ambulance services request the legal protection of involuntary treatment paperwork to protect themselves if the patient changes his or her mind en route. Under rare circumstances—for example, if the patient's insurance company does not cover ambulance transfers and the patient has come to the emergency department with reliable friends or family members—transportation by friends or family may be appropriate. Patients should never be allowed to transport themselves to psychiatric hospitals. The patient's belongings and any documentation from the patient's emergency department visit that has not already been sent to the accepting hospital, including any recommendations for psychiatric or nonpsychiatric treatment made from the emergency department, should be sent along with the patient.

Discharge to Outpatient Treatment

> Mr. F did not accept the offer of psychiatric hospitalization. Because he was
> not judged to be an immediate danger, involuntary hospitalization was not
> judged to be appropriate for him. The emergency department clinician began
> to develop an outpatient treatment plan with Mr. F and his mother.

Once the determination has been made that a patient does not require inpatient treatment, the objective of the emergency department intervention
shifts toward resolution of the crisis that led to the emergency department visit.
This step requires assessment of the presenting concern, as detailed in prior
chapters, and provision of medication and nonmedication interventions that
can address this concern. Moreover, follow-up psychiatric care is often warranted to assure a smooth course following emergency department discharge.

Many psychiatric conditions respond to psychotropic medications, as discussed in previous chapters. The patient may need to continue to take medications beyond the emergency department visit. In many cases, when the
patient has the capacity for self-monitoring, this step requires a simple prescription. However, some patients are sufficiently impaired by their condition
that their capacity for self-monitoring is debilitated. Determining whether a
patient has the capacity for self-monitoring is a matter of clinical judgment.
If the patient's presentation to the emergency department was secondary to
medication nonadherence, then the likelihood of impaired capacity for self-
monitoring with regard to medications is evident.

In the circumstance of impaired capacity for self-monitoring, it becomes
imperative to shore up supports around the patient to assure medication adherence. This step can be as simple as providing a better way to organize the
medications, such as a daily medication box, or as complicated as arranging for
daily "eyes-on" observation of medication administration. Contacting family
members, staff of residential programs, or other people who care for the patient can be critical in this step. These supportive individuals can assist with medication administration, as well as bring medication adherence issues to the
attention of the patient's mental health providers.

Psychiatric medications are often expensive, and patients often cannot afford these medications without assistance. The psychiatrist should take health
insurance concerns into account when prescribing a medication to the patient

on discharge from the emergency department. If the patient does not already have health insurance, it may be appropriate to assist the patient in obtaining health insurance. If the patient is being discharged with a prescription for medications, the clinician should consider providing him or her with a small supply of the medication. In general, and especially for a patient who may engage in suicide attempts by overdose, only enough medication should be provided to treat the patient until a follow-up visit can be completed.

In determining a disposition, the emergency department clinician should attempt to coordinate with the patient's primary outpatient treatment provider, if the patient has one. This individual will hopefully have a longitudinal formulation of the patient and may be able to inform the emergency department clinician about the current outpatient treatment plan and trajectory, as well as historical factors that may not be readily obtained from the patient. Moreover, the outpatient treatment provider may be able to accept responsibility for scheduling outpatient follow-up with the patient or may even provide the specifics of a follow-up appointment before the patient is discharged from the emergency department. It is always acceptable to attempt to contact a patient's outpatient treatment provider at any hour of day, even if the result is contact with an answering service. At least the contact from the emergency department ensures that the outpatient provider knows that the patient has been in the emergency department.

Many psychiatric emergencies are triggered by changes in interpersonal circumstances. For example, a patient may become depressed if a loved one dies, or a patient's paranoid psychosis may worsen if that patient is asked to move into a new residence. In these situations, the emergency department provider may be able to prevent a return to the emergency department by addressing such changes in interpersonal circumstances. The patient who "just needs someone to talk to" may have that need met just by experiencing the emergency department assessment and the support provided by the emergency department provider. This is an important factor to assess prior to discharging a patient from the emergency department.

Sometimes, the crisis in a patient's interpersonal circumstances may be too complex to address in a single visit with a single provider. In such a situation, the emergency department provider can rapidly assess the patient's interpersonal circumstances and help the patient develop the tools to ask for support from others in his or her life. Of course, only sufficiently self-confident and insightful patients will be able to do this for themselves. If considered necessary, even though it may not be appropriate in other psychotherapeutic circumstances, the emergency department provider should consider speaking to friends and family members on behalf of the patient to accomplish this task, but only as supported by the patient. One option is to hold an impromptu family meeting in the emergency department prior to the patient's discharge. Moreover, emergency department providers should be cognizant of community programs that may be of service to a patient in crisis, such as local churches that provide food and clothing, social clubs, free support groups for family members, drop-in centers, and Alcoholics Anonymous/Narcotics Anonymous (AA/NA) meetings.

Some patients require more support than can be provided by a single provider on a single visit and do not have the capacity or opportunity to get this support from already established treatment providers or friends and family. These patients require more support from mental health services allied with the emergency department or community mental health programs. In the following section, we discuss the Comprehensive Psychiatric Emergency Program (CPEP) of the Bellevue Hospital Center as an example of the extent to which emergency department or community mental health services can provide wraparound services for patients in crisis. Because the availability of these services varies from community to community, we advise our readers to familiarize themselves with services available in their respective communities. Even though the CPEP presented here serves New York City, readers may find analogous services within their own communities.

Comprehensive Psychiatric Emergency Program

Description

CPEPs were originally developed in response to increased demands for psychiatric emergency services in New York State. The original goal of CPEPs included alleviating overcrowding in emergency departments, minimizing the dependence on inpatient psychiatric admissions, and connecting patients to community mental health services appropriate to their needs (Allen 1995; Surles et al. 1994).

Each CPEP operates as a flexible, integrated emergency system that serves a particular patient population that requires a comprehensive level of care. A

CPEP's staff comprises several disciplines, including psychiatry, psychology, social work, substance abuse counseling, and nursing, working together in a team format to best serve the needs of patients. The disposition of patients varies depending on their psychiatric and psychosocial needs. For instance, patients may be treated and released with appropriate outpatient follow-up, admitted voluntarily or involuntarily to an inpatient unit, or placed on a 24-hour hold or in the extended observation unit (EOU). The latter two options allow clinicians the flexibility of observing patient behavior and evaluating risk on an ongoing basis, which can be especially useful when the clinician cannot obtain adequate clinical information about the patient, possibly due to intoxication, psychosis, cognitive limitations, or other factors. These options leave time for more thorough and detailed evaluation, observation for mental status changes, and contact with collateral informants, and can be useful in preventing unnecessary hospitalization.

The types of patients who are most likely to benefit from an EOU admission, rather than just a 24-hour hold, are primarily individuals with substance abuse problems, discussed in more detail later, and those with Axis II personality disorders (Clarke et al. 1997). Not only does EOU hospitalization allow for continued observation, but patients placed in the EOU will frequently respond to brief treatments aimed at resolving the immediate crisis, thereby fostering insight into diagnosis and current factors leading to the emergency department visit, as well as increasing motivation for continued outpatient care. Examples of short-term treatment interventions typically used throughout an EOU stay are containing, safe environment; supportive psychotherapy; motivational interviewing; psychoeducation; and psychopharmacology; as well as family meetings. The literature demonstrates that implementing certain dialectical behavior therapy strategies and techniques in the psychiatric emergency service can increase outpatient treatment motivation and compliance in patients with parasuicidal behaviors, such as those diagnosed with borderline personality disorder (Sneed et al. 2003). If further treatment and stabilization is warranted after 72 hours, patients can be admitted voluntarily or involuntarily to an inpatient unit, or if they are ready for discharge to an outpatient facility, they will be given appropriate referrals.

Referrals from a CPEP may include outpatient mental health clinics (freestanding or hospital-based clinics), substance abuse programs, dual-diagnosis programs, or specialty clinics (young adult or geriatric, cognitive-behavior therapy or dialectical behavior therapy, neurobehavioral). Patients are more likely to follow up with their referral if a specific appointment is given (Jellinek 1978). However, given the nature of the emergency department, this is not always possible and, therefore, additional wraparound services may be required.

Crisis Outreach Services or Wraparound Services

> Mr. F was discharged from the emergency department with a prescription for an antipsychotic medication. Even though he was skeptical about the utility of this medication in treating his jaw, his mother agreed to ensure that he started to take it. He was given a follow-up appointment in the Bellevue Hospital Center Interim Crisis Clinic (ICC). During his initial visits in the ICC, he continued to speak about his delusion, refused to take off his sweatshirt's hood or make eye contact, and struggled with the idea of having a psychiatric illness. He was still isolating himself at home, was not eating enough, often paced in his room, and did not sleep well. Psychoeducation and support were provided for Mr. F's mother. As the patient's symptoms improved with supportive brief therapy focusing on his strengths, he was able to gain some insight into his psychiatric and social situation. He was then referred to a specialty clinic whose staff came to the ICC for initial evaluation. The patient fully engaged in outpatient treatment after leaving the ICC and continued to improve.

One of the most challenging aspects of referring emergency department patients for outpatient care is assuring that patients get to the care that is recommended. Patients may not follow up because of noncompliance or because of difficulties navigating the complexities of the mental health system. Although patients discharged from the emergency department represent a high-risk population (Bruffaerts et al. 2004; Segal et al. 1998), their follow-up rates are low (Boyer et al. 2000; Bruffaerts et al. 2005; Del Gaudio et al. 1977). There has been an increasing focus in the United States and Europe on establishing crisis intervention and bridging services to address this problem (Bressi et al. 2000; De Clercq and Dubois 2001). Although the availability of such resources varies from setting to setting, one of the underutilized components of CPEP legislation is crisis services.

Bellevue Hospital Center's ICC is staffed by psychologists, psychiatrists, and trainees. Excluding prisoners, patients only requiring case management, and patients who have no intention of stopping their substance abuse, most patients discharged from a CPEP can be referred to the ICC. During daytime hours, appointments are scheduled by calling the clinic. At night and on weekends, the appointment book is placed in CPEP, and patients are scheduled directly by the evaluating clinician. Typically, patients receive an appointment within a week. However, depending on the clinical situation, an appointment can also be scheduled for the next day. Patients often feel relief leaving the CPEP when they know that they will be able to see someone quickly. The day before the appointment, the patient receives a reminder phone call.

During the first appointment, the patient is informed that he or she will be seen briefly, for three to six sessions, to address the precipitating crisis that led to CPEP presentation, and to find the most appropriate follow-up. The treatment focuses on continued evaluation and diagnostic clarification and psychotherapeutic interventions. Most patients receive psychopharmacological evaluation and treatment (if needed). They are typically provided with sufficient medication to last until the next appointment. They can also be referred for specialist consultations, laboratory studies, or other medical workup. Although a detailed description of the services provided is beyond the scope of this chapter, the treatment focuses on addressing the crisis and precipitating events, and on improving patients' coping skills, support network, and self-care. Patients and their families are also provided with psychoeducation. Occasionally, patients are referred back to the CPEP due to decompensation.

During their treatment in the ICC, continued psychiatric care is discussed. Recommendations might include outpatient psychotherapy and/or psychopharmacology, dual-diagnosis treatment, substance abuse treatment, or specialized treatment for a specific problem. Although a small number of patients are able to navigate the mental health and insurance system on their own, most patients require assistance. Most cases are closed only after a patient has an appointment in another setting. For a small number of patients, the services of the ICC adequately resolve their crisis, and they do not require an additional referral. Further services provided might include enrollment in health insurance or referral for intensive case management. If the patient does not show up for the ICC appointment, clinical staff make every attempt to reach him or her by phone, by letter, or by contacting family or other providers. If the patient has a history of self-harm or impulsivity and presents a risk, mobile crisis unit (MCU) services are used.

Mobile Crisis Unit

> Months later, Mr. F's mother called the emergency department requesting help for her son. Mr. F had stopped his medications, and his symptoms were returning. The MCU team went to Mr. F's apartment, but he refused to let the team in. The team then called Mr. F and explained that they were coming to provide help. Mr. F accepted the team on the second visit. After three visits, he began to trust the team and agreed to be referred back to the ICC. Mr. F returned twice to the ICC and was started back on medication. He then missed his third appointment, and the MCU team again visited him and took him to his next appointment. He responded very well to the medication and supportive psychotherapy and reengaged in outpatient treatment.

An MCU is an integral part of the CPEP. It can provide rapid psychiatric services outside of the emergency department setting. The MCU was established in 1967, after the deinstitutionalization of psychiatric patients in the 1960s, and was created to serve psychiatric patients who cannot leave or are afraid to leave their home, or otherwise could not arrange for clinic, hospital, or private psychiatric care outside the home (Chiu and Primeau 1991).

The MCU team can travel to the patient's home and meet with the patient, family members, and/or roommates, which allows for a more accurate assessment. During the assessment process, the team communicates with any other medical or psychiatric providers as appropriate. The involvement of the MCU at the early stage of decompensation and the ability to provide evaluation and crisis intervention in the natural surrounding of the patient can be very effective. In addition, the MCU has the resources to refer the patient to treatment facilities and educate family members and patients about their illness and resources in the community. Other agencies can also be contacted, including those that can provide delivery of food or that can help patients apply for home health aid if needed.

The main goal of the MCU is to keep patients in their community setting while assuring the safety of patients and others around them. This is achieved by engaging reluctant patients in treatment, conducting a more comprehensive assessment, and strengthening patient support networks. Studies show that MCU interventions prevent hospitalization (Guo et al. 2001; Hugo et al. 2002), provide the most help in the least restrictive environment, and are cost-effective.

Disposition of Challenging Populations

Although many patients evaluated by the emergency department present with complex psychiatric and psychosocial problems, certain groups of patients present particular disposition challenges. These include individuals who are homeless, those with substance abuse or dependence, and repeat presenters.

Homeless Patients

A significant relationship has been found between homelessness and severe mental illness (Folsom et al. 2005). Homeless individuals account for almost 30% of visits to the emergency department due to difficulty accessing ambulatory care and low compliance with outpatient follow-up (Kushel et al. 2006; McNiel and Binder 2005). In addition to having severe mental illness, these patients present with complex issues, including substance abuse, histories of violence, and medical complications related to their homeless status (Folsom et al. 2002). The challenge of the disposition of these patients is to be able to address their social problems in addition to their medical and psychiatric needs. An experienced multidisciplinary team that is aware of the complexity of the patient situation and of the resources available in the community is essential.

The first concern of the team when discharging a homeless patient is housing. In most large cities where homelessness is prevalent, a shelter system exists. Although shelters vary from city to city, most are gender or family status specific. Typically, a shelter has a certain number of beds available and specific policies and regulations about bed assignment. Food and certain social services are also available on the premises. Drop-in centers do not have beds but allow patients to stay in chairs overnight, to keep their belongings on site, and to use showers or other facilities. Some shelters can provide psychiatric treatment and assist with referrals to single room occupancy facilities, typically called SROs, or other housing options. SROs often have case managers and sometimes psychiatrists on the premises. Homeless patients with substance use problems can also go to nonmedical detoxification shelters or dual-diagnosis residential programs. Some hospitals have established agreements with outside facilities for crisis beds. Such beds are used as temporary housing options for patients whose main problems at that moment are related to housing, rather than deterioration in their psychiatric condition. At times, the emergency department staff is able to connect the homeless patient with family or with agencies with whom the patient was previously placed.

Before patients leave the hospital, the staff must also address food and clothing needs. Food is provided to the patient during the evaluation process in the emergency department. Upon discharge, patients get information needed to find free meals provided by the city or private facilities, such as soup kitchens, as well as procedures to apply for food stamps. Patients receive clean clothes, provided by the social services in the hospital. If the weather is extremely cold, patients can stay overnight in the emergency department, even if there is no other indication for hospitalization.

During evaluation in the emergency department, the staff also provide any medical care the patient needs. Homeless patients can present with a variety of medical complications, such as hypertension, coronary artery disease, skin infections, cellulitis, lice and scabies, and complications of diabetes, such as peripheral vascular problems. These problems can be addressed in the emergency department and treated appropriately before discharging the patient. If the patient does not present with an acute medical problem, he or she can still benefit from referrals to the medical clinic.

Substance Abusers

Patients who abuse alcohol and/or other drugs present to the emergency department with symptoms on a continuum from mild to severe. They may be irritable and/or dysphoric, or they may exhibit violent and/or suicidal behavior and major withdrawal symptoms. In addition, research has shown a significant incidence of psychiatric comorbidity with substance abuse (Anthony et al. 1994), which makes assessment and treatment, including facilitating appropriate dispositions for these patients, quite challenging in the emergency department.

The fundamental issue in treating patients who abuse substances is establishing whether other psychiatric illnesses, such as anxiety, depression, mania, or psychosis, are present and, if so, establishing whether substance use is the primary or secondary disorder. This is particularly difficult to do when a patient initially arrives at the hospital either intoxicated or experiencing withdrawal symptoms. As discussed previously, a longer-term assessment can be very useful in this circumstance.

After determining whether the patient has a psychiatric diagnosis unrelated to his or her substance use, the clinician will have a better idea of whether a patient requires primarily substance abuse treatment or treatment that is focused on both substance abuse and mental illness. When developing and implementing a plan for disposition, it is essential to evaluate potential obstacles a patient might face when transitioning to outpatient treatment. Issues of motivation should be assessed, because many substance abusers often feel forced into treatment by the legal system, family, or friends, which will likely affect eventual outcome. The importance of flexibility in the treatment approach should be emphasized. Specifically, more severe substance abusers may require a total-abstinence approach to treatment, such as AA/NA, whereas others will benefit from a harm-reduction model of treatment, which might be more acceptable to them (Moss et al. 2007). Other personal and environmental factors to consider that may interfere with successful referrals include lack of social and/or family supports, child care responsibilities, limited transportation, and difficulty taking leave from work. Table 13–1 details some options for disposition for patients with dual diagnosis.

Repeat Presenters

In recruiting for a study on reasons for repeat presentation to the emergency department, Bruffaerts et al. (2005) found that 14.3% of their clinical population had repeat presentations to the emergency department even after excluding those patients with an interval psychiatric hospitalization. These patients often elicit strong reactions from providers. They are called "frequent fliers" or "repeat offenders" and utilize considerable emergency department resources (Simon et al. 1999).

Typical repeat presenters include those with fewer social and financial resources and more severe mental problems, such as substance abuse disorders or dual diagnoses, psychotic illnesses, and/or personality disorders. Those who do not receive an appropriate disposition or do not comply with recommended follow-up are more likely to present to the emergency department within a short period (Bruffaerts et al. 2005).

As for any patient presenting to the emergency department, risk assessment is essential. Although these patients frequently self-present requesting psychiatric help only to refuse recommendations, it is important to examine the most recent course of illness. For example, a patient with a severe substance abuse

Table 13–1.   Disposition options and indications for dual-diagnosis patients

Setting	Indications and exclusion criteria
Medical detoxification units: Medical hospitalization for up to 7 days to observe and treat signs of withdrawal	Patient has risk factors for a medically complicated withdrawal. Patients cannot be dangerous to self or others, and should be motivated for ongoing sobriety.
Nonmedical detoxification: Community organizations that support the patient through withdrawal	Patient has no significant risk factors for a medically complicated withdrawal. Patients cannot be dangerous to self or others, and should be motivated for ongoing sobriety.
Community-based rehabilitation programs: Programs that provide support for patients as they enter sobriety and help patients develop skills for maintenance of sobriety (e.g., Alcoholics Anonymous)	Patient has completed withdrawal and does not require physical separation from substances to remain sober. Individual programs may have more specific indications and exclusion criteria.
Residential rehabilitation programs: Short-term (e.g., 28 days) or long-term (3–6 months) voluntary therapeutic communities	Patient has completed withdrawal and requires prolonged separation from substances to develop skills for maintenance of sobriety. Individual programs may have more specific indications and exclusion criteria.
Harm-reduction programs: Programs that prevent substance-related emergencies while recognizing that a patient may not yet be able to achieve sobriety (e.g., methadone programs or buprenorphine treatment)	Patient is unable to function without a substance or a substitute for the substance of choice. Enrollment in these programs may also provide additional time to work on the patient's motivation for sobriety.

problem may often present intoxicated, clear quickly, and request discharge. However, if the presentations increase in frequency, if identifiable psychosocial stressors contribute to the current presentation, and if the behavior begins to present a danger to self or others, voluntary or involuntary hospitalization or other interventions may be warranted.

Although repeat presenters are often unable to follow up with the emergency department recommendations, they should be continuously reevaluated for their motivation to seek treatment. Not doing so risks missing "intervenable moments" that, if used correctly, may eventually lead to interruption of the pattern of repeated presentation to the emergency department.

It is not unusual for those who repeatedly visit the emergency department to be seeking social or financial resources. As one homeless patient who frequently presented during bad weather stated, "I just need some food and a good night's sleep and I'll be OK." In addition to being homeless, these patients often have chronic psychotic illness and possible substance abuse. One must be aware that the initial request for sleep and food might also reveal acute psychosis and paranoia regarding the shelter system or police. If risk assessment reveals no immediate concerns, as noted earlier, the disposition should focus on meeting the patient's basic needs, such as food, clothing, and shelter referrals.

Another type of repeat presenter is a patient with chronic mental illness whose family seeks emergency department services as a respite from the patient. In these cases, the intervention should focus on the family and on obtaining appropriate respite services for them in the future.

Possible cognitive impairment can contribute to repeated presentations to the emergency department. Those with substance abuse problems, homelessness, or chronic psychosis may have difficulties with organizational abilities, learning and memory, and attention and concentration (Breier et al. 1991; McGurk and Mueser 2003). All of these difficulties may potentially impact the ability of patients to follow up with the emergency department recommendations and engage in outpatient treatment. Although a comprehensive cognitive evaluation is not possible in the emergency department, brief cognitive screening is useful (Cercy et al., in press; Simakhodskaya et al. 2005). When cognitive limitations are suspected, extra effort should be made to assist patients by making appointments, explaining medication regimen, and doing outreach.

Yet another type of repeat presenter, and perhaps the most difficult, is the patient who is suspected of seeking secondary gain. Although a full discussion of malingering is outside the scope of this chapter, examples of secondary gain include seeking housing after losing it because of drugs and/or alcohol abuse or conflicts at home, asking for letters or psychiatric evaluation to prove "illness" for financial or social needs, hiding from the law and responsibility, or simply claiming suicidal thinking as a way to get into the hospital. As noted earlier, it is essential to conduct a social assessment for these patients in addition to psychiatric evaluation of symptoms. One should be aware of inconsistencies in the patient's story, discrepancies between the patient's and any collateral information, and variability between the patient's self-report and actual behavior. For example, during the psychiatric interview, a patient might be tearful and complain of severe depression and suicidal ideation. However, the staff in the emergency department might observe the patient actively interacting with staff and other patients, watching television, and making phone calls that reflect clear future planning. Given such observations, the emergency department staff can discharge the patient with clear documentation of these discrepancies. Notably, patients frequently present both with a valid crisis or psychiatric problem and evidence for seeking secondary gain. The discharge plan must address the presenting problem if it is proven to be present.

Despite continued efforts to connect repeat presenters to mental health resources in the community, a significant proportion of frequent visitors will not enter formal treatment facilities other than the emergency department. However, considering that most of them are self-referred (Bruffaerts et al. 2005), it is possible that the emergency department becomes their regular treatment setting. Adopting a long-term treatment perspective, such as intensive case management, within the emergency department could be beneficial (A.M. Sullivan and Rivera 2000; P.F. Sullivan et al. 1993).

Key Clinical Points

- Assessment guides disposition. The severity of illness and multiple psychosocial factors determine whether the patient is transferred to another emergency department, an inpatient facility, or a different type of residential program, or is discharged from the emergency department with outpatient follow-up.

- The goals of emergency department care shift based on the disposition. The plan to transfer a patient to an inpatient psychiatric facility means that the goals of emergency department care shift to immediate maintenance and safe transfer, whereas the plan to discharge the patient to outpatient treatment means that the goals of emergency department care shift to crisis resolution and prevention of return to the emergency department.

- Multiple community-based mental health and non–mental health services can be used to shore up a patient's capacity to function in the face of a psychiatric crisis.

- The patient should always be assessed thoroughly, even if disposition will be difficult. Even the toughest of patients to treat have the potential for improvement.

References

Allen MH (ed): The Growth and Specialization of Emergency Psychiatry. San Francisco, CA, Jossey-Bass, 1995

Anthony JC, Warner LA, Kessler RC: Comparative epidemiology of dependence on tobacco, alcohol, controlled substances, and inhalants: basic findings from the National Comorbidity Survey. Exp Clin Psychopharmacol 2:244–268, 1994

Boyer CA, McAlpine DD, Pottick KJ, et al: Identifying risk factors and key strategies in linkage to outpatient psychiatric care. Am J Psychiatry 157:1592–1598, 2000

Breier A, Schreiber JL, Dyer J, et al: National Institute of Mental Health longitudinal study of schizophrenia: prognosis and predictors of outcome. Arch Gen Psychiatry 48:239–246, 1991

Bressi C, Amadei G, Caparrelli S, et al: A clinical and psychodynamic follow-up study of crisis intervention and brief psychotherapy in psychiatric emergency. New Trends in Experimental and Clinical Psychiatry 16:31–37, 2000

Bruffaerts R, Sabbe M, Demyttenaere K: Effects of patient and health-system characteristics on community tenure of discharged psychiatric inpatients. Psychiatr Serv 55:685–690, 2004

Bruffaerts R, Sabbe M, Demyttenaere K: Predicting community tenure in patients with recurrent utilization of a psychiatric emergency service. Gen Hosp Psychiatry 27:269–274, 2005

Cercy SP, Simakhodskaya Z, Elliott A: Diagnostic accuracy of a new cognitive screening instrument in an emergent psychiatric population. The Brief Cognitive Screen. Acad Emerg Med (in press)

Chiu TL, Primeau C: A psychiatric mobile crisis unit in New York City: description and assessment, with implications for mental health care in the 1990s. Int J Soc Psychiatry 37:251–258, 1991

Clarke P, Hafner RJ, Holme G: The brief admission unit in emergency psychiatry. J Clin Psychol 53:817–823, 1997

De Clercq M, Dubois V: Crisis intervention modes in the French-speaking countries. Crisis 22:32–38, 2001

Del Gaudio AC, Carpenter PJ, Stein LS, et al: Characteristics of patients completing referrals from an emergency department to a psychiatric outpatient clinic. Compr Psychiatry 18:301–307, 1977

Folsom DP, McCahill M, Bartels SJ, et al: Medical comorbidity and receipt of medical care by older homeless people with schizophrenia or depression. Psychiatr Serv 53:1456–1460, 2002

Folsom DP, Hawthorne W, Lindamer L, et al: Prevalence and risk factors for homelessness and utilization of mental health services among 10,340 patients with serious mental illness in a large public mental health system. Am J Psychiatry 162:370–376, 2005

Guo S, Biegel DE, Johnsen JA, et al: Assessing the impact of community-based mobile crisis services on preventing hospitalization. Psychiatr Serv 52:223–228, 2001

Hugo M, Smout M, Bannister J: A comparison in hospitalization rates between a community-based mobile emergency service and a hospital-based emergency service. Aust N Z J Psychiatry 36:504–508, 2002

Jellinek M: Referral from a psychiatric emergency room: relationship of compliance to demographics and interview variables. Am J Psychiatry 135:209–212, 1978

Kushel MB, Gupta R, Gee L, et al: Housing instability and food insecurity as barriers to health care among low-income Americans. J Gen Intern Med 21:71–77, 2006

McGurk SR, Mueser KT: Cognitive functioning and employment in severe mental illness. J Nerv Ment Dis 191:789–98, 2003

McNiel DE, Binder RL: Psychiatric emergency service use and homelessness, mental disorder, and violence. Psychiatr Serv 56:699–704, 2005

Moss HB, Chen CM, Yi H: Subtypes of alcohol dependence in a nationally representative sample. Drug Alcohol Depend 91:149–158, 2007

Salinsky E, Loftis C: Shrinking inpatient psychiatric capacity: cause for celebration or concern? National Health Policy Forum Issue Brief No. 823. August 1, 2007. Available at: http://www.nhpf.org. Accessed October 10, 2009.

Segal SP, Akutsu PD, Watson MA: Factors associated with involuntary return to a psychiatric emergency service within 12 months. Psychiatr Serv 49:1212–1217, 1998

Simakhodskaya Z, Cercy SP, Elliott A: Diagnostic accuracy of cognitive screening in an emergent psychiatric population. Paper presented at the annual meeting of the American Psychiatric Association, Atlanta, GA, May 2005

Simon JR, Dwyer J, Goldfrank LR: The difficult patient. Emerg Med Clin North Am 17:353–369, 1999

Sneed JR, Balestri M, Belfi B. The use of dialectical behavior therapy strategies in the psychiatric emergency room. Psychotherapy Theory, Research, Practice, Training 40:265–277, 2003

Sullivan AM, Rivera J: Profile of a comprehensive psychiatric emergency program in a New York City municipal hospital. Psychiatr Q 71:123–138, 2000

Sullivan PF, Bulik CM, Forman SD, et al: Characteristics of repeat users of a psychiatric emergency service. Hosp Community Psychiatry 44:376–80, 1993

Surles RC, Petrila J, Evans ME: Redesigning emergency room psychiatry in New York. Adm Policy Ment Health 22:97–105, 1994

Suggested Readings

Boyer CA, McAlpine DD, Pottick KJ, et al: Identifying risk factors and key strategies in linkage to outpatient psychiatric care. Am J Psychiatry 157:1592–1598, 2000

Bruffaerts R, Sabbe M, Demyttenaere K: Predicting community tenure in patients with recurrent utilization of a psychiatric emergency service. Gen Hosp Psychiatry 27:269–274, 2005

Sullivan AM, Rivera J: Profile of a comprehensive psychiatric emergency program in a New York City municipal hospital. Psychiatr Q 71:123–138, 2000

14

Getting Patients From the Clinic to the Emergency Department

Divy Ravindranath, M.D., M.S.

Rachel L. Glick, M.D.

Case Example

It is 3:30 P.M., and you are in session with Ms. R, a 63-year-old woman being treated for major depression. She reveals that she has had persistent suicidal ideation for the last 2 days secondary to the recent death of her husband. She has gone as far as to take a handful of ibuprofen out of the bottle. She did not ingest the pills because she was interrupted by a phone call. She feels very alone in her depression. She has not told anyone else and revealed it to you only because she knows she should be honest with her treatment providers. When asked whether she feels safe going home, your patient declines to answer.

Psychiatric emergencies rarely start in the emergency department. When a behavioral emergency occurs, the first issue is safe transfer to a location where the patient can be more effectively managed. This chapter addresses this situation. Given that the point of contact between a clinician and a patient is most often in an outpatient psychiatric setting, that setting is the focus for this chapter. However, many of the included recommendations may be equally applicable in other settings, including medical clinics.

Preincident Preparation

Preincident preparation can be critical for the efficient resolution of any psychiatric emergency. This prepping can start well before patients even enter the clinic. For example, the office can be constructed to allow escape from any room if a clinician is faced with someone who may be dangerous to the clinician or to allow for comfortable containment of patients who may be dangerous to themselves. Clinics can also be constructed to allow for observation of all areas from the reception desk, and the reception desk itself can be sufficiently high and broad that an agitated patient is prevented from jumping over the desk while still allowing for ease of communication (Wright et al. 2003).

Knowing the office layout is important in planning where to manage a psychiatric emergency in the clinic should one occur, and familiarity with one's surroundings is essential for being able to manage psychiatric emergencies safely. As discussed in Chapter 1, "Approach to Psychiatric Emergencies," personal safety should be assured when conducting a psychiatric assessment. This includes equal access to exits for both the clinician and the patient and awareness of items in the immediate area that may be used as weapons or shields.

Front desk staff members are often the first to witness a patient who may be agitated or escalating. Therefore, all front desk staff members should receive training in recognizing the warning signs of an impending emergency, including the signs of escalation of agitation listed in Table 14–1. Moreover, the training should include instruction on how to communicate concern about a potential emergency to the clinician responsible for the patient and to the remainder of the clinic staff. These techniques must be tailored to the individual clinic, given that the availability of alphanumeric paging, overhead paging, and other methods for communication vary from site to site. Each clinic should also have a protocol for contacting clinic security and/or local police officers for assistance if an emergency gets out of control.

Table 14–1.   Signs of escalation of agitation

Assessment	Signs of escalation	Signs of impending violence
Appearance	Clenching of jaw/hands	Clenched jaw/hands
	Narrowed eyes	Piercing stare
	Frowning	Narrowed, glaring, or darting eyes
	Anger/upset	Fearfulness/anger
	Anxiety	Anxiety
	Face becoming reddened	Veins standing out
	Beginning of perspiration	Reddened face
		Profuse perspiration
Speech	Tremulous	Inappropriate
	Muttering	Swearing
	Sarcastic	Shouting
	Loud	Repetitive
	Swearing	Rambling
Movements	Exaggerated movements	Exaggerated movements
	Wringing hands	Making fists
	Nervous energy	Pounding
	Pacing	Severe nervous energy
Behaviors	Demanding	Belligerent
	Intrusive	Threatening
	Crying	Pushing/punching/kicking
	Hostile	Throwing items
	Behaving strangely	

Source.   Courtesy of John Kettley and Judy Rizzo, Psychiatric Emergency Services, University of Michigan Health System.

Emergencies may develop in the course of a regular return visit. For example, a patient may reveal to a clinician profound and persistent suicidal ideation that has been hidden from everyone up to that point. Another patient may become agitated in the course of the interview. Thus, it is equally important for clinicians to understand clinic-wide mechanisms for communicating this distress to others and the need for any assistance in the immediate management of the crisis. Again, these techniques should be tailored to the specific clinic given the differential penetration of communication resources.

Training in verbal deescalation techniques using a formal program, such as the Crisis Prevention Institute (CPI) program (www.crisisprevention.com), can further enhance staff readiness for emergencies. The following elements should be considered: respecting personal space, not being provocative, establishing verbal contact, being concise, identifying wants and feelings, listening closely to what the patient is saying, agreeing to disagree, setting clear limits, and offering choices (Fishkind 2008).

Finally, training in preparation for an on-site psychiatric emergency should include assignment of roles to various individuals in the clinic. For example, some staff members can be responsible for directing other patients away from the area, whereas other staff members can be responsible for contacting on-site security or police services if needed. Moreover, practicing the emergency, as in a "mock code," can also be useful in cementing the roles assigned to individual members of the clinic. Training has been shown to reduce the frequency of assaults in the workplace (Petit 2005; Wright et al. 2003).

Acute In-Office Evaluation

Case Example *(continued)*

You identify Ms. R's situation as a potential emergency and tell her that you believe she should receive further evaluation in the emergency department. Your patient agrees. Per clinic protocol, you use the hotline to the front desk from your office phone to notify staff that your patient will need to be transferred by ambulance to the local hospital's emergency department for further evaluation and management of suicidal ideation. Your patient becomes upset that you broke her confidentiality. Your front desk staff hears her starting to escalate and asks whether you need security on standby. You respond affirmatively.

As soon as a psychiatric emergency is recognized, the clinician has two responsibilities. First, the clinician needs to assure the safety of everyone involved in the crisis, including the identified patient, and to determine whether the identified patient has any mental status abnormalities that imply an underlying psychiatric or medical condition warranting further evaluation and management in the emergency department.

Protection of the safety of other staff members and patients in the clinic depends on the nature of the emergency. A patient who is depressed and suicidal or quietly delirious may not pose much of a threat to other individuals. These patients can be safely contained in a comfortable and quiet room, such that other patients or staff members do not bother them. However, psychotic and agitated patients or individuals who are actively threatening others pose more danger to bystanders. As such, the prudent action is to clear the area of all bystanders prior to engagement of an individual in this state.

Although the task of assessing the patient is presented here after the discussion of preservation of safety, it is important to note that this is neither a subordinate goal nor a goal that must be met in sequence. More likely, the assessment of the individual will inform the clinician's decision about the degree to which the safety of others needs to be protected. This is a recursive process, wherein the more the clinician is able to assess about the identified patient, the more the clinician will be able to adjust the surroundings to facilitate further safe assessment.

The assessment for underlying psychiatric pathology should focus on those mental status abnormalities that may predispose a person to dangerousness to self, dangerousness to others, or inability to care for self. Findings may include disheveled appearance, psychomotor agitation, despondent mood, nonreactive affect, disorganized thought process, thoughts about hurting self or others, and/or poor insight. Certainly, this list is not exhaustive. The assessment in the clinic is intended to facilitate immediate management and disposition to a more secure area. It is *not* meant to provide definitive treatment. As such, the threshold for considering dangerous behavior as secondary to a possible psychiatric illness should be low.

Immediate Management

Case Example *(continued)*

You tell Ms. R that you needed the help of other people to make sure that she can be kept safe and that the front desk staff and all other health professionals involved are subject to the same privacy protections as you are. You reaffirm to the patient that your commitment is to her best interests and that in this case, the involvement of others to preserve her safety was in her best interests.

> After this explanation, Ms. R calms down and continues to be in agreement with going to the emergency department. You begin completing legal paperwork to force involuntary psychiatric evaluation, just in case the patient changes her mind or becomes upset again.

Immediate management of a psychiatric emergency in the clinic is similar to management of a psychiatric emergency in the emergency department, except that outpatient clinicians rarely have access to medications and, in most states, cannot legally implement seclusion or restraints. Outpatient clinicians have to rely on interpersonal techniques for defusing psychiatric emergencies. Again, the nature of the technique used depends heavily on the nature of the emergency. An individual who is not at great risk of dangerousness to others simply needs to be convinced not to depart the clinic until transportation to the emergency department can be secured. Alternatively, an individual who is at great risk of dangerousness to others should be addressed with the goal of decreasing the immediate risk.

Many verbal and nonverbal interventions can be useful in deescalation of an agitated and potentially escalating person. The person should be engaged verbally. The objective is to determine the reason why the patient is agitated and escalating, and empathize with his or her plight. The clinician's body language should reflect openness to the patient's perspective, while preserving ease of exit if needed. The clinician should remain calm and allow agitated individuals to resonate with this, thereby achieving calm themselves. Tone should be kept low, and the clinician should avoid all impulses to argue with an agitated individual (Petit 2005). As discussed previously, participation in a formal training program, such as the CPI program, can prepare the clinician for this task.

Agitated individuals should be offered choices, no matter how small, to help them remain in control of when and how they deescalate. An important point to negotiate here is for the agitated individual to give up any weapons he or she may have. If successfully accomplished, then this is strong evidence that the agitated individual is comfortable with the clinician's being in charge of the circumstances and it also minimizes risk of damage or injury if the agitated individual does become violent.

Simultaneous engagement by multiple clinicians—that is, a "show of force"—may at times be useful in deescalating an agitated patient. Moreover, an advisable practice is for different individuals to repeatedly attempt engagement of the patient, as long as it is safe to do so. The agitated individual may respond better to someone other than the first clinician.

As stated previously, clinicians in a clinic may not have access to psychotropic medications for management of agitation. The exception is if the patient has brought his or her medications to the office. In this circumstance, it may be advisable to ask the agitated patient to take an extra dose of an oral benzodiazepine or antipsychotic. Both of these medication classes are effective in the management of agitation, and oral administration can be just as effective as parenteral administration of the medication (Yildiz et al. 2003).

The tone of engagement changes if and when the patient becomes violent. At that point, concerns regarding safety trump the desire to meet the agitated individual's needs. The clinician should rapidly determine whether to flee or to allow the agitated individual to escape the immediate environment. In either circumstance, professionals with more training in management of hostile individuals (clinic security or police officers) need to be brought in to continue management of the situation. Hopefully, these professionals have already been contacted as part of the clinic protocol for management of psychiatric emergencies. If the agitated individual flees, then security or police officers should be given a detailed description of the individual and the circumstances so they can continue in pursuit. In all states, individuals who may be dangerous to themselves or others because of a psychiatric illness can be apprehended in the community and brought to an emergency room for further evaluation and management.

Disposition

Case Example *(continued)*

Ms. R asks whether she can drive herself to the emergency department. She is concerned about the cost of the transfer. You tell her that her mood state is too fragile to allow for transfer by any means other than ambulance and that you hope the cost of the ambulance transfer will be covered by her health insurance. Ms. R is upset by the lack of certainty about cost and decides to leave for home. By then, security officers have arrived and are standing outside your door. Their presence stops the patient from fleeing. The ambulance arrives shortly thereafter, and the patient is transferred to the emergency department.

Once stabilized, the identified patient may warrant further evaluation in the emergency department. This is especially valuable if the patient may require ongoing evaluation and management or perhaps psychiatric hospitalization to return to psychiatric baseline.

The question of transportation to the emergency department is an important one and requires consideration of the patient's mental status abnormality. The clinician may contemplate transportation by the patient or the patient's loved ones for patients who are potentially dangerous to themselves only. However, severe suicidal ideation does constitute a medical emergency, and the judgment of a patient experiencing severe suicidal ideation may be sufficiently impaired that transport by self or family members risks nonarrival to the emergency department. Moreover, patients who have made a suicide attempt prior to presentation to the clinic may appear medically stable, but this assessment cannot be guaranteed until a more thorough evaluation is completed. Most patients warrant at least transportation by emergency medical services (EMS). More agitated patients definitely warrant transport by EMS; however, given the escalated risk of dangerousness to EMS personnel (Brice et al. 2003), transportation by police may also be considered. Given that both EMS personnel and police respond to most emergency calls, this is often a decision that can be deferred to the professionals in question.

If the individual in crisis does not actually have evidence of underlying psychiatric pathology (e.g., the agitated individual is a family member or a friend of a patient), or if the identified patient is sufficiently stabilized by the interventions performed in the clinic and other follow-up plans can be arranged, then further evaluation in the emergency department may not be appropriate. These individuals can be asked to leave the clinic when the interaction is complete. If they continue to be agitated or repeat in their escalation with this request, then further intervention by security or police may be needed to escort the person off of the clinic premises.

Key Clinical Points

- Psychiatric emergencies often start outside the emergency department.
- Clinic preparation and planning for an emergency can be critical.

- Assessment in a clinic-based emergency should focus on protection of the safety of all involved and assessment for mental status abnormalities that might require further assessment and management in an emergency department.

- Immediate management of a clinic-based emergency relies on interpersonal interventions, rather than medications or physical techniques.

- Once the patient is stabilized, the clinician should determine disposition based on the ongoing needs of the patient.

References

Brice JH, Pirrallo RG, Racht E, et al: Management of the violent patient. Prehosp Emerg Care 7:48–55, 2003

Fishkind AB: Agitation II: de-escalation of the aggressive patient and avoiding coercion, in Emergency Psychiatry: Principles and Practice. Edited by Glick RL, Berlin JS, Fishkind AB, et al. Philadelphia, PA, Wolters Kluwer/Lippincott Williams & Wilkins, 2008, pp 125–136

Petit JR: Management of the acutely violent patient. Psychiatr Clin North Am 28:701–711, 2005

Wright NM, Dixon CA, Tompkins CN: Managing violence in primary care: an evidence-based approach. Br J Gen Pract 53:557–562, 2003

Yildiz A, Sachs GS, Turgay A: Pharmacological management of agitation in emergency settings. Emerg Med J 20:339–346, 2003

Suggested Readings

Forster JA, Petty MT, Schleiger C, et al: kNOw workplace violence: developing programs for managing the risk of aggression in the health care setting. Med J Aust 183:357–361, 2005

Petit JR: Management of the acutely violent patient. Psychiatr Clin North Am 28:701–711, 2005

Wright NM, Dixon CA, Tompkins CN: Managing violence in primary care: an evidence-based approach. Br J Gen Pract 53:557–562, 2003

15

Supervision of Trainees in the Psychiatric Emergency Service

Erick Hung, M.D.

Amin Azzam, M.D., M.A.

The psychiatric emergency service is often an intense, busy environment that provides assessments and care to severely ill psychiatric patients. It has become a main entry point into the mental health system for many patients and often the only treatment setting for many who are chronically mentally ill (Allen 1996; Schuster 1995). Because a busy psychiatric emergency service provides many opportunities to view a wide range of acute psychopathology, it is an excellent setting for trainees of mental health services. Beginning in the early 1980s, a number of articles appeared focusing on the exciting learning opportunities in the psychiatric emergency service and discussing ways to optimize learning experiences (Accreditation Council for Graduate Medical Education 2007; American Association for Emergency Psychiatry Education Committee 1998; American Medical Association 2002; Brasch and Ferencz

1999; Muhlbauer 1998). Furthermore, several groups, including the American Association for Emergency Psychiatry, have outlined model curricula for emergency psychiatry training (Brasch et al. 2004). As these curricula mature, psychiatric supervisors and educators must tend to how they supervise and teach emergency psychiatry. What makes emergency psychiatry supervision both exciting and challenging for the supervisor is the variety of settings, the vast array of professional interactions, and the diversity of roles that a supervisor must undoubtedly adopt.

Research confirms that the performance of students, as measured by knowledge and skills assessments, is directly related to the prowess of their teachers (Paice et al. 2002). Good teachers are recognized not only by their teaching abilities (i.e., organization and clarity of presentation, enthusiasm and stimulation of interest, group interaction skills) but also by their supervisory skills and "doctoring" qualities (i.e., competence, clinical knowledge, analytic ability, professionalism) (Kilminster and Jolly 2000).

Following principles of good supervision has a positive impact on both patient outcomes (Grainger 2002; Kilminster and Jolly 2000; McKee and Black 1992; Osborn et al. 1993) and trainee learning (Luck 2000). When more supervision is provided, patient satisfaction is higher, patients report fewer problems with care, and morbidity and mortality are lower. The effect of good supervision is greater when the trainee is less experienced and the cases are more complex (Kilminster and Jolly 2000). Good supervision reduces trainee stress and increases learning (Luck 2000). Trainees do not mind working long hours if they receive good support (Kilminster and Jolly 2000).

Work in medicine has many stressors, and failing to cope well with these stressors can lead to emotional exhaustion and burnout (Luck 2000; Willcock et al. 2004). Trainees who cannot cope with stress make significantly more errors (Jones et al. 1988). This leads to increased costs as a result of trainee absenteeism and litigation by patients against hospitals because of suboptimal care (Firth-Cozens 2003). The causes of poor performance may lie with the person, the system, or the supervisor (Lake and Ryan 2005). Supervision is often perceived to be inadequate by trainees, and lack of supervisors is one of their greatest stressors (Paice et al. 2002). The concept of supervision is more global than clinicians providing episodes of help with patient care (Kilminster and Jolly 2000). It requires planning to ensure that trainees provide high-quality patient care all the time, that their time in a particular clinical service provides a good opportunity for professional growth, and that potential problems are anticipated and prevented (Busari et al. 2005; Kilminster and Jolly 2000).

Psychiatric emergency settings vary based on 1) type of facility (e.g., independent community facility vs. academic teaching hospital), 2) proximity to medical emergency services, and 3) types of providers (e.g., psychiatrists, other physicians, psychologists, therapists, nurses, social workers, technicians). Consequently, the role of an emergency psychiatry supervisor is broad. As shown in Figure 15–1, a supervisor's duties include providing clinical care to patients, assuring that each patient receives a quality standard of care, abiding by legal statutes, working in complex systems and administration, and modeling professionalism. In addition, and perhaps most importantly, educating mental health trainees is a core responsibility.

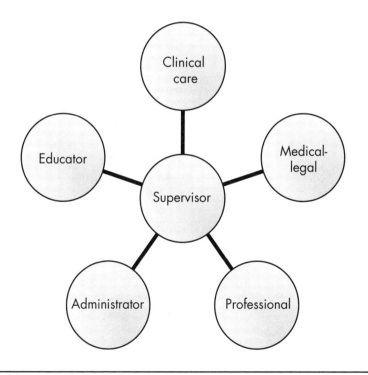

Figure 15–1. Roles of a psychiatric emergency setting supervisor.

Although the emergency psychiatry supervisor wears many hats, we focus in this chapter on the role of being an educator in a psychiatric emergency service (Figure 15–1). To be a competent clinician-educator in emergency psychiatry, the supervisor must first be able to diagnose and treat the patient, then diagnose and treat the learner, and finally diagnose and treat the supervision (see Figure 15–2).

Duties include understanding and assessing the learner and then teaching to the learner's level and his or her educational needs. To improve as educators, supervisors must be able to self-reflect, collaborate with colleagues, and solicit feedback from learners. In "diagnosing" the supervision setting, supervisors need to assess the strengths and weaknesses of the teaching encounter. In "treating" the supervision setting, supervisors need to improve on areas of confusion, modify styles of teaching, and address any tensions in the learning climate.

Diagnose and Treat the Patient

Other chapters in this book have addressed specific clinical issues in emergency psychiatry relating to the diagnosis and treatment of patients in the emergency setting. The challenge for supervisors in the psychiatric emergency training service is that they must diagnose and treat patients in a learning environment, tending to the dual and at times conflicting needs of patient and trainee. Consequently, supervision can take a variety of forms. One organizational schema for forms of supervision is based on the degree of learner autonomy (see Figure 15–3).

At the beginning of the spectrum, learners essentially shadow the supervisor as he or she provides direct clinical care in the psychiatric emergency service. At this stage, learning is through observation. The learner takes part in a discussion in which the supervisor discloses thoughts about the case, walking the learner through the decision-making process that led to a particular differential diagnosis or treatment plan. As a learner progresses to being more autonomous, the supervisor may ask the learner, after shadowing a clinical interview, what the learner's impressions are of the case. The supervisor increases the learner's autonomy and potential for learning by moving away from self-disclosure of his or her own thought process and toward questioning the learner to provide thoughts and impressions regarding the case.

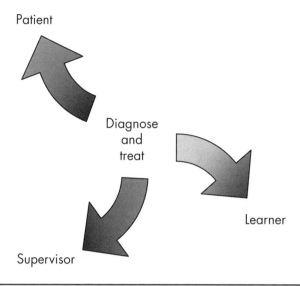

Patient

Diagnose
and
treat

Learner

Supervisor

Figure 15–2. Centrality of diagnosis and treatment.

Learner autonomy is further increased when the supervisor asks the learner to engage in the interview with the patient. At this stage, the supervisor is more of a direct observer in the room, allowing the learner to conduct the psychiatric interview independently. The supervisor may interject intermittently during critical teaching moments, but ultimately these should decrease in frequency as learner autonomy is maximized. Further autonomy is achieved when the learner independently interviews the patient in the psychiatric emergency service and then presents the case to the supervisor immediately following the interview. In this situation, the supervisor is present on the service and is immediately available to precept the case. Removing the supervisor from the physical vicinity of the learner allows the learner to interview the patient, formulate an initial assessment and plan, and then discuss the case immediately with the off-site supervisor. In this case, the real-time supervision provides opportunities to impact the formulation and direction of clinical care as it progresses, while simultaneously allowing for significantly more learner autonomy. Often, this stage of supervision takes place on call overnight in the psychiatric emergency service, where the supervisor discusses the

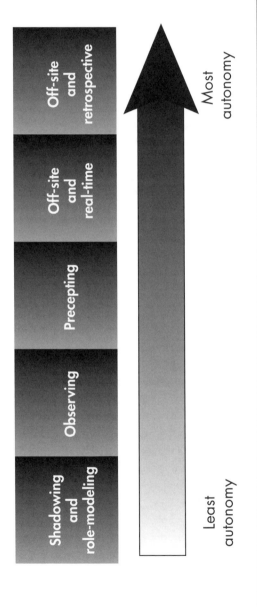

Figure 15–3. Spectrum of supervision.

case with the trainee over the phone and collaborates on the diagnosis and treatment plan.

In the final stage of the supervision spectrum, the supervisory experience is disconnected from the direct clinical care of the patient. At this stage, supervision takes place off-site and retrospectively. The supervision may occur the following day, week, or even month after the direct clinical care. Unquestionably, this stage of supervision maximizes the learner's degree of individual autonomy. In some cases, the learner may be a senior trainee with years of clinical experience. In others, the learner is a professional peer requesting supervision for consultation and self-growth.

Thus, the spectrum of supervision is broad and complex. Teaching and effective supervision inevitably take place at every stage on the spectrum. However, the essential point in creating a successful supervision encounter is not where a supervisor falls in the spectrum, but rather *how* he or she decides where on the spectrum to mold the supervision experience. Several factors influence this choice, including learner needs, clinical considerations, medicolegal considerations, and system constraints (see Figure 15–4). The tension between these factors and learner educational needs is always present in psychiatric emergency services with trainees. Because of this tension, it is also necessary to focus on the educational needs of the learner, to foster an effective supervision experience, as discussed in the following section.

Diagnose and Treat the Learner

Diagnosing and treating the learner can be a challenging yet exciting experience for the supervisor. How does a supervisor know if the learner is really learning from the teaching session? How does a supervisor assess the learner's needs? Even assuming accurate assessment, how does the supervisor best teach to that learner's level? Supervisors may accomplish aspects of diagnosing and treating the learner intuitively (particularly those who are "natural" teachers), but for many supervisors, clinical teaching skills are not innate. Most supervisors have experienced both effective and poor teaching styles during their own training and need to be sensitive to the impact these styles have on trainees' competence and confidence. The supervisor who is starting out in clinical teaching, however, can be uncertain about what constitutes a successful teaching interaction. Fortunately, over the past two decades, an explosion of re-

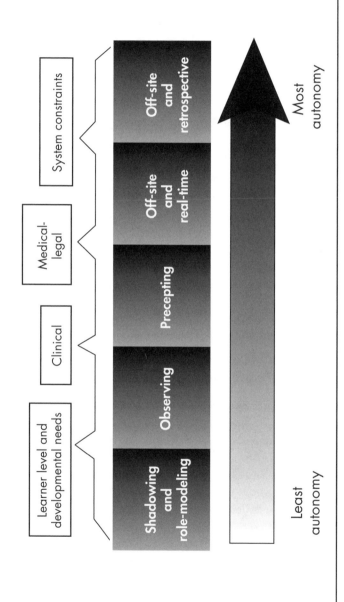

Figure 15–4.   Factors influencing spectrum of supervision.

search has occurred in medical education. Several easy-to-use models help supervisors elicit learners' educational needs, teach to their learners' level, and provide effective feedback (Neher et al. 1992, 2003; Pangaro 1999; Wolpaw et al. 2003). In this section, we highlight some of the most helpful models that can be useful in busy psychiatric emergency services for effective teaching, as well as for providing feedback.

RIME Model

Pangaro (1999) initially described the RIME model as a developmental framework for assessing learners in clinical settings. Pangaro described a progressive continuum of four performance levels: reporter, interpreter, manager, and educator. In 2002, Battistone et al. proposed observer as an introductory stage for the model.

Preceptors can use this model to assess the level of an individual learner's clinical performance during case presentations in the psychiatric emergency service. Learners at the observer level (e.g., early-first-year medical students) will not yet have the skills to take a pertinent history or present a patient. Learners at the reporter level (e.g., second-year medical students) will be able to reliably, respectfully, and honestly gather information, write basic notes, differentiate normal from abnormal, and present their findings. Interpreters (e.g., early-third-year medical students) will be able to present a patient case, select the important issues, offer differential diagnoses, and support arguments for or against various diagnoses. Learners at the manager level (e.g., most late-third-year medical students) will be able to present the case, offer a differential diagnosis, and formulate diagnostic and therapeutic plans. Learners who have reached the educator level will be able to do all of the above, as well as define important questions, research information regarding the topic, and educate others. Some students attain educator-level skills by the time they graduate from medical school, whereas others may not achieve this level until they are residents.

The value of the RIME model is that it provides a common descriptive terminology that is highly acceptable to learners and preceptors (Ogburn and Espey 2003). The RIME descriptors are nonjudgmental and assist supervisors in giving meaningful feedback. This model could easily be introduced during an orientation to the psychiatric emergency service for learners at any level of training, and will establish a shared vocabulary for feedback.

Table 15–1 provides an example of the use of the RIME model in a clinical scenario—that of a young woman with an acute manic episode who pre-

Table 15–1.   RIME model: a young woman with an acute manic episode

RIME level	Description	Case presentation by RIME level	Preceptor coaching response
Observer	Understands only what is happening	"Ms. V is a 26-year-old female. She was brought into the psychiatric emergency service by the police on an involuntary hold."	"Good. Now, go in and ask the patient herself to describe to you what she is feeling."
Reporter	Understands "what" is wrong	"…and the police report that she was running down the main street, half-naked, screaming that God has given her the power to fly.…She endorses feeling on top of the world, racing thoughts, pressured speech, grandiose ideas, decreased need for sleep, and impulsively using street drugs. She denies psychotic or anxiety symptoms."	"Excellent report. Now, 'interpret' these symptoms for me. What do you think could be going on? Let's come up with a differential diagnosis."
Interpreter	Understands "why" it is wrong	"Based on her symptoms and past psychiatric history, I believe she has an acute manic episode in the context of a bipolar illness secondary to recent medication nonadherence. Other possibilities include schizoaffective disorder, substance-induced mood disorder, drug intoxication, or delirium."	"Excellent differential diagnosis. Now, how will we proceed to 'manage' the workup?"

Table 15–1.   RIME model: a young woman with an acute manic episode *(continued)*

RIME level	Description	Case presentation by RIME level	Preceptor coaching response
Manager	Understands "how" to address the problem	"…I'll complete the workup by ordering a set of baseline labs including lithium level and urine toxicology screen. I'll also assess her orientation by completing the Folstein Mini-Mental State Examination. I plan to treat her with drug X to target her manic symptoms. I also think we should put her in an open seclusion room to minimize stimulation from other patients."	"That sounds like a first-class workup and an excellent plan. Why would you choose this particular drug instead of drug Y?"
Educator	Committed to self-learning and education of the team	"This case seems representative of a typical manic presentation. According to the Texas algorithm for acute mania, we should also consider starting an atypical antipsychotic or mood stabilizer. Also, the algorithm suggests that drug X is more cost-effective and efficacious than drug Y."	"Good job. You are right on top of the latest literature. Now let's get you a more complicated case."

sents for mental health evaluation and care. This same clinical scenario will be used with subsequent educational models so the various models can easily be compared and contrasted.

One-Minute Preceptor Model

Often, after presenting a patient to a preceptor, learners tend to end their presentations and wait for the preceptor to formulate the case and discuss an assessment and plan for the patient. In a busy emergency care setting, preceptors may be tempted to "jump right into the case" and discuss their thoughts and opinions immediately after hearing the case. The unfortunate danger in this approach is that the preceptor does not assess the learner's knowledge or skill level. Because this is typical of many teaching encounters (Irby and Papadakis 2001; Parsell and Bligh 2001; Tiberius et al. 2002; Ullian et al. 1994), preceptors may feel as if they are being effective teachers when in essence they have not fully engaged their learners in "owning" the learning process. The one-minute preceptor model, originally developed by Neher et al. (1992) and subsequently modified (Neher et al. 2003), is a five-step model that helps supervisors assess the learner and teach to the learner level. The five parts or microskills of the model are get a commitment, probe for supporting evidence, teach general rules, reinforce what was done right, and correct mistakes.

By asking the learner specific questions based on the model, the preceptor can effectively understand the learner's current knowledge and skill level, tailor teaching to teach toward specific learning needs, and provide formative, specific feedback to the learner. The model has been studied in outpatient settings in multiple specialties, with both learners and preceptors describing significant improvement and confidence in their teaching skills after using the model (Aagaard et al. 2004; Furney et al. 2001; Irby et al. 2004; Neher and Stevens 2003; Parrot et al. 2006; Salerno et al. 2002).

Using the five steps in the one-minute preceptor model will help the supervisor assess the learner more effectively, provide more targeted teaching, create a culture of positive reinforcement and constructive feedback, and ultimately improve the teaching encounter on behalf of the learner and the educator. The model can easily be delivered in busy psychiatric emergency services with trainees. Table 15–2 provides an example of the use of the one-minute perceptor model in the previously cited clinical scenario of a young woman with an acute manic episode.

SNAPPS Model

In busy emergency settings, learners have a tendency to become relatively passive reporters focused on presenting history and objective findings to the preceptor (Wolpaw et al. 2003). Foley et al. (1979; cited in Wolpaw et al. 2003) directly observed teaching encounters and found that students were passive and received a preponderance of low-level, factual information. Learners were seldom asked questions and rarely asked to verbalize their problem-solving efforts. Based on work in cognitive learning and on reflective practice for educators, the SNAPPS model is a collaborative model for case presentations in an outpatient setting that can easily be translated to the emergency setting. The SNAPPS model for case presentations follows a mnemonic consisting of six steps: summarize, narrow, analyze, probe, plan, and select (see descriptions of steps and sample questions in Table 15–3).

This model links learner initiation and preceptor facilitation in an active learning conversation. It focuses on what supervisors can do to empower learners and enable trainees to contribute more to the clinical encounters. Rather than passively awaiting the preceptor's assessment of the learning climate, learners are expected to identify their own learning goals. The learner-driven educational encounter in the emergency setting emphasizes the role of the learner and the supervisor in a collaborative learning conversation. In this teaching and learning "dance," one partner may lead, but each must know the steps. Wolpaw et al. (2003) advocated that the learner can and should be taught to lead. The preceptor or supervisor may coach the learner until the steps become automatic but should avoid taking over the conversation.

SNAPPS makes learners do most of the work, through justifying their thinking and exploring what they do not know (rather than having the preceptor question them on what they do know). A pilot study of SNAPPS showed that learners were more actively involved and readily came up with questions, unlike in more traditional interactions (Wolpaw et al. 2003). Supervisors could respond to learners, rather than thinking up novel questions (Wolpaw et al. 2003).

When teaching, clinicians often ask questions aimed at elucidating low-level knowledge. In 1933, John Dewey, one of the most influential thinkers

Table 15–2. One-minute preceptor model: a young woman with an acute manic episode

Microskills	Description	Preceptor questions	Common pitfalls
Get a commitment	After hearing a presentation or seeing a patient together, ask the learner what he or she thinks. *Rationale:* Learners should be involved in processing and problem solving as opposed to just collecting data.	"What do you think is going on with this patient?" "What do you think is the most important issue to address today?" "What would you like to accomplish during this evaluation?" "What do you think led to the patient's current manic episode?" "What do you think has been contributing to this patient's medication nonadherence?"	Quickly offering your own opinion Asking for more data only Jumping straight into a mini-teaching session
Probe for supporting evidence	Ask the learner for evidence that supports his or her opinion. *Rationale:* Asking learners to reveal their thought processes allows you to identify what they do and do not know.	"What were the major findings that led to your conclusion?" "What else did you consider?" "What facts led you away from acute mania...?"	Grilling the learner Giving away the answer too quickly

Table 15–2. One-minute preceptor model: a young woman with an acute manic episode (*continued*)

Microskills	Description	Preceptor questions	Common pitfalls
Teach general rules	Make one or two brief teaching points tied to the case. *Rationale:* Teaching is more memorable and transferable when it is offered as a general rule and when it is tied to a clinical experience.	"Like we see in your patient, most patients with acute mania have these core features…"	Trying to accomplish too much in a single teaching encounter Providing unsupported, idiosyncratic personal opinions
Reinforce what was done right	Comment on specific work that was done well and what effect it has on patient care. *Rationale:* Skills in learners are vulnerable and become well established with reinforcement.	"You did a good job asking specific and detailed questions about the patient's sleep patterns throughout the night." "Excellent detailed and nonjudgmental history taking on the patient's recent substance abuse."	Giving feedback that is too general (i.e., "Great job!")
Correct mistakes	Identify mistakes to the learner as soon as possible in an appropriate setting, and discuss how to avoid or correct the error in the future. *Rationale:* Mistakes left unattended have a good chance of being repeated.	"Given the patient's recent suicide attempt, we'll need to get more information from a family member and therapist instead of just relying on today's visit for all the information."	Providing judgmental feedback (e.g., "Terrible job—even a high school kid would have known to ask about current suicidality!")

Table 15–3. SNAPPS model: a young woman with an acute manic episode

Step	Description	Example questions (asked by the learner)
Summarize	Summarize briefly the history and findings	The patient is a 26-year-old woman who was brought into the psychiatric emergency service by the police on an involuntary hold. Her current symptoms include euphoria, grandiosity, racing thoughts, pressured speech, decreased need for sleep, and impulsively using street drugs. She has not been adherent to medications prescribed to her for bipolar disorder.
Narrow	Narrow the differential to two or three relevant possibilities	"The patient's clinical presentation is consistent with an acute manic episode. This episode could be explained by several possibilities: 1) an exacerbation of her bipolar disorder in the context of medication noncompliance; 2) a substance-induced mood disorder secondary to recent stimulant intoxication; or 3) a delirium secondary to electrolyte abnormalities."
Analyze	Analyze the differential by comparing and contrasting the possibilities	"I think that the most likely possibility is an exacerbation of the patient's bipolar disorder in the context of medication noncompliance. The supporting evidence for this possibility is that the patient's family told me that she has not been taking her medications at home over the past month. A substance-induced mood disorder is less likely because the patient denies any recent substance use. A delirium seems less likely because the patient is fully oriented and does not have any medical risk factors for electrolyte abnormalities."

Table 15–3. SNAPPS model: a young woman with an acute manic episode (*continued*)

Step	Description	Example questions (asked by the learner)
Probe	Probe the preceptor by asking questions about uncertainties, difficulties, or alternative approaches	"I am uncertain as to how much I should believe the patient when she says that she has not used any substances recently. I have been mistaken in the past. I do not know what objective clinical examination findings I could observe in patients with a stimulant intoxication." "I also am not sure how to structure an interview with a manic patient. In this interview, I feel that the patient controlled the questioning, and I had difficulty redirecting the patient."
Plan	Plan management for the patient's psychiatric issues	"I would like to gather more collateral information from the patient's outpatient mental health clinic. Given that the patient is acutely manic right now, I would like to order a urine toxicology screen and basic labs. Additionally, I would like to minimize the patient's stimulation in the milieu and start an atypical antipsychotic and a benzodiazepine. What do you think about this management plan?"
Select	Select a case-related issue for self-directed learning	"I am not entirely sure what algorithms have been developed for the management of acute mania. I have heard about the Texas algorithm but would like to read more about it. Maybe I will look up a flowchart and present it to you on our next teaching encounter."

on education in the twentieth century, proposed that thinking and problem solving occurred not when answering a question posed by a teacher, but when attempting to solve a problem important to the learner (Irby and Papadakis 2001). We learn more from what we "don't know" than what we "do know." Therefore, shifting from asking "What is the cause of …?" to "What are you uncertain about?" moves away from simple factual recall and promotes thinking. SNAPPS is a strategy to introduce this approach.

Tips for Effective Feedback

Giving feedback is an essential skill for all supervisors, yet techniques for giving *effective* feedback are rarely taught in clinical medical education. By definition, feedback is the ongoing appraisal of performance based on direct observation aimed at changing or sustaining behavior (Aagaard et al. 2004). The literature on effective feedback focuses on several strategies, including creating a safe learning environment for feedback, reviewing educational objectives, providing a format for delivering feedback, and dealing with poorly performing trainees (Gordon 2003). The following guidelines, summarized in Table 15–4, can improve a supervisor's effectiveness in providing meaningful feedback to trainees.

1. *Understand educational goals and objectives from the beginning.* Before a trainee begins working in the psychiatric emergency service, it is essential for supervisors to give a brief orientation, outlining the educational goals and objectives during the time spent on the service. Educational learning goals and objectives often overlap with the expectations and needs of the service, but to the greatest extent possible, educational goals should be highlighted separately from the service needs. For effective feedback to occur, learners need to understand what the actual educational goals and objectives are, because these are the markers against which they will be measured.

2. *Maintain a safe learning environment.* Provide a safe setting for students to experience autonomy in data gathering and initial evaluation of patients. For patients on the service whose cases are less acute, learners are encouraged to be the first "clinician" beyond the triage desk. For patients whose cases are more acute (e.g., those requiring emergent medications, seclusion, or restraint), learners are often involved in more

Table 15–4. Ten tips for effective feedback

 1. Understand educational goals and objectives from the beginning.
 2. Maintain a safe learning environment.
 3. Foster mutual respect.
 4. Provide feedback in a timely manner.
 5. Provide feedback that is specific.
 6. Limit feedback to a few objectives at a time.
 7. Provide feedback in a specific format.
 8. Label feedback as feedback.
 9. Limit feedback to behaviors that are remedial.
 10. Solicit feedback rather than impose it.

peripheral tasks or observer status; however, supervisors must ensure that learning issues and learners' performance are addressed once the patient has been stabilized.

 3. *Foster mutual respect.* Supervisors should show learners the respect they would give to any other colleague. Anything that helps the trainee see feedback as an informed, nonevaluative, objective appraisal of performance intended to improve his or her own clinical skills (rather than as an estimate of his or her personal worth) will help in the process. When feedback fails, it is usually because it led to trainee anger, defensiveness, or embarrassment.

 4. *Provide feedback in a timely manner.* Feedback should not necessarily be restricted to a scheduled session designed solely for the purpose of performance appraisal. In fact, the most effective feedback often is that which occurs on a day-to-day basis, as part of the flow of work on the service and as close to the event as possible. This maximizes both trainee and supervisor capacity to remember specific aspects of the clinical and teaching interaction. Furthermore, it provides ample opportunity for trainees to improve skills and to demonstrate their improvement to the supervisor. Of course, the pace of events in the emergency psychiatry setting can be challenging to seasoned preceptors and daunting to trainees. Despite this challenge, feedback can be effectively done "on the run" as the supervisor reviews how a case is progressing or the communication skills of a trainee in conveying only essential information.

5. *Provide feedback that is specific.* Feedback should deal with specifics, making use of real examples. Generalizations, such as references to a trainee's organizational ability, efficiency, or diligence, rarely convey useful information and are far too broad to be helpful as feedback. For example, saying, "Gee, what a great job you did," may bolster the learner's self-esteem but does not really provide a meaningful assessment of his or her performance.

6. *Limit feedback to a few objectives at a time.* The supervisor can often give a lot of very useful feedback to the learner after a clinical encounter. However, even the most well-intentioned and informative feedback session can be diminished if the supervisor provides an exhaustive, all-inclusive list. Limiting feedback to a few pearls at a time (generally one to three points) not only allows the learner to digest the information appropriately but also forces the supervisor to establish more frequent feedback sessions. Additionally, limiting feedback encourages the supervisor to actively determine what his or her two or three most important teaching points should be.

7. *Provide feedback in a specific format.* Many educators like the "feedback sandwich" technique: 1) start with acknowledging something that the learner did well, 2) offer constructive critique of an area for growth, and 3) finish with another area of strength. Other educators believe that overemphasis on the positive may undermine appreciation for and attention to the deficiency. Regardless of the specific format, the crucial element in providing feedback is that it should be descriptive and nonjudgmental.

   Information that is shared with the trainee should focus on actions rather than interpretations or assumed intentions. Data based on actions not only are more accurate but also allow for psychological distance, a critical component when the feedback is negative or the trainee insecure. Subjective data are also perfectly appropriate for feedback about clinical skills. When included as part of the feedback, subjective data should be clearly labeled as such. When dealing with personal reactions and opinions, "I" statements should be used. When the supervisor says, for example, "In watching this videotape, I began to feel that you were not comfortable talking about the patient's recent suicide attempt," the trainee is allowed to view the assessment as one person's reaction. Even more preferable are statements such as, "I saw your hand shaking; you abruptly changed the subject," which allow the trainee to interpret the behavior.

8. *Label feedback as feedback.* Unless feedback is explicitly labeled, learners will fail to recognize feedback and supervisors will not be recognized for their efforts. Supervisors need to clearly identify their comments as constructive or formative feedback on the performance for that shift or clinical encounter. Helping learners understand that the comments to come are intended to foster their improvement rather than serve as an evaluation reduces the likelihood that a learner will receive the feedback in an emotionally charged fashion.

9. *Limit feedback to behaviors that are remedial.* The supervisor should limit feedback to behavior that the learner can correct or improve. If observed behaviors are not within the trainee's power to change or are far beyond his or her developmental level, then these should not be included as feedback. Such deficits, if they are substantial, mean that the trainee should alter his or her goals, not the process by which he or she attempts to meet a goal. Preceptors who find themselves frustrated with a trainee should take a 5-minute time-out before providing criticism.

10. *Solicit feedback rather than impose it.* Feedback works best when it is solicited rather than imposed. By first soliciting feedback from a learner on his or her own performance, the supervisor conveys a positive message that both learner and supervisor can improve their communication and performance. Furthermore, the trainee should take an active part in the process, and the supervisor's open-ended questions can help break the ice. If both parties can reach agreement on these questions, they will have an agenda for the remainder of the discussion.

Diagnose and Treat the Supervision

Supervisors need to assess their own teaching skills. There are times when educational efforts fail, and lack of assessment of the teaching in those moments guarantees that the learner will continue to flounder. This section explores crucial elements of supervision, mechanisms to be reflective in teaching, and ways to troubleshoot an unsuccessful teaching experience by evaluating structural and teacher-learner dyadic barriers to good teaching.

Qualities of a Good Supervisor

A good supervisor does the following:

- Ensures that both supervisor and trainee are clear about their respective roles and responsibilities for the encounter, particularly with regard to patient care.
- Informs the trainee how supervision will occur (e.g., that time will be set aside to observe the trainee's performance).
- Provides feedback in a positive way. Unless weaknesses are tackled in a clear, unambiguous way, trainees will not get the message.
- Makes time to get to know the trainee as a person, as someone who has a life outside medicine as well. It can be interesting and impressive to learn what trainees can do, along with letting them learn something of the supervisor's own life.
- Recognizes that power factors (e.g., age, gender, sexuality, race) may influence the relationship. If any of these cause a problem that cannot be satisfactorily resolved, a different supervisor should be found for the trainee.

Another way of considering the qualities of a good supervisor is to examine the factors that are associated with a happy trainee (Firth-Cozens 2003; Jaques 2003; Jones et al. 1988; Lake and Ryan 2004a, 2004b, 2004c, 2005; Luck 2000; Paice et al. 2002; Willcock et al. 2004). Among these factors are the following:

- Being supported, especially out of hours
- Being given responsibility for patient care
- Being involved in good teamwork
- Receiving feedback
- Having a supportive learning environment
- Being stimulated to learn
- Having a supervisor take a personal interest in him or her

Being Reflective in Teaching

Improvements in a supervisor's teaching can occur only if he or she reflects on how each encounter went (Irby and Papadakis 2001; Wall and McAleer 2000). The supervisor can do this in simple ways, such as these:

- Ask oneself, "How did that go? What went well? If I did it again tomorrow, what would I change to make it better?" Too often supervisors rush on to the next busy task and never do this, then find themselves doing the same thing year after year.
- Ask the learners for both verbal and written feedback. Ask them what they thought went well and what could be improved. Ask them to write down any points that were not clear, then collect and read the comments to find out what still confuses them. Also, ask learners to fill in an evaluation form.
- Review the learners' progress. Next time, consider whether they remembered the lessons taught and whether they performed well in assessments. Don't ask, "What did I teach?" but rather "What did they learn?"
- Ask a colleague to observe one's teaching and provide structured feedback.

Although it may not seem possible, "just-in-time" teaching can be thought of as a planned learning activity (Cantillon 2003; Gordon 2003; Kaufman 2003; Lake and Ryan 2004a, 2004b; Morrison 2003). Supervisors in psychiatric emergency services know 1) they will be busy, 2) they will be teaching, and 3) certain topics are likely to recur. Therefore, planning is critical. By being reflective about teaching, an instructor can refine his or her lessons so that each iteration will be better than the one that preceded it. With experience, supervisors build up teaching scripts on common topics (e.g., acute mania), including components related to diagnosis, management, social circumstances, and so forth (Kaufman 2003). Supervisors can then draw on these scripts in the context of assessing the patient, to guide them in covering the essential teaching points. This can be in a 5-minute opportune moment, a 20-minute interactive tutorial, or a 1-hour lecture, as appropriate.

Troubleshooting an Unsuccessful Teaching Event: Structural Barriers

Supervisors cite several factors that can lead to poor teaching encounters, each of which can be overcome with personal efforts, such as reading about education in book chapters such as this one, as well as preparation, such as the tips and suggestions offered in the previous two subsections (see "Qualities of a Good Supervisor" and "Being Reflective in Teaching"). The factors that lead to poor teaching encounters include the following:

- *Lack of time:* The single most important factor clinicians cite is lack of time, due to increased patient and administrative loads. The fact that there are shorter hospital stays, sicker patients, and fewer patients that may be appropriate "teaching cases" also contributes to the problem. These pressures are unlikely to be resolved in the near future (Spencer 2003).
- *Lack of training:* Most clinical educators have never been taught how to teach, supervise, or assess, regardless of whether the trainees are students, junior doctors, or other health professionals in training (Gibson and Campbell 2000).
- *Criticism of teaching:* Although most educators diligently try to teach well, they often learn that their trainees rated them poorly, which leads to diminished motivation to improve teaching. Clinical supervisors have been found to teach by humiliation and sarcasm, provide poor supervision and assessment, teach in variable and unpredictable ways, and provide insufficient feedback (Irby 1995). An inquiry into the clinical services at a tertiary hospital noted poor supervision and training and recommended that all senior doctors should partake in "train-the-trainer" courses (Douglas et al. 2001).
- *Lack of rewards:* Material rewards and recognition for teaching remain inadequate. To cope with these challenges, educators need both knowledge and skills (Spencer 2003; Wall and McAleer 2000) to teach effectively in the clinical setting.

Despite a supervisor's best efforts, there will still be barriers that will diminish the quality of teaching. Supervisors need to recognize that not all "moments" in the clinical setting are good teaching moments. Enhancing the number, length, and frequency of good teaching moments requires the supervisor to consider the following (Douglas et al. 2001):

- Are the learners (or supervisor) distracted by other duties, time constraints, tiredness, or hunger?
- Is the location busy, noisy, too public, or uncomfortable?
- What is the atmosphere? Do the learners feel comfortable demonstrating their lack of knowledge and asking questions, or are they fearful of being humiliated?
- Do the learners feel as though they belong? Do they believe that their opinion is valued?

- Do the patients know what is expected? Have they agreed to be involved? Is their dignity respected?

In the emergency department, where patients may be agitated and dangerous to others, the safety of the environment is a critical factor to assess when determining why an educational effort was less than successful. If the environment is not safe (e.g., in the case of threatening behavior by the patient), then fear will preclude this autonomy and the learner will be less able to engage in and learn from the clinical situation. Assurance of safety may even require specific instruction in how to remain safe in the face of dangerous situations.

Troubleshooting an Unsuccessful Teaching Event: Dyadic Barriers

If the environment was right and the instructor was appropriately positioned to teach, then perhaps something in the instructor-learner relationship led to failure in the educational intervention. To address this possibility, the instructor should be aware of two critical theoretical concepts: 1) the psychological distance between an instructor and a learner and 2) basic adult learning theory.

The teacher-learner relationship has an enormous impact on the quality of teaching and learning, with interpersonal variables accounting for half the variance in teaching effectiveness (Tiberius et al. 2002). Positive interpersonal relationships between teachers and learners increase the quality of teaching (Deci et al. 1991). The concepts of psychological size and psychological distance are crucial for understanding what aspects in the interpersonal environment contribute to a successful learning climate (Vaughn and Baker 2004). *Psychological size* is defined as the perceived status one person has relative to another (e.g., the difference between trainee and teacher). *Psychological distance* relates to the degree of positive and negative emotional connectedness in a relationship. Vaughn and Baker used these concepts in examining 45 pediatric preceptor-resident pairs engaged in longitudinal continuity training experiences. They demonstrated that both residents and preceptors perceived the residents as having a smaller psychological size compared with the preceptor, and that residents perceived greater psychological distance in the relationship than did preceptors. This distance was significantly related to both residents' satisfaction with particular preceptors and their perception of the preceptors' effectiveness. Teachers who are able to capitalize on specific strategies to emphasize their interpersonal relationships (i.e., by reducing the psychological size difference and distance in the relationship) can facilitate the learning process in general and simultaneously increase learners' sense of self and their professional and personal competence. Some specific strategies to consider include using first names reciprocally, sharing one's own experiences as a trainee, self-disclosure as appropriate, and taking time to learn about trainees' hobbies or other professional and personal obligations.

The trainees in psychiatric emergency services are adults who want to learn. If it appears that learning is not progressing, supervisors should consider whether their teaching style and their trainees' learning styles are congruent, as well as whether the clinical setting is conducive to learning. Adults like to have an input into their learning. Adult learning principles are not evidence based, but should be regarded as "models of assumption about learning" (Deci et al. 1991; Kaufman 2003; Neuman and Piele 2002). Questions to consider in optimizing a learning climate are provided in Table 15–5.

As educators, supervisors in psychiatric emergency services need to be flexible to suit the learners and the circumstances. Learning is about creating knowledge based on integrating new information with old, an active process that challenges the learner's prior knowledge (Peyton 1998; Vaughn and Baker 2001). As each learner progresses, a shift often occurs from being dependent (where the learner needs substantial input and direction) to being interested (where the learner needs some guidance) to being self-directed (where the learner takes personal responsibility for his or her own learning). A supervisor's teaching style needs to take into account trainees' prior knowledge and stage of learning (Hutchinson 2003; Parsell and Bligh 2001; Vaughn and Baker 2001).

Expecting a struggling trainee to define his or her own needs or presenting a mini-lecture to an experienced trainee will discourage both. Nevertheless, a degree of mismatch can challenge a learner and be a good thing. Shifting teaching styles from authoritarian (telling students what to learn) to delegating (getting them to decide what they need to know) shifts the workload away from the supervisor and makes teaching and learning more fun. Also, learners like to learn in different ways at different times; sometimes a didactic presentation is perfectly appropriate. The key is targeting the teaching to the "learning edge"—wherever that may be for each learner and at that specific moment.

Table 15–5. Questions to optimize learning climate

Category	Specific questions
Personal motivation	Are trainees interested and eager to learn (internal motivation) or do they want to learn simply to pass an exam (external motivation)?
Meaningful topic	Is the topic relevant to trainees' current work or future plans? Have you made it clear why it is important?
Experience-centered focus	Is learning linked to the work trainees are doing and based on the care they are giving patients?
Appropriate level of knowledge	Is learning pitched at the correct level for a trainee's stage of training?
Clear goals	Have you articulated the anticipated outcome goals so that everyone knows where you are heading?
Active involvement	Do trainees have the opportunity to be actively involved in the learning process, and to influence the outcomes and process?
Regular feedback	Do trainees know how they are doing? Have you told them what they are doing well (positive critique), as well as what areas could be improved?
Time for reflection	Have you given trainees time and encouragement to reflect on the subject and their performance (self-assessment)? Shifting from thinking about what you want to teach to what trainees want to learn (e.g., asking what areas they are unclear about) shifts from a teacher-centered to a learner-centered approach.

Figure 15–5 provides a framework to minimize the degree of mismatch between a teacher's style and specific student's stage of learning such that the teaching encounter can be optimal.

Conclusion

The psychiatric emergency service provides a rich environment for patient encounters, rapid clinical decision making, and opportunities for trainees to experiment with a variety of interventional strategies. Although emergency psychiatry supervisors wear many hats on a psychiatric emergency service, the educational role is a crucial hat in any teaching service. In this chapter, we discussed the three components to being a good supervisor for trainees on the service: knowing how to diagnose and treat 1) the patient, 2) the learner, and

Learner stages	Teaching styles		
	Authority	Motivator/Facilitator	Delegator
Dependent learner	**Match**	Mild mismatch	Severe mismatch
Interested learner	Mild mismatch	**Match**	Mild mismatch
Self-directed learner	Severe mismatch	Mild mismatch	**Match**

Figure 15–5.   Matching learner stages to teacher styles.

3) the supervision setting itself. In practicing the strategies and suggestions outlined for each of these three components, supervisors will be able to be effective, meaningful, and influential educators for trainees. Good teaching not only helps satisfy the clinical work in the emergency setting but also is essential in the training of future mental health providers.

Key Clinical Points

- An effective educator needs to be able to diagnose and treat the patient in a supervision framework that matches the clinical demands and the learner's needs.

- Effective teaching involves understanding and assessing the learner and teaching the learner at his or her educational level.

- The RIME model is useful to assess the level of an individual learner's clinical performance.

- An effective educator needs to reflect actively on the teaching method before, during, and after every teaching encounter.

- In assessing the teaching encounter, educators should improve on areas of confusion, modify styles of teaching, and address any tensions in the learning climate.

- The one-minute preceptor and SNAPPS models are methods for efficient and effective teaching.

- Providing effective feedback to learners is an important teaching skill that should be done in a timely, specific, limited, behaviorally oriented, and learner-solicited manner.

References

Aagaard E, Teherani A, Irby DM: Effectiveness of the one-minute preceptor model for diagnosing the patient and the learner: proof of concept. Acad Med 79:42–49, 2004

Accreditation Council for Graduate Medical Education: Common program requirements: general competencies. February 13, 2007. Available at: http://www.acgme.org/outcome/comp/GeneralCompetenciesStandards21307.pdf. Accessed October 10, 2009.

Allen MH: Definitive treatment in the psychiatric emergency service. Psychiatr Q 67:247–262, 1996

American Association for Emergency Psychiatry Education Committee: A model curriculum for psychiatric resident education in emergency psychiatry. Emergency Psychiatry 4:18–19, 1998

American Medical Association: Graduate Medical Education Directory, 2001–2002. Chicago, IL, American Medical Association, 2002, p 317

Battistone MJ, Milne C, Sande MA, et al: The feasibility and acceptability of implementing formal evaluation sessions and using descriptive vocabulary to assess student performance on a clinical clerkship. Teach Learn Med 14:5–10, 2002

Brasch JS, Ferencz JC: Training issues in emergency psychiatry. Psychiatr Clin North Am 22:941–954, 1999

Brasch J, Glick RL, Cobb TG, et al: Resident training in emergency psychiatry: a model curriculum developed by the education committee of the American Association for Emergency Psychiatry. Acad Psychiatry 28:95–103, 2004

Busari JO, Weggelaar NM, Knottnerus AC, et al: How medical residents perceive the quality of supervision provided by attending doctors in the clinical setting. Med Educ 39:696–703, 2005

Cantillon P: ABC of teaching and learning in medicine: teaching large groups. BMJ 326:437–440, 2003

Deci E, Vallerand R, Pelletier L, et al: Motivation and education: the self-determination perspective. Educational Psychologist 26:325–346, 1991

Douglas N, Robinson J, Fahy K: Inquiry into the obstetric and gynaecological services at King Edward Memorial Hospital 1990–2000. Perth, Department of Health, Government of Western Australia, 2001

Firth-Cozens J: Doctors, their well-being, and their stress. BMJ 326:670–671, 2003

Foley R, Smilansky J, Yonke A: A teacher-student interaction in a medical clerkship. J Med Educ 54:622–626, 1979

Furney SL, Orsini AN, Orsetti KE, et al: Teaching the one-minute preceptor: a randomized controlled trial. J Gen Intern Med 16:620–624, 2001

Gibson DR, Campbell RM: Promoting effective teaching and learning: hospital consultants identify their needs. Med Educ 34:126–130, 2000

Gordon J: ABC of learning and teaching in medicine: one to one teaching and feedback. BMJ 326:543–545, 2003

Grainger C: Mentoring: supporting doctors at work and play. BMJ Classified (Career Focus) 324:s203, 2002

Hutchinson L: ABC of learning and teaching in medicine: educational environment. BMJ 326:810–812, 2003

Irby DM: Teaching and learning in ambulatory care settings: a thematic review of the literature. Acad Med 70:898–931, 1995

Irby DM, Papadakis M: Does good clinical teaching really make a difference? Am J Med 110:231–232, 2001

Irby DM, Aagaard E, Teherani A: Teaching points identified by preceptors observing one-minute preceptor and traditional preceptor encounters. Acad Med 79:50–55, 2004

Jaques D: ABC of learning and teaching in medicine: teaching small groups. BMJ 326:492–495, 2003

Jones JW, Barge BN, Steffy BD, et al: Stress and medical malpractice: organizational risk assessment and intervention. J Appl Psychol 73:727–735, 1988

Kaufman DM: ABC of learning and teaching in medicine: applying educational theory in practice. BMJ 326:213–216, 2003

Kilminster SM, Jolly BC: Effective supervision in clinical practice settings: a literature review. Med Educ 34:827–840, 2000

Lake FR, Ryan G: Teaching on the run tips, 2: educational guides for teaching in a clinical setting. Med J Aust 180:527–528, 2004a

Lake FR, Ryan G: Teaching on the run tips, 3: planning a teaching episode. Med J Aust 180:643–644, 2004b

Lake FR, Ryan G: Teaching on the run tips, 4: teaching with patients. Med J Aust 181:158–159, 2004c

Lake FR, Ryan G: Teaching on the run tips, 11: the junior doctor in difficulty. Med J Aust 183:475–476, 2005

Luck C: Reducing stress among junior doctors. BMJ Classified (Career Focus) 321:2, 2000

McKee M, Black N: Does the current use of junior doctors in the United Kingdom affect the quality of medical care? Soc Sci Med 34:549–558, 1992

Morrison J: ABC of teaching and learning in medicine: evaluation. BMJ 326:385–387, 2003

Muhlbauer HG: Teaching trainees in turbulent settings: a practical guide. Emergency Psychiatry 4:28–30, 1998

Neher JO, Stevens NG: The one-minute preceptor: shaping the teaching conversation. Fam Med 35:391–393, 2003

Neher JO, Gordon KC, Meyer B, et al: A five-step "microskills" model of clinical teaching. J Am Board Fam Pract 5:419–24, 1992

Neuman P, Piele E: Valuing learners' experiences and supporting further growth: educational models to help experienced adult learners in medicine. BMJ 325:200–202, 2002

Ogburn E, Espey E: The R-I-M-E method for evaluation of medical students on an obstetrics and gynecology clerckship. Am J Obstet Gynecol 189:666–669, 2003

Osborn LM, Sargent JR, Williams SD: Effects of time-in-clinic, clinical setting and faculty supervision on the continuity clinical experience. Pediatrics 91:1089–1093, 1993

Paice E, Rutter H, Wetherall M, et al: Stressful incidents, stress and coping strategies in the pre-registration house officer year. Med Educ 36:56–65, 2002

Pangaro L: A new vocabulary and other innovations for improving descriptive in-training educations. Acad Med 74:1203–1207, 1999

Parrot S, Dobbie A, Chumley H, et al: Evidence-based office teaching: the five-step microskills model of clinical teaching. Fam Med 38:164–167, 2006

Parsell G, Bligh J: Recent perspectives on clinical teaching. Med Educ 35:409–414, 2001

Peyton JWR: The learning cycle, in Teaching and Learning in Medical Practice. Edited by Peyton JWR. Rickmansworth, UK, Manticore Europe, 1998, pp 13–19

Salerno SM, O'Malley PG, Pangaro LN, et al: Faculty development seminars based on the one-minute preceptor improve feedback in the ambulatory setting. J Gen Intern Med 17:779–87, 2002

Schuster JM: Frustration or opportunity? The impact of managed care on emergency psychiatry. New Dir Ment Health Serv 67:101–108, 1995

Spencer J: ABC of learning and teaching in medicine: learning and teaching in the clinical environment. BMJ 326:591–594, 2003

Tiberius RG, Sinai J, Flak EA: The role of teacher-learner relationships in medical education, in International Handbook of Research in Medical Education. Edited by Norman GR, van der Vleuten CPM, Newble DI. Dordrecht, The Netherlands, Kluwer Academic, 2002, pp 463–497

Ullian JA, Bland CJ, Simpson DE: An alternative approach to defining the role of the clinical teacher. Acad Med 69:832–838, 1994

Vaughn L, Baker R: Teaching in the medical setting: balancing teaching styles, learning styles and teaching methods. Med Teach 23:610–612, 2001

Vaughn LM, Baker RC: Psychological size and distance: emphasizing the interpersonal relationship as a pathway to optimal teaching and learning conditions. Med Educ 38:1053–1060, 2004

Wall D, McAleer S: Teaching the consultant teachers: identifying the core content. Med Educ 34:131–138, 2000

Willcock SM, Daly MG, Tennant CC, et al: Burnout and psychiatric morbidity in new medical graduates. Med J Aust 181:357–360, 2004

Wolpaw TM, Wolpaw DR, Papp KK: SNAPPS: a learner centered approach for outpatient education. Acad Med 78:893–898, 2003

Suggested Readings

Neher JO, Gordon KC, Meyer B, et al: A five-step "microskills" model of clinical teaching. J Am Board Fam Pract 5:419–424, 1992

Pangaro L: A new vocabulary and other innovations for improving descriptive in-training educations. Acad Med 74:1203–1207, 1999

Wolpaw TM, Wolpaw DR, Papp KK: SNAPPS: a learner centered approach for outpatient education. Acad Med 78:893–898, 2003

16

Working With Medical Students in Psychiatric Emergency Settings

Tamara Gay, M.D.

Laura Hirshbein, M.D., Ph.D.

During psychiatry rotations or in other clinical clerkships, third- and fourth-year medical students often encounter patients with behavioral emergencies. Regardless of their ultimate specialty choice, students would be well served to learn about the management of behavioral emergencies because they must be able to deal effectively with them in their future careers (Townsend 2004). Specific training in the basics of the approach to behavioral emergencies can be a valuable component of students' psychiatry rotation (Brasch 2008).

Medical students may train in a variety of settings, including the medical emergency department, specialized psychiatric emergency services, or advanced comprehensive psychiatric emergency programs (Breslow 2002). At their level of undergraduate medical education, clerkship students are equipped with the interview, assessment, and treatment planning skills needed to assist in evaluating patients. However, most settings that provide urgent or acute care are bustling busy places. A tension can exist between the need for physicians and other emergency clinicians to work quickly and efficiently and medical students' needs for quality learning and teaching opportunities. We believe that with careful planning, thorough orientation of students to their psychiatric emergency experience, and some careful thought about ways in which students can be integrated into emergency care, these competing agendas can be harmonized.

Medical Student Orientation

General Considerations

Insufficient orientation of medical students to any new service often occurs, because of either time constraints or failure to recognize students' unfamiliarity with the setting. Psychiatric emergency settings are no exception. A careful review of usual emergency operating procedures is essential for the student to become a valued member of the treatment team as well as a well-informed adult learner. One method that can be extremely useful is to develop a short patient vignette that illustrates a patient's journey from arrival in the emergency space to discharge, along with points at which students may intervene or be of assistance. The following case example describes a typical presentation of a patient to a psychiatric emergency service (PES).

Case Example 1

Mr. L is brought to the PES by his case manager. As he begins to fill out paperwork, his vitals are obtained and he is triaged by a nurse (opportunity for student to observe/participate in triage process). The patient denies any thoughts of wanting to hurt himself or others and he is not agitated, so he is permitted to stay in the waiting room (instead of going into seclusion or restraints). His case manager comes into the staff room to give a report about the patient's noncompliance with medications and his worsening thought disorganization, paranoia, and inability to attend to his basic needs. The patient's available chart information is reviewed and indicates that Mr. L is a man with chronic paranoid schizophrenia who has a long history of noncompliance. According to the chart, he has no history of violence toward others.

A clinician is assigned to see the patient (opportunity for student to either interview patient alone or accompany clinician; in some settings, the primary interview is done by a social worker, and a student may substitute for social worker if the student feels comfortable). After the initial interview, additional information is obtained from the patient's mother, who confirms that Mr. L has not taken his medications in several weeks. Laboratory values are obtained to double-check on medication levels and to rule out any physical illness (opportunity for student to contact family or other significant individuals for information). The patient needs to be checked periodically to make sure he or she remains stable while a hospital bed is located (opportunity for student to take ownership of case by doing follow-up checks). The patient is admitted to the hospital (opportunity for student to participate in admission process).

This vignette can be adapted to the particular training site. A vignette approach works well because medical students usually retain information best when it is linked to patient encounters (Howe et al. 2007; Rees et al. 2004).

Safety Orientation

As part of the orientation, special attention must be paid to the physical safety of the medical student. A tour of the facility, with an emphasis on security and student safety, is imperative. The student needs to know where panic buttons are located and observe demonstrations of appropriate seating arrangements that ensure equal patient and clinician or student access to a door. Each psychiatric emergency setting is unique, and students must be well versed in the specific protocols, resources, management, and operations of their institution. Also, although students have been taught throughout much of their medical education that they should ignore or minimize their own feelings and reactions to patients (Bosk 1981; Klass 1994), students in psychiatric emergency settings need to learn to pay attention not only to their patients' clinical presentations but also to their own strong emotional reactions or subconscious feelings of discomfort (Shea 1998).

Approaches to Integrating Medical Students Into Psychiatric Emergency Care

Various methods have been used to allow the active participation of medical students across clinical sites. We examine four models that are appropriate in psychiatric emergency settings.

Tag-Along Method

In the tag-along method, following a brief discussion of the patient's presenting symptoms with the teaching clinician, the student accompanies the clinician into the interview room. The student takes an observer-only role and has limited involvement in the interview (although he or she may have an opportunity to ask questions at the end of the interview). This arrangement may be necessary in several situations: when a student is very inexperienced, when a patient's presentation is exceptionally complicated, or when law enforcement is involved. This model presents learning limitations: being placed in a passive role will impede knowledge acquisition for medical students, although it does give the student an opportunity to witness management of acutely agitated or potentially aggressive patients.

Case Example 2

Ms. S is a 39-year-old single female registered nurse brought by the police to a psychiatric emergency room of a community hospital because of erratic driving and paranoid statements when stopped by the police. She is followed by a local psychiatrist for major depressive disorder with psychotic features but is unknown to PES personnel. She has been unable to work for the past 18 months secondary to treatment-resistant symptoms, especially paranoia. The primary evaluator is the resident on call in the emergency department. He makes the decision to use the tag-along method with his medical student. After reviewing the available information and briefly interviewing the police officer, the resident and medical student go together to evaluate Ms. S. The patient is initially cooperative with the resident's questioning, but she begins to become agitated after explaining "I've been bugged." She elaborates her history in a disorganized way and becomes convinced as she talks that the interviewers are part of the conspiracy that has planted listening devices on her person. The interview must be abruptly terminated after the patient threatens the resident in a loud voice and gets out of her chair and stands over the medical student. Ms. S is then medicated with an intramuscular haloperidol-lorazepam combination. After 1 hour, the patient becomes much calmer and can resume the evaluation.

The resident wisely decided to be the primary evaluator but allowed the student to be a passive observer of the interview. This decision was based on the fact that PES personnel had little background knowledge of this paranoid patient.

Sequential Interviewing

The sequential interviewing method allows a medical student more active participation and some autonomy in the evaluation of an acute patient. Prior to beginning the interview, the primary evaluator and the student briefly discuss the case and settle on a time limit for the student-directed portion of the interview (e.g., 15–25 minutes). Then the student and primary interviewer do the evaluation together in a sequential format. Both are present for the entire interview. Advantages of this sequential interviewing model are that it allows for a substantial amount of student participation without sacrificing much in clinical efficiency. The primary clinician is present for the entire evaluation and therefore hears in real time the portion of the history conducted by the student. This is also the only model in which the student can be given specific feedback as to his or her interview skills and technique (Gay et al. 2002).

Case Example 3

Mr. K is a 29-year-old single male accountant who presents to the PES of an academic hospital. Two weeks earlier, he was seen for a new patient evaluation, by a psychiatrist working in the institution's outpatient clinic, with complaints of depression and anxiety. A selective serotonin reuptake inhibitor (SSRI) was initiated at that visit. When Mr. K presents to PES, he reports sudden onset of racing heart, shortness of breath, and other physiological symptoms consistent with a panic attack. He reports five similar episodes in the past 10 days. After reviewing the medical record, including a recent workup by a cardiologist that is negative for cardiac pathology, the resident and medical student decide to interview the patient sequentially, with the medical student performing the first 20 minutes of the interview. The patient appears initially anxious but is very cooperative with the interview. The medical student asks good open-ended questions and comments to Mr. K that he must be very relieved to have learned that "you've had a negative cardiac workup, so you know there is nothing seriously wrong with you." The resident continues the evaluation of Mr. K and makes a diagnosis of panic disorder. Low-dose clonazepam is prescribed three times daily, and Mr. K is discharged home to continue follow-up with his outpatient treater.

In the postencounter educational wrap-up session, the resident is able to give specific constructive criticism to the medical student regarding her portion of the interview. This includes explaining that although it might appear validating to tell someone experiencing panic symptoms that nothing is seriously wrong with him or her, this reassurance is well-meaning but misplaced, because the patient *is* experiencing troublesome symptoms. This teachable moment for the medical student could only have occurred with the sequential evaluation model.

Collateral Information Gathering

A third method for integrating the medical student into the emergency evaluation of the patient is to assign him or her the job of obtaining collateral information from the family or care providers. This information is often vital to appropriate decision making in psychiatric emergencies, but it is sometimes difficult to obtain because of time limitations or because patients feel that the psychiatrists are listening too much to family and not enough to them. By separating the individuals who conduct the interviews with different parties, the primary psychiatrist can still maintain the alliance with the patient while the student talks with the family. A further benefit of this separation is that students are at a stage of training in which their active listening skills are particularly appreciated by families.

Case Example 4

Ms. T, a 34-year-old stay-at-home mother, has been brought to the PES of an academic hospital. She is accompanied by her husband, who says that he is worried about her because she has seemed really depressed and is not showing much interest in their 2-year-old son. She had an episode of depression when their son was an infant and responded well to sertraline (which she discontinued over a year ago).

The faculty psychiatrist interviews Ms. T, who reports that she has been feeling anxious and is having difficulty sleeping. She appears only superficially engaged with the interview but denies that she is suicidal. She says she wants to stay out of the hospital because she has to take care of her son. She agrees to get engaged in outpatient treatment and states that she is willing to restart sertraline.

With the patient's permission, the medical student talks separately with the patient's husband. He reports that his wife has been perseverating about the fact that she is a bad mother and saying that her son would be better off without her. He also reports that her twin sister died by medication overdose when she was a teenager. Of most significant concern was that the husband found a large quantity of unidentified pills on his wife's bedside table (prompting the emergency evaluation).

In this case, the additional information provided by the separate interview with the husband provides vital collateral information that makes a huge difference for the decision about the next intervention for the patient (hospitalization vs. outpatient treatment). Obviously, good clinical care requires obtaining collateral information whenever possible. In this area, a medical student can significantly contribute to the gathering of information in a way that might be less likely to antagonize patients (because the discussion with family is being done by someone other than the primary clinician).

Traditional Medical Clinic Model

A fourth method, which can be especially effective for a more advanced medical student (late-third-year or fourth-year student), is the traditional medical clinic model. The one-minute preceptor (Neher and Stevens 2003) and/or SNAPPS (Wolpaw et al. 2003) methods will bring much added value to this model (see Chapter 15, "Supervision of Trainees in the Psychiatric Emergency Service"). After a brief review of the presenting symptoms and historical information with the primary evaluator, the student goes alone into the interview room and evaluates the patient. Afterward, the student presents the case to the primary clinician. Then the student and clinician return to the patient and complete the evaluation. This method requires the primary treater to have a high level of confidence in the medical student's capabilities and to be well versed in active listening to student presentations, particularly listening for sins of omission. This model ensures that the patient benefits from a thorough and complete evaluation, while giving the student the opportunity to function at a higher level with significantly more autonomy.

Case Example 5

Mr. R is a 40-year-old married father of two, employed as an assistant principal of a junior high school. He presents alone to the PES for worsening symptoms of anxiety and depression. The fourth-year medical student and resident on call review the patient's record and decide to have the student conduct the initial interview by himself and then present his findings, assessment, and plan to the resident. Mr. R is a cooperative and excellent historian who explains that his symptoms began approximately 6 months ago after his wife had a near-fatal heart attack. He immediately took on almost all of the parenting and caregiving roles in the family but now feels he has "no more to give." The medical student carefully assesses the patient's risk for self-harm and decides he is at low risk. Mr. R. experiences a great sense of relief from being able to tell his story. He wonders aloud for the first time whether his overprotective strategy regarding his family has been the most effective one. He agrees to call his wife and explain the reasons for his trip to the PES. The student then presents Mr. R to his resident, with a diagnosis of major depressive disorder, single episode. The student's plan includes referral to an outpatient provider for combination treatment with antidepressant medication and short-term psychotherapy (interpersonal relationship–focused treatment).

After briefly evaluating the patient herself, the psychiatric resident concurs with the student. The resident does her own risk assessment screening for suicidality and finds low risk. Mr. R has benefited from a comprehensive evaluation and a well-designed treatment plan. The educational goal of increasing independent practice for an advanced medical student has also been fulfilled.

Common Factors

All four of the previously described medical student integration models can be effectively used in evaluation of behavioral emergencies. It is crucial to follow sound educational principles, particularly taking into account each student's psychiatric knowledge base and interviewing skills. Also, including a postencounter student debriefing and making several key teaching points satisfactorily close the educational loop.

Intended Learning Goals and Objectives for Medical Students

General Principles

Medical students require very specific learning objectives. However, in clinical settings, particularly those involving delivery of emergency care, it is challenging to consistently cover specific topics (Brasch et al. 2004). The emergency psychiatry portion of the rotation does provide opportunities for two elements that are sometimes not addressed in other settings: safety and rapid decision making.

Although violence is a potential risk in any clinical encounter, the psychiatric emergency setting allows students an opportunity to formally discuss safety issues. A preliminary discussion of safety will have taken place during the students' introduction to the shift or rotation experience. Any encounters with potentially or actually aggressive patients will provide teachable moments to reinforce issues such as the importance of maintaining good personal space boundaries with patients. Emergency settings can help students recognize the differences among acute agitation, violent intent, and short- and long-term risks to self or others. An emergency rotation can also be the appropriate setting to dispense with the myth that a patient's "contracting for safety" provides sufficient reassurance that the patient is not at risk for suicide (Simon 1999).

In addition to understanding safety issues, students need to be able to see that different treatment settings require different ways to approach diagnosis and treatment. One particularly challenging concept for students is that assessments in a PES setting often cannot yield a definitive discrete diagnosis. Students may have to be satisfied with a lengthy differential diagnosis. However, treatment planning that takes into account patient safety and the safety of others must be very specific and individualized. Students may become focused on long-term treatment planning for a given patient and must be redirected to acute crisis intervention strategies that properly match the behavioral emergency setting.

Although safety issues and crisis management can consistently be addressed within most shifts, educators realize that available patient encounters do not always provide a comprehensive and complete set of patient problems that perfectly match specific psychiatric emergency learning objectives. If an emergency setting has low patient volume or if students can only be assigned a few shifts per rotation, then other steps must be taken to ensure adequate knowledge acquisition. One way to overcome this deficiency is to use paper case vignettes to supplement actual clinical exposure (Hirshbein and Gay 2005). Teaching cases can be constructed with history provided sequentially and questions interspersed at appropriate decision points. Each case can be concluded with a discussion section explaining the rationale for assessment and treatment decisions. A similar format of teaching cases can be developed using educational computer programs, one example being Professional Skillbuilder (Mangrulkar et al. 2008). This program provides video vignettes of patient interviews, punctuated by question screens that allow students to mimic actual patient encounters and clinical decision making. Feedback regarding correct or incorrect answers is a valuable part of these types of self-study exercises. These computer enhancements to education can be built into emergency settings (Pusic et al. 2007).

Specific Behavioral Emergencies

In clinical settings, supervisors need to ensure that students are taught certain principles about specific behavioral emergencies.

1. *Agitation/potential for violence.* Know risk factors for violence in the PES setting; know appropriate interview and management techniques to decrease the potential for violence.
2. *Suicidal ideation.* Learn risk assessment and determination of when hospitalization is necessary.
3. *Psychotic symptoms.* Be able to prepare a medical and psychiatric differential diagnosis for psychotic symptoms; be able to describe common and serious side effects of antipsychotic medication.
4. *Delirium.* Be able to recognize, assess, and manage the delirious patient.
5. *Substance abuse/withdrawal.* Know signs, symptoms, clinical course, and treatment of intoxication and withdrawal regarding alcohol and other common drugs of abuse.
6. *Self-harm and self-mutilation.* Be able to assess and differentiate between these behaviors and a suicide attempt.
7. *Panic/anxiety.* Be able to recognize symptoms of a panic attack and understand the importance of acute treatment for symptom improvement.
8. *Children's issues.* Be able to use a developmental approach for assessment and treatment; know the legal requirements and procedure for reporting suspected child abuse or neglect.
9. *Legal issues.* Understand state commitment laws for involuntary treatment; be able to assess a patient's capacity to give informed consent.

Conclusion

Although faculty and residents may sometimes have the perception that student teaching will take away from either clinical operations or resident teaching, in fact the effort taken to instruct students can increase the educational benefit for all (Hoellein et al. 2007). Within psychiatric emergency settings, effective integration provides the opportunity for students to learn how to handle behavioral emergencies—a skill they will need in their future regardless of specialty—and the opportunity for enhancing the clerkship because responsibility and direct patient care are available student opportunities in these settings (Clardy et al. 2000).

Key Clinical Points

- **Tag-along method** (student goes with supervisor and observes the interview): Advantages include the opportunity for inexperienced students to obtain real-time exposure to a case. This method works well with a potentially dangerous patient. However, the student has little opportunity to interact directly with the patient.

- **Sequential interviewing method** (student begins the interview while supervisor is present): This method provides an opportunity for the student to talk to the patient while the supervisor observes and builds on the interview and allows feedback on the student interview. This method can be difficult with agitated patients and perhaps more time consuming.

- **Divide and conquer method** (student interviews family or friends and obtains collateral information): Advantages include the student's making a tangible contribution to case management. The family and friends feel that they have an advocate who is listening to them, whereas the primary evaluator maintains a therapeutic alliance with the patient. A drawback of this method is that the student does not directly interact with the patient.

- **Traditional medical clinic method** (student performs interview alone, then presents case to supervisor): The student learns from this method by taking charge of the case and having the opportunity to be the primary clinician. Supervision opportunities exist around case presentation and clinical decision making. The student needs to have substantial experience before assuming this role in the psychiatric emergency setting.

References

Bosk CL: Forgive and Remember: Managing Medical Failure. Chicago, IL, University of Chicago Press, 1981

Brasch JS: Education and training in the psychiatric emergency service, in Emergency Psychiatry: Principles and Practice. Edited by Glick RL, Berlin JS, Fishkind A, et al. Philadelphia, Lippincott Williams & Wilkins, 2008, pp 485–495

Brasch J, Glick RL, Cobb TG, et al: Residency training in emergency psychiatry: a model curriculum developed by the education committee of the American Association for Emergency Psychiatry. Acad Psychiatry 28:95–103, 2004

Breslow RE: Structure and function of psychiatric emergency services, in Emergency Psychiatry. Edited by Allen MH. Washington, DC, American Psychiatric Publishing, 2002, pp 1–33

Clardy JA, Thrush CR, Guttenberger ML, et al: The junior-year psychiatric clerkship and medical students' interest in psychiatry. Acad Psychiatry 24:35–40, 2000

Gay TL, Himle JA, Riba MB: Enhanced ambulatory experience for the clerkship: curriculum innovation at the University of Michigan. Acad Psychiatry 26:90–95, 2002

Hirshbein LD, Gay T: Case-based independent study for medical students in emergency psychiatry. Acad Psychiatry 29:96–99, 2005

Hoellein AR, Feddock CA, Wilson JF, et al: Student involvement on teaching rounds. Acad Med 82:S19–S21, 2007

Howe AV, Dagley V, Hopayian K, et al: Patient contact in the first year of basic medical training—feasible, educational, acceptable? Med Teach 29:237–245, 2007

Klass P: A Not Entirely Benign Procedure: Four Years as a Medical Student. New York, Plume, 1994

Mangrulkar RS, Chapman C, Westfall J, et al: The Professional Skillbuilder: A Web-Based Tool to Promote Clinical Skills Improvement for Medical Students. Password authenticated Web site for University of Michigan medical students. Ann Arbor, Regents of the University of Michigan, 2009

Neher JO, Stevens NG: The one-minute preceptor: shaping the teaching conversation. Fam Med 35:391–393, 2003

Pusic MV, Pachev GS, MacDonald WA: Embedding medical student computer tutorials into a busy emergency department. Acad Emerg Med 14:138–148, 2007

Rees C, Sheard C, McPherson A: Medical students' views and experiences of methods of teaching and learning communications skills. Patient Educ Couns 54:119–121, 2004

Shea SC: Psychiatric Interviewing: The Art of Understanding. Philadelphia, PA, WB Saunders, 1998

Simon RI: The suicide prevention contract: clinical, legal, and risk management issues. J Am Acad Psychiatry Law 27:445–450, 1999

Townsend MH: Emergency psychiatry training for third-year medical students as reported by directors of medical student education in psychiatry. Teach Learn Med 16:247–249, 2004

Wolpaw TM, Wolpaw DR, Papp KK: SNAPPS: a learner-centered model for outpatient education. Acad Med 78:893–898, 2003

Suggested Readings

Brasch JS: Education and training in the psychiatric emergency service, in Emergency Psychiatry: Principles and Practice. Edited by Glick RL, Berlin JS, Fishkind A, et al. Philadelphia, PA, Lippincott Williams & Wilkins, 2008, pp 485–495

Townsend MH: Emergency psychiatry training for third-year medical students as reported by directors of medical student education in psychiatry. Teach Learn Med 16:247–249, 2004

17

Afterword

Gregory W. Dalack, M.D.

You have come to the end of this handbook, perhaps thinking about ways to integrate and solidify the information to which you have been exposed in the preceding chapters. Your journey has taken you through a unique offering: one that has focused on clinical situations, as opposed to diagnostic categories, combining the approach of an accomplished psychiatry trainee with the sage view of a senior practitioner in the field. This pairing provides a richly integrated perspective, which we trust will be useful to those in training as well as those supervising trainees.

In a book that nicely offers "take-home" points at the end of each chapter, there are several broad take-home points that are clearly applicable to the psychiatric emergency service (PES) setting, and are best never forgotten in any clinical setting:

1. *Pay attention to the patient's chief complaint and think broadly about the clinical presentation as you develop a differential diagnosis and plan for treatment.* One should never assume that the patient seen in a psychiatric set-

ting has solely a primary psychiatric disorder any more than one should assume that all patients presenting to a cardiology clinic have problems with their hearts. Many of the chapters in this book have underscored the potential for "medical mimics" to cause the presenting complaints, including symptoms of anxiety, depression, psychosis, catatonia, and cognitive impairment. In addition, the recognition that comorbid conditions are often present is critical to the complete assessment of patients presenting for care.

2. *Partner with your colleagues to access and interpret information.* This is particularly necessary when collaborating to complete a medical workup as part of a PES assessment. In addition, input from social work staff, legal staff, and security staff may be critically important when approaching cases of suspected child abuse, or circumstances in which the safety of patients, staff, or bystanders in the PES is at issue, or cases in which involuntary commitment to care may be indicated. There is considerable wisdom contained in this volume to guide you as you assess the risk for violence in patients, consider the need for seclusion and restraint, and face the legal and ethical issues that arise in the emergency setting.

3. *Watch for, seek to create, and make the most use of "teachable" moments.* Crisis sometimes creates the opportunity for a patient, parent, or other family member, previously disinclined to participate in treatment, to be engaged and motivated to understand the patient's condition and the steps recommended to address it.

4. *Think about the PES contact as an important link in a continuing chain of care.* Thoughtful attention to developing an effective disposition is key to more completely addressing the presenting complaint and reducing the chances of a return visit, in crisis, to PES.

5. *Take the opportunity to teach: teach patients, families, students, and colleagues.* Chapter 15, on emergency psychiatry supervision, and Chapter 16, on working with medical students, are particularly rich, outlining the approaches to educating the adult learner and suggesting ways to use specific opportunities in the emergency setting to teach and solidify clinical skills and medical knowledge.

As an entry point for care or a safe haven during an exacerbation of a chronic condition, the emergency setting is often a tense and high-stakes setting. Patients and families are anxious and fearful; available clinical information may seem sparse or feel overwhelming. We trust that the guidelines and approaches outlined in this handbook will be useful to you as you work to make sense of the clinical situations you encounter, supporting your roles as clinician, educator, and lifelong learner.

Index

Page numbers printed in **boldface** *type refer to tables or figures.*